NUTRIFY
AND
DETOXIFY

MANAGE
TODAY'S HEALTH
CHALLENGES

Linda Lieb Peterson

"Nutrify and Detoxify," by Linda Lieb Peterson. ISBN 978-1-62137-936-2 (softcover); 978-1-62137-937-9 (eBook).

Published 2017 by Virtualbookworm.com Publishing Inc., P.O. Box 9949, College Station, TX 77842, US. ©2017, Linda Lieb Peterson.

Library of Congress Control Number: 2016920877.

TABLE OF CONTENTS

Notice to Readers

The material in this book is **not** intended to replace the services of a physician nor is it meant to encourage self diagnosis and treatment of illness or disease. The focus of this book is to educate each person to understand his/her body, the roots of disease, and to give each person tools for wellness.

The information herein is not a substitute for professional medical treatment. The author has made every effort to give the reader the most accurate information available at the time of publishing. Any application of the recommendations set forth in the following pages is at the reader's discretion and sole risk. The author and publisher cannot accept legal responsibility for any problem arising out of experimentation with the methods described herein.

If you are under a physician's care for any condition, he or she can advise you whether any changes you wish to make after reading the following material are suitable for you. Working with a trained practitioner is always wise when considering major changes in diet, exercise, or lifestyle.

DO NOT STOP medications you are taking without a physician's approval and assistance.

About the Author

Linda Lieb Peterson almost died at age five from Bright's Disease. Throughout the next years she was plagued with one infection after another. At death's door again in 1993, she began to question what was really wrong with her body and started the search for options outside conventional medicine. Learning the reasons for her ill health became her passion.

During Linda's many years as a public school teacher, she also became concerned about the increasing numbers of unhealthy or damaged children who were being prescribed drugs to control their behavior. After being drugged they seemed to lose their childhood, their creativity, and their hope.

She became convinced that the underlying causes of her ill health were related to the problems of those children and also to the maladies of other chronically ill people, including many elderly.

Linda Lieb Peterson is currently working as a Wellness Educator teaching classes on healthy living including: nutrition, herbs, and homeopathy. Her professional training includes:
- BA in Education from the University of Montana plus graduate credits
- Chartered Herbalist Certificate (CH) from Dominion Herbal College in British Columbia
- Diploma in Homeopathy (D.I. Hom.) from the British Institute of Homeopathy in the United Kingdom
- Certified Nutritional Consultant (CNC), Member American Association of Nutritional Consultants (AANC)
- Board Certified Holistic Health Practitioner, American Association of Drugless Practitioners

Linda is an avid champion of our right to choose the health care we need.

Dedication

To Cousin Ray, who taught me to appreciate the birds of the air, the plants of the earth, the beauty of the masters, and to thirst for knowledge.

To my sons, Brian and Kevin, you are my reason for living. You allowed me to grow up with you and encouraged me to do whatever I needed to do. I hope you will use this book as a guide for your health.

To my sister, Cecilia, who educated me about the world.

To God, my Creator, Friend, and Guide, Who has provided the people to teach and guide me through thick and thin, so I could experience the lessons I needed to grow and evolve.

Acknowledgements

Words cannot convey the gratitude I feel for two friends without whom this book may never have been finished. They both selflessly gave time to edit and support the process for this to be published. Linda Kittle has been the editor and driving force behind this book and Kathy was editing at my side for my first book, which never got published, but from which much of this material was gleaned.

My thanks to Kris Sampson for the photo of the author.
Food basket on cover from
https://www.pexels.com/search/food/

Too many people have edited and given suggestions during the writing of materials that have culminated in this book to name. I appreciate the support of loyal friends who have encouraged my efforts even when it looked hopeless.

A special thanks to the many health practitioners who have been significant in guiding me in my personal journey to find wellness.

I want to thank the many great researchers and authors who have blazed the trail to help us return to natural methods for wellness. They all contributed to my education as you will see throughout the book.

PREFACE

We all want to be well, regaining health and avoiding illness. Can we? Could illness be the result of mostly manageable circumstances? Can we ordinary folk manage our own health and minimize illnesses?

I have spent over 20 years analyzing and studying health issues, and I have found that the answer to these questions is **YES!**

It is my goal to guide you to find what you need to build your body to prevent disease and to deal with whatever diseases come along.

We each need to create our own individual plans for wellness. Specific features such as certain nutrients, herbs, and homeopathic remedies can be added to each plan as needed. However, determining what is available and appropriate can be time consuming and confusing. I have extracted what I think are the best choices and practices, along with reference citations, to help you in your search for health.

How did I get involved in finding healthy solutions? I've had a lifetime of sickness and disease. I was sick with infections much of the time from age 3 to age 50. Medical science kept me alive with antibiotics, though I never got well. At age 51 the antibiotics no longer were working for the infections. Now what? I was like many of you, frustrated and scared because my health was deteriorating quickly. I realized it is not any doctor's responsibility to keep me well. It is my responsibility.

I turned to traditional holistic health. The first alternative practitioner I visited was an herbalist who taught me that detoxifying my body would set it free to heal. Then I could use nutrients found in herbs and other healthy foods to regain and maintain my health. I was hopeful, as I had finally found a path that made sense to me. Following that path, though, was more complicated than I had imagined.

Over the last few decades science has provided vast amounts of information concerning health. I find much confusion and contradiction among authors. What should we believe? Where should we start?

Health begins with NUTRIFYING and DETOXIFYING the body.

It took me a long time and much study to realize thatmost chronic diseases are basically the result of the body's struggle with:

- lack of necessary nutrients
- toxicity, often resulting from the environment
- underlying infections
- stress
- lack of rest and sleep

Therefore, my beginning protocol for dealing with any disease is the same.

1. Detoxify the body systems using nutrients, herbal cleansing, homeopathy, and physical manipulation such as massage and acupuncture. Consider these cleanses:

- colon cleanse with liver support herbs
- blood cleanse with lymphatic herbs
- heavy metal cleanse

2. Rebuild the immune system. This will involve healing the gut by restoring gut flora balance with probiotics and eating prebiotic foods and herbs.

3. Eat a nutrient-dense diet based on vegetables, good fats, lean meats, fruits, and herbs. Avoiding processed food, artificial ingredients, and wheat is important.

If you are going to take charge of your health you will also need to:

- think out of the conventional box and ignore critics
- embrace individuality—find what works for you
- increase rest, decrease stress, and surround yourself with people who will support your journey
- filter everything through common sense

This book is an attempt to filter the writings of many authors to create a common-sense guide for finding optimal health and preventing disease. I have discussed a number of common chronic conditions and included lists of nutrients and healthy foods for you to consider.

Information keeps changing, so as we study we each need to decide what makes sense to and for us.

I wish you well on your journey!

PART A: THINKING OUT OF THE BOX

1 We Were Created to be Well

<u>Humans, as all creatures, were created to live in a natural environment and eat foods as found in Nature</u>.

Now our bodies are continually trying to compensate to survive in a much different world, the world of toxic substances and denatured foods.

Most people are functional but not really well. If you have to take an OTC (Over–The-Counter), prescription, or recreational drug to function, or if you need to visit the doctor often, you are not well. Being well is thriving with energy, vitality, and enthusiasm without unnatural stimulation.

The body will be well if the cells receive the nutrients they need and if the body can detoxify the toxins received from foods and the environment.

Each animal has a diet that is optimal for it. A seal wouldn't live long on a diet of greens; while a giraffe would not live long on a diet of meat.

I find it interesting that pet food companies are changing their ingredients to fit the natural diet of dogs and cats. We need to listen to what that says about what our bodies need. We were meant to eat foods as found in Nature for our type, not man-made ingredients packaged as food.

What is the diet Man needs to thrive? Our early ancestors focused on hunting and gathering food. This simple act involved several key elements:

- They were obtaining whole foods of many varieties, usually raw and in season, straight from their environment.
- Their only drink was water.
- They covered a large area of land to find food, so they were getting regular exercise.
- Their lives revolved around the amount of daylight. (1)

Early man lived on what was in his environment: meat, fish, nuts, fruits, roots, and above ground plants.

1

Approximately 10,000 years ago a significant change occurred in the diet of some of the early people. Gradually they learned to cultivate grasses for their seeds and made breads, thus ensuring a steady food supply.

Bread has been a staple of many cultures, but many people in the US are having difficulty digesting wheat or gluten today. **It's important to realize that the wheat available today is not the same as it was in early times or even 60 years ago**. Modern wheat was introduced around the year 1960. It was developed via cross-breeding and crude genetic manipulation, which changed the nutrient and protein composition of the plant. Modern wheat is less nutritious.

Dr. William Davis, in his book, Wheat Belly says, "Modern wheat varieties contain up to 40 times more gluten than heirloom varieties, as selective breeding, hybridization and even genetic modification techniques have been applied over the years to improve wheat yields. This means the types of wheat consumed by people today are far different than the types traditionally consumed by ancient societies." This altered wheat is found in many food products and may be a greater part of our diet than we realize.

See more on wheat in "Proteins, Fats, and Carbohydrates."

What is the diet that is optimum for Man? Experts don't agree as to what that should be, but I believe it is best described by Loren Cordain in his book, The Paleo Diet, "We were genetically adapted to eat what the hunter-gatherers ate." (1) I translate that to mean to eat a variety of foods found naturally in season.

Common herbs have been a part of Man's diet from early times. The herbs parsley, sage, rosemary, and thyme were mentioned in the old English folk song, "Scarborough Fair."

In medieval times such herbs were commonly used in tonics. Today, we know these herbs are loaded with nutrients and medicinal properties. Adding these common herbs to your diet could improve your health and lower your risk of disease.

Parsley	Garlic	Cayenne peppers
Sage	Ginger	
Rosemary	Oregano	
Thyme	Dill	

When Man decided he was smarter than Nature and discounted the value of natural foods and herbs, the natural balance within our bodies was altered. Our bodies no longer received what they needed for optimum health.

When Man decided to alter Nature by creating chemical substances, conditions within the human body began to change, causing new diseases and malfunctions. Why is it we think humans can live on ingredients created in a test tube? Why do we put artificial ingredients in our bodies? We'll explore specifics throughout the book.

Man has created chemical substances and technology, often with little research as to how they would affect the body. These include:

- Creating artificial additives which are added to packaged foods
- Over-processing foods so that their nutritional content is changed
- Growing foods using chemicals as fertilizer and pesticides on land that is often stripped of the natural minerals and organic material.
- Using chemical preservatives to extend the shelf life of foods
- Fluoridating water, tooth paste, mouthwash. *Fluoride is a poison.*(2)
- Using mercury in our dental fillings & vaccines. (2)
- Genetically modifying food seeds with no idea what the long term effects will be
- Combining chemicals to create innumerable products such as:
  - personal care products which we slather on our bodies

-cleaning supplies which we touch & breathe
- pesticides and artificial fertilizers
- industrial and workplace products

- Creating innumerable prescription and over the counter drugs
- Flooding the body with electromagnetic fields created by microwaves, transmission lines, smart meters, x-rays, mammograms, CT scans, and cell phones and their towers. (3)

Drugs have become the answer for every malady for many folks. Drugs can be life saving in emergency situations, but they are too often used merely to relieve symptoms when the source of the problem needs to be found. Symptoms should lead us to the underlying cause, where the body needs help. The body wants to be well. Drugs may be necessary in specific situations, usually for short periods of time, but can they repair the body?

Drugs and chemicals are NOT in our food chain.

Nutrients nourish, rebuild, and detoxify the body. We need nutrients, sunshine, joy, exercise, and a clean environment for a healthy body.

Our health is our responsibility, but we have NOT been taught how to stay well. We are in charge of our own health. No one else should choose for us, but we need guidance.

Knowing When to Get Help—Listen to Your Body

It is very important to understand your body well enough to know when you need medical attention. I have a damaged body as a result of many years of eating incorrectly, vaccines, chemicals, and too many infections for which I was prescribed antibiotics. Therefore I need to carefully manage my life to include the most nutritious food, avoid chemicals, use various detoxifying procedures, and balance my emotions.

If I have a serious medical problem, I temporarily use the physician-prescribed drugs until I can deal with the underlying cause naturally. For example, when I couldn't

4

lower my blood pressure with natural foods and remedies, I consulted a medical doctor.

Conventional medicine has some very good diagnostic tools which have revealed some things I could not diagnose myself. For example, when a major joint was painful and no longer functioning well, tests showed the joint needed to be replaced.

When we have medical procedures, we need to understand that we may need drugs for a while to avoid another problem, such as a blood clot. Usually we can return to our drug-free state if we understand the use of foods, herbs, and homeopathy in our healing process.

<u>Symptoms</u> are your body's cry for help.

Learn the difference between when a symptom may be telling you something is serious (requiring immediate medical attention) or that simply a change in diet or lifestyle is indicated.

When a symptom comes on suddenly, lingers longer than usual, or just seems different, it calls for medical attention.

According to the American College of Physicians, "these symptoms require immediate medical attention. These do not represent every medical emergency." (4)

Emergency symptoms:
- Sudden numbness or weakness of the face, arm or leg, especially on one side of the body, which may be symptoms of a stroke.
- Difficulty breathing, shortness of breath
- Chest or upper abdominal pain or pressure lasting two minutes or more
- Fainting, sudden dizziness, weakness
- Changes in vision
- Difficulty speaking
- Confusion or changes in mental status, unusual behavior, difficulty walking
- Any sudden or severe pain
- Uncontrolled bleeding

5

- Severe or lasting vomiting or diarrhea
- Coughing or vomiting blood
- Suicidal or homicidal feelings
- Unusual abdominal pain
- Poisoning
- Drug overdose
- Loss of consciousness
- Major burns
- Spinal, head, or brain injury
- Severe allergic reaction

Other signs which may need medical attention:
- Blood in the urine or bowels
- Unusual sores or bumps
- Leg pain with swelling (4)

Learn to read temporary symptoms, such as general discomfort, headache, dizziness, temporary visual distortions, muscle weakness, or stomach ache to find if there might be a simple explanation. Ask yourself these questions, as any of these can cause the body to react with symptoms:

- Was there MSG (monosodium glutamate) in something I ate? If you ate fast food or processed food, it likely contained some form of MSG. We'll learn some of the hidden sources of MSG and how it affects the body.
- Was there artificial sweetener such as aspartame in something I ate?
- Were there artificial colors or flavors in something I ate?
- Did I eat food prepared in a microwave oven? Microwaves are suspected to change the molecular activity of food. (See more later).
- Have I eaten adequate protein for healthy brain function?
- Have I drunk six to eight glasses of pure water each day to flush my system?
- How much sugar or high fructose corn syrup have I consumed which may have been hidden in foods and drinks?

6

- Is my diet mostly packaged, prepared food with little nutrition? Is my body crying for nutrients?
- What cosmetics and other personal care products have I slathered on my body that could have toxic ingredients?
- Is there new carpet, paint, furniture, or cabinets in my environment? They often give off toxic gases causing many symptoms.
- Are air fresheners sending chemicals into my air?
- Is there an air-conditioning system circulating toxins in my workplace?
- Did someone just spray some chemicals on the landscaping near me?
- What cleaning products are being used in my environment?
- How much time do I spend in vehicles on crowded streets and highways absorbing the petrochemical residues?
- What prescription, OTC, or recreational drugs have I put in my body? What are their side effects and how are they interacting with one another or with herbs or foods such as grapefruit?
- What is the source and purity of nutritional supplements I have taken?
- Have I recently had a vaccination or flu shot?
- Do I have amalgam fillings in my teeth that may be leaking mercury?
- Could I have undetected food allergies or other allergies?

***When in doubt, seek medical help.
In an emergency, call 9-1-1 or go to the nearest ER.

The body reacts to created ingredients in foods, synthetic drugs, vaccines, and foreign substances in our environment as enemies that it doesn't understand. It may store the toxic substances if it cannot eliminate them, and symptoms of disease may result. Evaluating the above questions can help you make positive changes.

Disease is NOT an ACCIDENT

From my experience I have come to understand that malfunctions of the body and the diseases we face are mostly created by our lack of nutrition, toxicity from foreign substances, underlying infections, and the stress of dealing with our complex world.

We have been following the scientific medical model for the last 70 years and are getting sicker by the decade. WHY? We often hear that we are living longer, but what is life if you are in an Alzheimer's unit, hooked-to life-support machines, or surviving on a cocktail of drugs which creates miserable side effects?

With the use of vaccines and antibiotic drugs, medical science thought the world would be free of infectious disease. Today, the death rate from infectious disease is rising. (5)

It seems obvious that two problems have hastened the destruction of the body's ability to thrive.

1. The proliferation of chemicals and drugs in our lives has overworked the liver and the elimination systems.
2. Much of the food in today's American diet is processed and doesn't provide the nutrients our cells need.

Nutrients are the master key between you and disease.

2 Most Disease is Preventable

The body wants to be well and will be well if we give it what it needs.

Degenerative disease is touching the lives of all of us. The Free Dictionary defines degenerate disease as: "Any disease in which deterioration of structure or function of tissue occurs. Kinds of degenerate diseases include arteriosclerosis, cancer, and osteoarthritis..."

Most degenerative disease is avoidable. According to former U.S. Surgeon General Dr. C. Everett Koop, **of the 2.4 million deaths that occur in the United States each year, 75% are the result of avoidable nutritional factor diseases.** That number is conservative. (6)

Statistics keep changing, but we know **infectious disease is on the rise** as the microbes continue to mutate, making them resistant to the available drugs. http://www.webmd.com/news/20080220/new-infectious-diseases-on-the-rise
According to the National Institute of Health (NIH):
- Approximately nine million Americans suffer from cancer annually.
- 22 million suffer from heart disease.
- Autoimmune disease beats them both with an annual number of 23.5 million and rising. (7), (8)
- It is estimated that 1 in 68 children in the US has autism. Some estimate higher. (9)
- Babies in the United States have a higher risk of dying during their first month of life than do babies born in 40 other countries, according to a new report. (11)
- Americans suffer from an estimated 45-50 million adverse effects from prescription drugs—of which 2.5-4 million are serious, disabling, or fatal. (11)

The philosophy of health and medicine of the 20th century was like going up a hill backwards. Each time we were ill, a new drug was prescribed. We took the drug, which relieved symptoms, and we gradually climbed to a level of feeling better. In time we slid backwards, needing another drug for the same or different symptoms, often from side effects of the first drug. Again we climbed a bit higher as symptoms were relieved. Life for many of us has been that repeated process of taking a drug, feeling better, then sliding back as we have more symptoms. Sometimes that process continued with ever more serious symptoms and new drugs prescribed for a diagnosis of cancer, an auto-immune syndrome, diabetes, Alzheimer's, or some other dysfunction.

Only foods can feed and repair the body.

In the early 1900s life was simpler. There were few chemicals in our lives, no genetically modified foods, few vaccines, and limited chemicals and pollution. The addition of fluoride to water systems wasn't instituted until the 1940s. The use of chemicals in foods, personal care products, cleaning supplies, and yard pesticides has increased and industrial pollution has grown substantially through the years.

Our country was once very rural and the food supply was natural. When the soils were healthy, there was no need for the chemicals that are used in today's agriculture, and the food crops were more nutritious.

Starting in the 1940s we thought the new antibiotics would save the world from disease. Unfortunately, their use in humans and animals has been abused, causing a whole new set of problems. Microbes want to survive, so they are mutating faster than science can create drugs to control them. However, there are answers to be found in nature. Many herbs have amazing properties which will work where drugs are no longer effective. http://www.indieherbalist.com/journal/herbal-antibiotics-what-you-really-need-to-know

The U.S. has the most expensive health care system on the planet, yet we are a very sick nation. In 2000 WHO (World Health Organization) ranked the US health system as 37th in the world. A recent stat said we have dropped to 41st in the world. (12)

Being healthy in the 21st century will depend on our ability to return the planet to a healthful state.

3 Why We Are Sick

How do these conditions develop? They may develop from a single incident, but often they develop over time through a combination of factors, as we will see.

The scope of disease today is a great challenge for conventional medicine, because most disease is not easily solved with a prescription pad. <u>We need to think differently</u>. It doesn't work just to alleviate symptoms temporarily. <u>We need to know what caused the symptoms</u>.

Conditions like cancers, autoimmune disorders, and neurological diseases are strongly linked to infections by viruses, bacteria, or fungi. These infections can trigger the onset of a chronic disease.

Numerous studies have demonstrated a high incidence of chronic infections in chronic fatigue syndrome. These include viral infections of Epstein Barr (EBV), cytomegalovirus (CMV), human herpes virus-6, (HHV-6), and bacterial infections such as mycoplasma, Chlamydia pneumonia (CP), and Borrelia burgdorferi (Lyme disease). (13)

We have been taught to think that as soon as we have a symptom or feel sick, we need to pop a drug. In our "quick fix" mentality, we haven't learned how the body functions. It functions and heals based on the nutrients each cell receives.

We need to know WHY we are getting sick. Why do some people get a virus and others don't? I wondered as a child why I had repeated strep infections and no one else was sick.

Why do some people have chronic disease and others don't? Except for infections which are obvious, why do we get sick?

Often disease is a gradual process caused by many factors. It may start with our genetics, our weaknesses. The solution may involve correcting nutritional deficiencies, discovering food or other allergies, and

11

balancing excess acidity. It could be as general as heavy metal poisoning and as specific as needing to remove amalgam fillings from your teeth.

Usually disease is a combination of factors that cause the body to malfunction.

Disease doesn't just happen.

We need to help the cells heal by feeding them what they need and detoxifying them.

We will feel more in control of our health if we understand why we get sick.

We have neither been taught the importance of **preventing disease nor been given the knowledge needed.** Our culture today teaches us to depend on the doctor to **fix our problems.**

As a culture, we are impatient people who want everything as quickly as possible, so we follow whatever seems to get us to our goals as fast as possible, often without questioning the safety. We are taught that the government agencies will protect us from harm.

We followed because we thought everything was safe, healthy and for our good. Sadly, I have learned it was mostly for profit.

We've been programmed to:
- Do whatever the medical doctor says because he is the expert.
- Trust the doctor when CT scans, x-rays, mammograms, prostate biopsies, colonoscopies, prescription drugs, or surgery are recommended without researching the outcome.
- Reach for a pain killer without giving much thought as to WHY we have a headache. *Headache is a symptom of something wrong in your body.*
- Take a laxative never realizing that constipation is our body's signal that the intestinal tract is not working properly.
- Eat whatever is fast and convenient, thus filling our bodies with calories and toxins but <u>few nutrients</u>.

12

- Use the microwave to heat up something from the freezer, not considering the possible dangers.
- Clean our houses with a variety of products filled with unknown ingredients that may be <u>toxic or allergenic</u>.
- Use a fertilizer/herbicide formula and maybe a pesticide for the lawn <u>WITHOUT considering what effect the chemicals may have on our health, the aquifer, or the quality of the air. We do it because advertising says it works.</u>
- To be appealing, we use various products on our bodies not realizing many of the <u>ingredients may cause health problems</u>.
- Ignore the warnings about radiation and electromagnetic fields (EMFs) which are attacking our bodies daily from our new technology. <u>We ignore the danger warnings because we depend on the convenience.</u>

<u>We have blindly followed</u>. Now we must face the diseases that have manifested from the toxic environment, the toxic foods, the drugs, the lack of nutrients, and the lack of emotional stability and grounding in our lifestyle.

Big Government: As the United States grew in physical size and population, it was determined that the central government needed to form organizations to protect the businesses and people. The roots of the USDA and the FDA reach back to the mid 1800s.

As drugs were introduced to our world to help in trauma and infections, we trusted the FDA to make sure that pharmaceutical companies or the FDA tested all drugs to ensure their safety. In recent history some have begun questioning the integrity of both FDA and pharmaceutical companies.

<u>Prescription drugs</u>: <u>Severe side effects</u> of drugs are very prevalent, especially <u>those caused by using several drugs simultaneously</u>, or by certain drugs interacting with certain foods such as grapefruit.

<u>What baffles me is that people take prescriptions when</u>

often the side effects are worse than the condition for which they are prescribed. Reading Byron Richards' book, Fight for Your Health, is an eye-opener that will change your life. I will mention only a few of the most commonly used drugs. I hope you will research whatever you are . taking. (14)

1. Statins: It is interesting how the levels of acceptable cholesterol have been manipulated. Before 1984 it was thought that a middle aged man with a cholesterol reading over 240 with other risk factors may be at greater risk of heart disease. After the Cholesterol Consensus Conference of 1984 it was decided that men and women with a cholesterol reading over 200 should receive medication to lower cholesterol. Recently, the safe level has been lowered to 180. What evidence do they have?

Recent research is showing the level of cholesterol is not a prominent factor in cardiovascular disease (14), but doctors are still prescribing statins because that's what the protocol suggests. Many people have been coerced into taking statin drugs and have no idea how those drugs are affecting their bodies. Cholesterol is needed by the body for many processes. Inhibiting that production interferes with the body's natural synergy. Statin drugs inhibit not just the production of cholesterol but also a whole family of intermediary substances and processes. (14)

2. Anti-depressant drugs: I'm sure you have heard about the rising rate of suicide in young people who are taking anti-depressant drugs. Research shows that the very first week you start taking antidepressant drugs, your risk of committing suicide quadruples. (15)

The recent school shootings and other random acts of violence can often be connected to the medical use of drugs. According to PDR Health, "in clinical studies, antidepressants increased the risk of suicidal thinking and behavior in children and adolescents with depression and other psychiatric disorders." (16)

We have been coerced into thinking that drugs solve all

14

our problems, when often the drug creates more and worse health issues or even death.

We are all on drugs! Does that sound preposterous?
Drugs are being found in our water supplies. We are being medicated whether we want it or need it. Painkillers, antibiotics, antidepressants, and other prescription drugs are being detected in tap water and in rivers downstream from sewage plants. Pharmaceuticals have now become environmental pollutants. (17)

3. While some drugs claim to increase bone density, we know nutrients can. Bone is composed of protein, collagen, calcium, magnesium, phosphorus, and other nutrients. If you understand how the body functions, then it makes no sense to think that drugs can build strong bones.

4. Drugs are often prescribed to deal with autism, ADHD, and the many other syndromes that our children are developing. Once we understand that the body will heal itself when given the right nutrients and when it can eliminate the toxins, we will be better equipped to evaluate the protocols that are often recommended.

How safe and accurate are the testing procedures used by the medical profession?

We are not told the dangers of x-rays, CAT scans and many other tests. John Gofman, M.D., Ph.D., nuclear physicist, a medical doctor and one of the leading experts in the world concerning the dangers of radiation, presents evidence in his book, Radiation from Medical Procedures in the Pathogenesis of Cancer and Ischemic Heart Disease, which **strongly indicates over 50% of the death rate from cancer and over 60% of the death rate from ischemic heart disease today, is x-ray-induced.** (17) Much more information on the dangers of CAT scans, x-rays, mammograms, and other tests can be found on the Internet. (17) Sometimes we may need these tests, but only when there is a serious problem.

Are mammograms safe? In my late forties and following my doctor's advice, I had a mammogram which ended in a

15

medical crisis. It caused physical damage to me, as well as the need to use antibiotics to cure the recurring infection, which caused further complications. I started searching to find out if I really needed mammograms to safeguard against breast cancer. Maybe some women need testing, but are mammograms the answer?

I found mammograms are not the preventive the medical establishment would have us believe they are, and they can be extremely dangerous. There is new research from several countries of the dangers of mammograms and their lack of deterring death from breast cancer. <u>Here are some of the facts I found which justify my never having another mammogram.</u>

• The squeezing of women's breasts during mammograms may damage the tissues. If cancer is present, the rupturing of blood vessels may cause the cancer to spread to other parts of the body, increasing a patient's risk of death. (18)

• Compression isn't the only mammogram danger. A mammogram delivers many times more radiation than a chest x-ray and may increase the risk of cardiovascular damage. (19)

• Studies show that mammograms fail to detect cancer 30 percent of the time in women aged 40 to 49. In addition, it can take eight years before a breast tumor is large enough to detect, by which time the cancer could have spread to other parts of the body. (20)

• Some doctors conclude that mammograms offer no health benefits whatsoever. (21)

There are other options to detect breast cancer.
Thermography - Digital Infrared Imaging (DII) is a simple, non-invasive procedure that uses infrared cameras to detect patterns of temperature change in tissue. DII can catch cancer cells at work long before a tumor forms. It can't pinpoint the exact location of cancerous cells, or determine if a mass is present, so additional procedures such as an MRI or ultrasound are still necessary to determine if a tumor has already formed. (22)

16

Magnetic Resonance Imaging (MRI) is a noninvasive imaging technique that uses no compression, x-rays, or radiation. An MRI creates a detailed picture of the internal architecture of your breast tissue. (23)

Ultrasound is another diagnostic tool. It uses sound waves to produce sharp, high-contrast images. In dense breast tissue, the ultrasound can create an image that often allows a doctor to distinguish between a fluid-filled cyst and a solid mass. Mammograms do not make this distinction as accurately, though they are better than ultrasounds at detecting micro-calcifications, which can be an early sign of breast cancer. (24)

Beware of biopsies: We are learning about the dangers of needle biopsies. A June 2004 report on a rigorous study at the John Wayne Cancer Institute in Santa Monica, Calif., concluded that a needle biopsy may indeed increase the spread of the disease by 50 percent, compared to patients who receive the more traditional excisional biopsies or lumpectomies. (25)

Always get a second opinion. Do research, then ask yourself whether what is being recommended makes sense to you. I hope that after reading this book and using the references, you will have the tools to make good decisions about your health.

Petrochemicals, heavy metals, and other toxic wastes are changing the human body.

In 2005 when Dr. Doris Rapp MD, author of Our Toxic World–A Wake Up Call, was interviewed by Greg Ciola in *Crusader Health Publication*, she said there were something like 80,000-85,000 chemicals on the market. Less than 10% of these have been checked for safety. Today, it is estimated there are over 120,000 chemicals that have been unleashed on our planet. (26)

Every day we're all exposed to toxic chemicals coming from a wide variety of sources such as our air, water, food, cosmetics, toothpastes, deodorants, shampoos, household cleaners, vaccines, pharmaceutical drugs, plastics, carpets, paints, industrial solvents, insulation, pesticides, herbicides, fertilizers, gasoline and other petroleum by-products, to name a few.

Certain chemicals mimic hormones in our bodies. The documented decline in human sperm counts has been linked to environmental toxins. E.g., the sperm count in humans in 1932 was about 125 million per milliliter. By 1970 it was 100 million per milliliter. By 1990 it was 50 million per milliliter. A common insecticide that has been sprayed in an attempt to control West Nile Virus is known to cause a decrease in animal sperm count and cause abnormal chromosomes. (26) (27)

Many different chemicals are used in food processing and preservation. A scary fact comes from a Centers for Disease Control (CDC) scientist, Dr. James Pirkle: "If you gave a sample of blood or urine to us, we could find all sorts of things you didn't think you had. We are regularly, every day, exposed to 50,000 chemicals. Only a fraction of these chemicals have been studied for their effects on humans. There have been no studies at all showing the consequences of using these agents in varying combinations. Living in such a toxic environment places our bodies under constant bombardment from every conceivable angle." (28)

We know many chemicals are carcinogenic, but we have no idea how the devastation quotient rises when our bodies have to fight combinations of toxins.

4 The Root of Disease - Cellular Terrain

"Cellular terrain" is a term originated by an early scientist, Antoine Bechamp, who believed "the cause of disease is not germs themselves, but rather the inner condition of the patient's cellular terrain at the time of exposure." I feel this is the key to health we have been missing. (30) The overall health of the cells and our genetics determines how our bodies will react to our environment, stress, and what we put into our mouths.

All disease originates at a cellular level.

Do we make the connection between how we think, what goes in our mouths, what we slather on our bodies, and what we breathe, with how it is affecting our bodies? It is very basic:

Start with healthful molecular-building materials (foods and drinks)
> to create healthy cells so those cells
>> will build healthy tissues
>>> which form strong, healthy organs
>>>> which create healthy systems so you
>>>>> will have a healthy body.

All systems must work in harmony for optimum health.

Vital Force or vitality is the measure of how well our systems are working. As the Vital Force lowers we become increasingly vulnerable to dysfunction and disease.

We need a constant supply of the basic building materials for cellular growth, maintenance, and repair. These building materials need to be from natural sources. To quote Gary Tunsky again, **"We were born in a garden, not a laboratory."** (29)

We need these building materials every day for healthy cells:
1. Oxygen—breathe deeply
2. Water—the body is 2/3 water; water is needed for all body processes
3. 24 amino acids (The essential amino acids must be derived from food, others can be made in the body.)
4. Carbohydrates or glycogen

19

5. Fats (including saturated fats and essential fatty acids)
6. Phytonutrients (antioxidants and other necessary nutrients from plants)
7. 16 vitamins
8. 72 minerals
9. Enzymes
10. Glyconutrients
11. Sunshine (29)

EAT TO PREVENT DISEASE

Much of this book is devoted to helping you discover how foods contribute nutrients to your body.

You need variety in your meals and snacks to make sure you get all the nutrients. All foods should be organic or naturally grown without chemicals.

Many herbs are high in nutrients as well as having specific health promoting properties. I include many herbs in my daily diet.

Nutrients come from:

-Greens, other vegetables, and herbs which provide phytonutrients, vitamins, minerals and enzymes.

-Proteins from grass-fed poultry, eggs and meat; legumes, non-gluten grains, seeds, and nuts, and dairy—preferably raw or cultured.

-Carbohydrates which are not created equal! Complex carbohydrates are those with higher fiber and/or fat content and metabolize more slowly.

-Fats have been misunderstood for many years. In the last decade we are beginning to understand which fats are necessary and which are damaging.

A healthy gastrointestinal tract is necessary for proper digestion and absorption of nutrients. **When we understand the immune system originates mostly in the small intestine, we have a new respect for what we put in our mouths**. Often the intestinal walls become damaged allowing undigested food to pass into the blood stream causing a toxic condition.

"Death begins in the colon" is a phrase often used by alternative healers. The Greek physician Hippocrates is credited with using the phrase as early as 400 BC. (30)

Taking an antibiotic at any time in your life can set up an imbalance in your intestines. The balance of good bacteria is crucial to a healthy intestinal tract. To balance the bacteria, we can start by eating fermented or cultered food such as sauerkraut or by taking a good probiotic supplement before bedtime to repopulate the intestinal tract. By taking the probiotics at bedtime the good bacteria can populate all night without being impeded by having to deal with a new burst of food. It is also impotant to eat foods with adequate fiber and prebiotic foods that feed the good bacteria.

Healthy cells are the key to a strong immune system. The toxins from today's environment and the foods we eat constantly burden our immune systems; thus, we are very vulnerable. When the immune system is functioning optimally our bodies would normally kill millions of cancer cells and other invaders.

Factors that can injure the immune system:

1. pH - A constantly acidic cellular environment sets the stage for disease. When the body starts to become acidic, it deposits acidic substances (usually toxins) in the blood cells, which causes other cells to become more acidic and toxic. This results in a decrease in their oxygen levels and harms their DNA.

2. Dehydrated body - The lack of pure water for all the processes of the body causes toxic build-up and lack of proper functioning of the organs. Only pure water will wash the toxins from the body and provide what the organs need. We've already discussed the body's need for water.

3. **Nutritional deficiencies** such as:
- inadequate intake or reserves of vitamins.
- insufficient mineral intake or imbalance of mineral intake. For example, selenium deficiency increases the risk of developing malignancies, infections and heart disease. Minerals are used in rebuilding and detoxifying. Balance is important.
- lack of phytonutrients, especially antioxidants which keep free radicals in check.
- lack of good fats. The body needs a variety of natural fats, including saturated fats and a balance of essential fatty acids for crucial functions. Most diets have too much Omega 6 and are lacking in Omega 3 and 9.
- lack of enzymes. Raw vegetables and herbs are our best source of enzymes.
- lack of good quality protein, which provides the building blocks for the cells.

4. Food toxicity - Consumption of unhealthy dietary trans-fats, preservatives, artificial sweeteners, artificial colors, sodas, and other highly processed foods can cause an acidic condition. Eating and drinking non-nutrient foods causes a toxic environment in the body.

In Natural Strategies for Cancer Patients by Russell Blaylock, M.D., he discusses the following:
- **Refined sugar, high fructose corn syrup, and white flour** products all increase insulin production. Too much insulin is a stressor.
- **Food additives** can promote cancer growth and development. These include nitrites, nitrates, MSG, other sources of glutamate, aspartate, and carrageenan. (31)
- **Excitotoxins:** Aspartame, an artificial sweetener, and Monosodium Glutamate (MSG) a flavor enhancer are common ingredients in our processed food products. That may sound innocent, but they are brain toxins that can destroy neurons. We will discuss this subject in depth in Part B.

5. Stress from electromagnetic radiation and ionizing radiation: Injury to DNA and bone marrow may follow

22

radiation, leading to malignant changes in cells and greater opportunity for infections to occur. Examples include cell phones, CT scans, x-rays, wireless Internet, computers, microwaves, electric blankets, clock radios, high-tension power lines, and office machines. (32)

6. Home and workplace toxins include ingredients from personal care products, cleaners, air fresheners, pesticides, off-gassing of carpet and furniture, petroleum products for auto and yard use, workplace glues, inks, and other chemicals. (3)

7. Environmental toxins include heavy metals, pesticides, fluoride, and other chemicals. (3)

8. Emotional instability: Accepting oneself is basic to all other relationships, including those with partners, family, friends, and in the workplace. We live in a world where technology has replaced face-to-face interaction among people. Looking people in the eye and connecting with them on a deeper level is very important to our human nature.

9. Stress: The Oxford Dictionary definition of stress is "a state of mental or emotional strain or tension resulting from adverse or very demanding circumstances." When prolonged stress occurs, the body steadily releases cortisone that causes suppression of the immune system, death of nerve cells, failure to kill abnormal cells, increased free radicals, and increased risk of infection.

10. Excesses & addictions: The obvious addictions include: Nicotine, alcohol, drugs of all types, sugar, aspartame, foods with additives. Even toxic relationships can be addictions.

11. Lack of good sleep: We often don't respect the need for good sleep. Researchers say, "Loss of less than half a night's sleep can impair memory and alter the normal behavior of brain cells." (33) Sleep deprivation alters immune function, including the activity of the body's killer cells. Lack of sleep affects learning and memory, metabolism and weight control, mood, cardiovascular health, and safety. (34) The brain detoxifies as we sleep.

In a paper published in Science Translational Medicine scientists from the University of Rochester Medical Center dubbed this the "glymphatic system," because it acts like the body's lymphatic system but is managed by brain cells known as glial cells. The glymphatic system clears away toxins or waste products that could be responsible for brain diseases, such Alzheimer's and other neurological disorders. (35)

12. Vaccines: There are several ingredients in many vaccines that are considered by some to be carcinogenic, and compromise the immune system. (36)

13. Aging: As we age it becomes more difficult to activate the immune system.

14. Infection: Serious infections can deplete phagocytes (cells within the body capable of engulfing and absorbing bacteria and other small cells and particles) and cause a breakdown of many of the processes in the body. **Parasites** often host viruses, and many diseases and tumors originate from **viral infections. Underlying infections from whatever source** keep the body under stress. **Candida** or other systemic fungal infections are thought to cause or contribute to the development of malignant tumors. Maintaining a healthy balance of intestinal flora is one of the best ways to build strong digestive and immune systems. (37)

Avoiding infections may be more important than we thought.

Dr. Russell Blaylock and other sources say that stealth germs and hidden infections cause chronic disease. We are all familiar with the common cold, flu, or the occasional bladder infection, strep, or toenail fungus. These usually go away after a period of time with or without drugs. We think if the symptoms of the infection are gone it is cured, maybe not. (37)

There is evidence that remnants of viruses, bacteria, or fungus may be lurking in your body. These **lurking microbes could be causing a chronic type of infection that does deadly damage to your health and can last a lifetime without realizing you have it.** The damage to

24

the body is real and can be debilitating. There may be no outward signs of illness for a long time, but when triggered these silent infections can cause devastating disorders and lead to severe disability, even premature death.

Because these infections are insidious, often the person doesn't feel well and the reason isn't diagnosed. The number of these silent infections is growing. They are often precursors of cancer, autoimmune diseases, Alzheimer's, and Parkinson's diseases. In fact, there is growing scientific interest in the idea that even psychiatric disorders are triggered by persistent infections. An ordinary person would not connect any of these diseases to an underlying infection. (37)

Let's get back to preventing infections naturally.

Why do some people in a family become ill from a virus and others don't get sick? The health of each person's cells, tissues, and body systems (cellular terrain) will determine whether the virus or bacterium can occupy the host. All systems, especially the immune system, must be working well to reject invading microbes.

Why do we get infections? If the body is healthy it will resist many of the microbes that invade your cellular terrain, unless...

- your immune system becomes weakened and loses its ability to control outside factors
- your body's pH is too acidic
- you're not getting good sleep/rest, affecting all systems
- your cells lack nutrients to function properly
- lack of cleanliness/sanitation has allowed viruses and bacteria to enter the body
- your body is weakened from toxic overload
- you have experienced a physical or emotional trauma

A number of conditions, such as fever, stress, immune deficiency, nutritional deficiency, acidic conditions in the body, glutamate, mercury, fluoride, and pesticides, can activate a latent virus. Vaccinations can increase the risk of infections. (37)

5 Infections—Our Greatest Threat

Today, it seems the most life-threatening force may be infections. There is considerable concern and research in the scientific community about the speed at which microbes are mutating and proliferating. Why, you ask? Microbes want to survive, too, so they are mutating to become resistant to drugs and other chemicals which man has created to annihilate them. Since microbes seem to be mutating quickly, the research to create new drugs for the new "bugs" can't keep up.

The immune system is the major player in combating infections. When the immune system becomes stressed, it affects all body systems, often initiating or compounding chronic disease.

Only recently have biofilms become an area of research connected with infections. Bacteria build biofilms, thin armored fortresses, where they can live, breed and hide inside your body. Biofilms are often slimy or sticky and shield bacteria from the outside environment. You might find them on your pet's water dish, as plaque on your teeth, or sticking to tissues or medical implants in the body. Biofilms protect the bacteria from being attacked by antibiotics; thus, they are linked to many types of stubborn recurring staph infections such as MRSA. (38)

Studies suggest that some natural antimicrobials such as Manuka honey have shown activity against biofilms. It is believed that some herbs may also be effective against biofilms. (39) For more information see Stephen Harrod Buhner's books.

A World Without Antibiotic Drugs! What will we do?

There is light in this dilemma. Many herbs with antibiotic, anti-viral, anti-fungal, and anti-parasitic properties are still effective. Why won't the microbes become immune to the herbs? Drugs are created for specific microbes, while herbs have many constituents which work in synergy to help the body fight anything it doesn't recognize.

Infections can be life threatening, so we must understand what our options are and have access to them. Eating nutrient-dense food and using herbs or other natural remedies is the place to start, but **realize that when the infection is getting serious** you need to see a doctor.

We must reserve antibiotic drugs for use in serious infections. We can help by:
1. staying well, keeping a healthy cellular terrain which will naturally combat microbes
2. not asking our doctors for antibiotics when there is another solution
3. eating only grass-fed, free-range meat and eggs to avoid antibiotics in the meat
4. advocating that antibiotics not be given regularly to food producing animals
5. using herbs and other natural methods to stop or slow an infection

I avoid antibacterial soaps. Triclosan is a common ingredient used in many products to kill bacteria. An article in the Townsend Letter says, "Triclosan is a chlorophenol, a class of chemicals suspected of causing cancer in humans. The companies that manufacture and use triclosan claim it is safe; however, it is registered as a pesticide with the United States Environmental Protection Agency (EPA). Pesticides are chemicals designed to kill some life form. The EPA considers triclosan a high risk for human health and the environment." (40)

Some tips to avoid spreading viruses:
- I regularly sanitize my toothbrush and cup with hydrogen peroxide. (Never to be ingested.)
- Each person should have his/her own cup in the bathroom.
- Change the hand towel in the kitchen and the bathroom often.
- Sanitize telephones, computer keyboards, door knobs, and other commonly touched surfaces. Using natural sanitizers made with essential oils works well.

Is it a viral or bacterial infection? A patient can experience generalized, whole-body effects from either a bacteria or a virus—nausea, chills, vomiting, body aches, and fever. A virus typically causes symptoms that involve many organs at the same time, whereas a bacterial infection will usually become localized in one organ or organ system.

It is important to note that viruses can become bacterial infections very quickly if conditions are right.

Viruses need a host. To quote *Microbe World*, "Viruses can't metabolize nutrients, produce and excrete wastes, move around on their own, or even reproduce unless they are inside another organism's cells. They aren't even cells. When viruses come into contact with host cells, they trigger the cells to engulf them, or fuse themselves to the cell membrane so they can release their DNA into the cell. Once inside a host cell, viruses take over its machinery to reproduce. Viruses override the host cell's normal functioning with their own set of instructions that shut down production of host proteins and direct the cell to produce viral proteins to make new virus particles." (41)

Parasites

My introduction to parasites as a common health hazard was when I went to an herbalist in 1994 and he said I had high levels of parasites. I protested, but after the parasite cleanse, I realized he was right. The idea that parasites were feeding on me was really repulsive.

I had much to learn, so I began reading about Hulda Clark, who had done years of research on the relationship between parasites and disease. She has written many books making connections for us between the toxins in our environment, parasites, and diseases such as cancer. (42)

Leo Galland, M.D. in the Townsend Letter for Doctors said in 1988, "I strongly believe that every patient with disorders of immune function, including multiple allergies (especially food allergy), and patients with unexplained fatigue or with chronic bowel symptoms should be evaluated for the presence of intestinal parasites." (43)

Dr. Hazel Parcells, distinguished researcher, said, "Make no mistake about it, worms are the most toxic agents in the human body. They are one of the primary underlying causes of disease and are the most basic cause of a compromised immune system." (44)

"The combination of environmental toxins, an unhealthy diet and parasites poses a grave danger to humans. In fact, **parasites have killed more humans than all the wars in history,**" reported National Geographic in its award-winning documentary, *The Body Snatchers.*

A practitioner friend of mine says that 60-70% of his patients have parasites and many have candida yeast overgrowth and parasites. Some researchers state that as high as 85% of the population has parasites. Parasites and candida yeast overgrowth are often found together, causing double havoc.
http://www.fungusfocus.com/html/parasites_general_info.htm

How do humans get parasites?
- In food and water which has become infested
- From your pet. Often the eggs of parasites are on the coats of animals and certainly in their feces.
- From your fingers, which you may without thinking put in your mouth. Your hands may touch something that somebody touched after they touched feces or some parasite-infested animal or other object.
- By inhaling contaminated dust
- Through sexual contact
- From fleas, mosquitoes or other vectors
- From skin exposure
- By flying on an airplane through the air system and by touching what a contaminated person has touched.

The following are very common herbs, which, taken together, are effective against over 100 types of parasites. Cleansing is easy and usually has few, if any side effects.

When using herbs consult a practitioner or a good book.

Wormwood - Artemesia absinthium (capsules or tincture)
   Caution: Wormwood can be toxic if used internally in large doses or over long periods of time. Pregnant and breastfeeding women <u>should not ingest wormwood</u>.

Black walnut hull - Julans nigra (capsules or tincture)

Cloves—Syzygium aromaticum (capsules, must be freshly ground) (42)

The black walnut hull and the wormwood will kill the adults and developing stages while the cloves kill the eggs. Do this for at least three weeks, then continue only the cloves for another rwo weeks. **Only if you use them together will you rid yourself of all stages of parasites**.

You won't usually feel any changes unless you are very infested, then you might notice a bit of headache or nausea for a few days as they are dying off.

Since I travel and eat in restaurants so much, I do a parasite cleanse a couple times a year. It is very important that your colon is functioning well and you are having several eliminations per day. If not, do a colon cleanse before starting the parasite cleanse.

Garlic and pumpkin seeds are foods which are anti-parasitic. I regularly include them in my diet for their nutritional value and to help keep my intestinal tract free of nasty invaders.

<u>Plants which contain berberine also have anti-parasitic properties. These include:</u>
   • Goldthread—Coptis chinensis
   • Goldenseal—Hydrastis canadensis
   • Oregon grape—Berberis aquifolium
   • Barberry—Berberis vulgaris (45)

Consult a good medicinal herb book or a practitioner when using any of the above herbs, and take probiotics, because these herbs not only kill the bad critters but may also kill some of the good bacteria.

Grapefruit seed extract (GSE) is a broad-spectrum natural antibiotic capable of killing a wide variety of pathogens. It has been found to be very effective in the treatment of parasitic infections. It is also highly active against protozoa, bacteria, yeast, and some viruses. Grapefruit seeds contain a high content of proanthocynanin antioxidants and a wide array of flavonoids and minerals. It can be consumed internally or used topically. (46) I make a dilution in a spray bottle and carry it when I travel to disinfect hard surfaces, wash veggies and fruit, and spray on surface skin cuts. It's also great to spray in the mouth and throat to deal with any infection.

Fungus Infections

Candidiasis (Candida Albicans – a yeast infection) is a condition with which I have had plenty of personal experience. Candidiasis is found to be an underlying cause of many diseases. A vaginal yeast infection or thrush in the mouth may just seem annoying, but when candidia becomes systemic, it is debilitating. Research is finding that fungus and yeast overgrowth, which have been largely overlooked by conventional medicine, may be significant factors in chronic disease, even cancer. (47)

Candida albicans normally lives in balance with other bacteria in our intestines and is needed to protect the intestines from pathogenic bacteria. A healthy immune system depends on a balance between candida albicans and friendly bacteria like lactobacillus acidophilus, B. bifidum, Lactobacillus bulgaricus, and other friendly bacteria. If this balance is upset by antibiotics, pesticides, stress, or various chemical toxins, the immune system is weakened and conditions for candida albicans proliferation occur, causing a condition called candidiasis. The yeast may shift from a mycelia fungal form and start to invade the body in various ways. (48)

Candida produces dozens of toxins, which are released into the body and induce inflammation, which then leads to other symptoms. These toxins can suppress immune function and are an underlying problem in many chronic diseases.

If you have taken many antibiotics and feel sick all over and no one has been able to tell you what is wrong with you, see if you have some of these symptoms. Symptoms of candida will vary from person to person and may come and go.

- Visual disturbances may include blurring, sensitivity to light, and eye pain
- Incapacitating fatigue, drowsiness, achy muscles, loss of coordination, weakness, dizziness
- Unrefreshing sleep, never feel rested
- Mental fogginess, problems with concentration and short-term memory
- Flu-like symptoms such as pain in the joints and muscles and swelling
- Extreme tightness in the shoulders and neck
- Wheezing, coughing, tightness or pain in the chest, shortness of breath
- Skin rashes, itching, ringworm, psoriasis, athlete's foot, or toenail fungus
- Nasal or sinus symptoms such as headache, post-nasal drip, congestion, itching in the nose, burning or itching eyes, tearing eyes, ear pain, ear congestion, recurrent ear infections, sore throat, chronic sinus infections, visual changes
- Digestive issues such as bloating, belching, flatulence, diarrhea, or constipation
- Depression, anxiety, or irritability
- Dark circles under the eyes
- Crawling skin
- Genital irritation, itching, or burning; mucus-like or white discharge, pain during intercourse, menstrual cramps, burning during urination, urinary urgency, endometriosis, impotency
- Craving sugar and breads
- Sensitivity to strong smells such as tobacco smoke, perfumes, and chemicals. (47) (48)

If you have many of the above symptoms you will want to visit a natural practitioner who will be experienced in dealing with yeast overgrowth. It can be difficult to control, but I have found natural methods very effective.

Some dietary changes you could start would be to **avoid**:
- all yeasts, yeast breads, and alcohol—you don't want anything connected with yeast
- all sugars and products made with sugar—sugars feed candida
- artificial sweeteners and colors, and preservatives— they attack the immune system
- vinegars, as most are made with a yeast culture
- aged and moldy cheeses
- processed, dried, smoked, and pickled meats (49)

Do eat:
- foods high in fiber and complex carbohydrates like legumes, quinoa, brown rice, grains except wheat
- foods high in anti-oxidants to help fight infection -dark green, orange, yellow, and red vegetables
- organic or grass-fed meats and eggs
- all types of good fats (see Part B)
- limited fruits (a couple of servings of raw berries or apples per day - fruits contain sugars)
- prebioctic foods, which are listed later, and take a probiotic supplement such as acidophilus or bifidus.

<u>Herbs to help control candida</u>:

Berberines:	Pau d'Arco
Barberry root	Oregano oil
Goldenseal root	Olive leaf extract
Oregon grape root	Black walnut hull
Coptis (45)	Coconut oil
Garlic	Neem oil (50)
Mugwort (an artemesia)	

Dr. Doug Kaufman and David A. Holland have been researching the connection of yeast and fungus to the serious conditions of our time for many years. To learn more, find their books, <u>Fungus</u> by Doug Kaufmann and

33

The Fungus Link Volume 2: Tracking the Cause (Volume 2) by Doug A. Kaufmann and David Holland.

"Cancer is a fungus" says Dr.T. Simoncini of Italy in his book, Cancer Is a Fungus, published in 2007. He considers all cancers to be the result of a common fungus known as candida. Dr. Simoncini has been very successful in treating cancer with simple sodium bicarbonate, which would support the theory that when our bodies are too acidic we are more likely to become diseased. We've already discussed the importance of keeping the body slightly alkaline. For a very understandable explanation of Dr. Simoncicni's theory, see www.curenaturalicancro.com.

There are other fungi which give off toxins called **mycotoxins** in our environment. You may have heard of Aspergillosis, a condition caused by the Aspergillus fungus in connection with sinus or lung problems. It likes the slightly wet mucosal habitat. Aspergillus is commonly found growing in food, especially stored grain, in dirty air conditioning units, damp or flood-damaged housing, dead leaves, compost piles, or in other decaying vegetation, but Aspergillus fumigatus is a fungal species commonly found in bed pillows. It often affects people whose immune systems have been compromised, including those with leukemia, chemotherapy patients, transplant patients, and people using steroids or suffering from cystic fibrosis, HIV or AIDS, COPD, or any other chronic immune weakness. (51)

Black mold (which can be a variety of colors) may cause a variety of immune responses: runny noses, itchy-watery eyes, coughing, sneezing, and throat irritation, and more severe symptoms such as chronic sinusitis and asthma. (52)

You may have heard of "sick building syndrome," which can be caused by several factors including molds. You may need professional help with this situation, but be aware of whatever chemicals are being used to cure any mold problems.

Toenail fungus (onychomycosis). Doctors say toenail fungus is very common because the feet are often subject to the dark, warm, moist conditions that fungi favor. Some things that have helped people are:

- going barefoot if you can or wearing sandals when you can. Walking barefoot along the seashore where salt is in the sand or swimming in the salt water can be helpful.
- soaking your feet in sea salt water every night—about ½ c of sea salt to 1 gallon of warm water.
- using essential oils topoically. Tea tree oil (Melaleuca), peppermint (mentha piperita), camphor (Cinnamonum Camphora), and oregano (Origanum vulgare) all help heal nail fungus naturally because they are antifungal (antimicrobial) in nature. Mix an essential oil with a bit of olive oil, castor oil, or jojoba oil so it will not burn the skin around the nail. Adding DMSO (Dimethyl sulfoxide) to an essential oil will help the benefits of the oil to be absorbed by the nail faster.

The most serious food mold is Clostridium botulinum, better known as **botulism.** It forms in canned or wet-pack foods that are not properly processed and sealed. (53)

If food appears slimy, has tiny spots of any color, if there is a fuzzy surface, or if it smells bad, **toss it**. When opening canned food make sure you hear the air "whisp" as the seal is broken. If a can is bulging at all on the top, toss it. Obviously moldy food should be discarded in such a manner that your animals and children won't be able to get into it.

Mycotoxins are every bit as bad for your animals as they are for you. Aflatoxin is a type of mycotoxin produced by Aspergillus molds. Aflatoxin commonly grows on beans, rice, tree nuts, and wheat. It grows less often on other grains and nuts. Chlorophyll seems to be an antidote to aflatoxin exposure, so consuming green foods and green drinks often may help keep the less serious molds in check. (54)

<u>If I'm sick with symptoms that could be viral or bacterial, what should I do</u>?

- Rest. Sleep is very important to immune function.
- Drink plenty of water and herbal teas.
- Increase vitamins C and D.
- Avoid sugars, sodas, and other junk food.
- Eat only light, nutrient-dense foods. Include vegetable juices.
- Avoid dairy products, as they produce mucus. (55)

Determine whether the symptoms are general or specific. If the symptoms are specific to an area or an organ you may want to consult your doctor.

In either case I would start dosing with extra vitamin C (1000 mg twice daily), echinacea and/or astragalus root tinctures to help the immune system. If you feel comfortable that it is not serious, choose other herbs from the following material to continue the healing. If you use any kind of drugs, beware of interactions with herbs or grapefruit seed extract.

Nature has provided many plants with the properties to destroy bacteria and other harmful microorganisms. If you are going to rely on herbs during infections it is best towork with an experienced holistic health care practitioner when using herbs as medicines.Having a couple of good herb books as a reference is important. My favorites are:

<u>Herbal Antibiotics</u> by Stephen Harrod Buhner
<u>Herbal Antivirals</u> by Stephen Harrod Buhner
<u>Herbal Healing for Children </u>by Demetria Clark (It is very applicable for adults and has good recipes for herbal products.)
<u>Today's Herbal Health </u>by Louise Tenney, MH

Herbs with **Antiviral and/or Antibacterial** properties:

- **Aloe vera** (fresh juice or gel), external: antibacterial, antimicrobial, antiviral anti-inflammatory. <u>Use internally only under a practitioner's supervision.</u>
- **Andrographis paniculata:** antiviral, antibiotic, antiparasitic, immune stimulant

36

- **Astragalus root:** antiviral, antibacterial, anti-inflammatory, immune stimulant
- **Calendula petals:** antibacterial, antiviral
- **Cat's claw:** antiviral, antibiotic
- **Chamomile:** antiviral, antibiotic
- **Cryptolepsis**: antibiotic
- **Echinacea:** antiviral, antibiotic, immune booster
- **Elderberry:** antiviral, antibacterial, immune booster
- **Eucalyptus:** antibiotic
- **Garlic:** antiviral, antibiotic, antibacterial, antifungal
- **Ginger root:** antiviral, antibacterial, antifungal, anti-inflammatory
- **Goldenseal:** antiseptic, antibacterial, antifungal, anti-inflammatory
- **Grapefruit seed extract:** antiviral, antibacterial, antimicrobial, antifungal
- **Green tea:** antiviral effect of catechins on influenza
- **Honey** (raw): antiviral, antibiotic, antifungal, anti-inflammatory, immune stimulant
- **Juniper berries:** antibacterial, antimicrobial, antiseptic, antifungal
- **Lemon balm:** antiviral
- **Licorice root:** antibiotic
- **Lomatium root:** antiviral, antibacterial
- **Mullein:** antiviral, antiseptic
- **Myrrh gum:** antiviral, antibiotic, antiseptic
- **Olive leaf extract:** antiviral, antimicrobial
- **Oregano oil:** antiviral, antibacterial, antifungal, antiparasitic
- **Oregon grape root:** antibiotic
- **Peppermint:** antiviral, antimicrobial
- **Propolis:** antibacterial, antiviral, antifungal
- **Sage:** antibacterial, antiseptic
- **Usnea:** antiviral, antibiotic, antifungal, immune stimulant
- **Wormwood:** antibiotic, antifungal

Using herbs or essential oils is **not recommended for women who are pregnant or nursing** unless working with a qualified practitioner. (56)

6 How Does Disease Progress in the Body?

Most disease, unless it is an infection, does not happen quickly. Major signs the body is out of balance include:

- congestion
- constipation
- dehydration
- inflammation
- pain

The progression of disease often looks like this:
We inherit weaknesses and...

- if the body isn't supplied with the nutrients to tame the weaknesses...
- this allows vaccinations, infections, and drugs (especially antibiotics) to damage the immune system and the gut flora which creates a lack of good bacteria, thus...
- damaging the intestinal track so nutrients are not being properly absorbed and constipation keeps the toxins and undigested food in the intestines to putrefy or leak back into the body, causing...
- congestion in other organ systems...
- resulting in various dysfunctions which we call disease.

As you read earlier, I've had a lifetime of sickness and disease. Medical science kept me alive with antibiotics, but I was never well. In later years the maladies became more complicated as my body was rebelling against so many things. In recent years high blood pressure and an aneurysm developed, my joints became almost dysfunctional, herpes recurs as soon as I'm stressed, and an autoimmune syndrome has developed. Why?

For me it started many years ago. I hope my story will help you understand how disease can develop one layer at a time. We all need to write our health history for our evaluation, as well as, to have information to give our practitioners. The more information they have, the more quickly they will see your health picture.

LITTLE FOIL PACKAGES

It was in 1946 in rural America that a small girl lay on a gurney surrounded by a flurry of doctors and nurses. A very concerned mother watched while they worked over her sick little girl. "Mrs. Lieb, we don't know if we can save her. She is very sick and we don't have a cure for Bright's Disease." The doctor explained that her kidneys were damaged and not functioning properly. He was filled with despair as he tried to explain their lack of understanding of the disease.

As he fumbled with a small foil package, the doctor said, "We will try this new drug which was used on our soldiers overseas. It's a long shot!" This was just after World War II, when knowledge of diseases was limited and options for cures were few.

This farm mother took her five-year-old girl home with only the little foil packages standing between her daughter and death. There was only one other case of Bright's Disease in the entire area. A girl nearly the same age had just died of Bright's Disease, so my family was extremely worried. No one understood why there were suddenly two isolated cases of Bright's Disease in this rural community.

I can remember the months with no salt and taking the little wonder pill in the foil packages. I was the girl on the gurney, and the precious pill in the foil package was penicillin. Penicillin was new to general medicine but had been used in the military. I was lucky my doctor had access to it in 1947. Gradually I got better, but from that time I was never healthy. It was the beginning of constant illness.

Actually, it had begun a year before when I was four. My tonsils had become so infected that I required emergency surgery. Why did my tonsils get so infected when we hardly ever left the farm? What caused the change from healthy baby to a sick little girl? Were the infected tonsils and the Bright's Disease connected to the same cause? Do these things just happen or is there a cause? From my research and study, I have come to see how each

39

happening affects our health for the rest of our lives.

My mother was 42 and my father was 43 when I was born. They had just gone through the Depression and drought. Food had been meager. There was little variety and practically nothing fresh, resulting in vitamin and mineral deficiencies in everyone's diets. I was breast-fed and seemed to be a healthy baby in spite of it all. My father died of a heart attack at age 43, just 7 months after I was born. He had recently been diagnosed as having diabetes, about which they knew very little at the time. The family said he had "blacked out" in the field several times in the weeks before he died. We speculated his death was related to the diabetes. At that time few understood anything about hereditary health characteristics, but now I see that I could be carrying the genetic tendency for diabetes which is often related to a somewhat weaker immune system.

The exact age of my regular immunizations is unknown, as the records were so old they had all been destroyed before I started my search. Information on any immediate reactions to immunizations is unavailable, but I started being sick at two years old; about the time of the first immunizations. At age four I was rushed to the hospital choking from very infected tonsils, which required that immediate tonsillectomy. Infected tonsils in a child so young is a sign of a compromised immune system, so if I was born with a somewhat weak immune system I could have been more vulnerable than most children to whatever was in the vaccines.

It was a mystery why two children of the same age in a small community who had not been in contact became victims of Bright's Disease. The only connecting link I have found after much study is that we were probably vaccinated from the same batch of vaccine(s). There may have been something in the vaccines that acted as an antigen violator. In recent years we have significant research connecting vaccines to immune weaknesses. http://www.historyofvaccines.org/content/articles/huma n-immune-system-and-infectious-disease

The Merck Manual of Medical Information describes the origin of Nephritis (also known as Bright's Disease). "Nephritis is inflammation of the kidneys. Inflammation of the kidneys generally is caused by an infection, or an immune reaction that goes awry and injures the kidneys. An abnormal immune reaction can come about in two ways: (1) An antibody can attack either the kidney itself or an antigen (substance that stimulates an immune reaction) attached to kidney cells, or (2) an antigen and antibody can combine somewhere else in the body and then become attached to cells in the kidney."(57)

Since the medical records are long gone, the connection between our developing Bright's Disease and having received vaccines from the same batch is an educated guess. Most of us never questioned how vaccines were made, the culture on which they are grown, or what other materials were added to stabilize and preserve the vaccine. Today, we know there are multiple connections of many factors in vaccines to disease, disabilities, and death. (58)

The bottom line is that something caused my severely infected tonsils and the Bright's Disease.

Throughout my childhood I was always sick. It seemed I had no resistance. My immune system was weakened and the tonsils, which are the first line of defense of the immune system, had been removed, so my body was very vulnerable. Very likely there was also a significant lack of vitamins and other nutrients in our diets.

In first grade I had measles, and I remember our house being quarantined when I had scarlet fever in second grade. Scarlet fever is a very contagious disease caused by streptococcus bacteria. The high fever, sore throat, swollen glands and thick, red rash lasted for a couple of weeks. It had spread to epidemic proportions in our little town, so quarantining the infected houses was mandated to hopefully control the epidemic. No one could even come to the door, the mail and groceries were delivered to the edge of our yard where Mother retrieved them. At the end of three weeks, we had to leave the house while the health department fumigated it to kill the germs. Everything that could be washed was washed and they burned the books and papers.

It was after the scarlet fever that I had recurring bouts of strep throat. It became almost comical as my brother, who had come home from serving in the army and was going to college, would call and ask, "Is Linda sick? Is it safe to come home?" I had the biggest Christmas ever in third grade when I had the chicken pox and everyone felt sorry for me, so I got more presents than usual. I remember sitting in my bed with all my new toys while the festivities were going on in the rest of the house. (That chickenpox is the reason I have been dealing with shingles recently.)

I seemed to be on the circuit for the mumps, flu, colds, or whatever virus came to town. A couple of times it would turn into bronchitis or pneumonia, which became a more serious problem. Strep throat seemed to be my doom. I can't begin to tell you how many times I had strep infections. Of course, the answer to all these infections was antibiotics, which kept me alive, but we had no idea the harm they were doing to my body. It wasn't until years later that I questioned why I was the only one in the community that had strep throat so often. Now I understand that the strep was never killed by the antibiotic, so when my immune system was weak it recurred.

At age eight or nine I started to gain weight, even though there was no change in diet. It was a puffy weight. In analyzing it now, it was possibly toxic load from drugs and my body's own wastes from infection, which were not being properly eliminated by the lymph and circulatory systems. The amount of antibiotics I had taken most likely created yeast overgrowth, which impairs digestion and elimination. In addition, I was always constipated, which was a sign no one heeded in those days.

At age ten I remember being taken on a very frightening trip through a North Dakota blizzard with a dishpan in my lap. I was heaving profusely, and when we arrived at the hospital they found I needed an emergency appendectomy.

It took several hours and many nurses to find a vein so they could type my blood and prep me for surgery. After the surgery it took much longer than usual for the massive scar to heal.

Why did they have such a hard time finding a blood vessel? What caused the appendix to become diseased? Why wouldn't the scar heal? I now understand these were all signs that my immune system wasn't functioning as it should have and that I had major nutrient deficiencies. In those days we never heard about the immune system.

We now know constipation and congestion are signs of disease. At that time we didn't know taking antibiotics would kill the good bacteria in our systems as well as the bad. I had had many penicillin shots, and the doctors tried each new antibiotic as it was available. Of course they damaged my gut. It's obvious to me now that I had candida albicans (yeast overgrowth), which contributed to the constipation and congested intestinal tract as well as interfering with the normal absorption of nutrients. Constipation was a warning sign the intestines were not able to eliminate completely. The appendix is a part of the lymph system, which is the circulatory system for the immune system and whose task it is to protect the body. When one is chronically constipated the toxic wastes are not properly eliminated; therefore, the appendix becomes engorged and infected as it tries to deal with the toxic waste which was not eliminated by the colon.

When prepping me for surgery the nurses couldn't find a vein for an IV. What caused that? Looking back at the diet of the times, it would seem I was probably deficient in many vitamins and minerals, causing the blood vessels to be weak and unstable. The scar was slow healing and when it did, it was thick and ugly. Lack of healing response would indicate the immune system wasn't working well and there were probably multiple nutritional deficiencies, especially of vitamins C and E.

I do recall a doctor in the early 1950's recommending that Mother give me a multi-vitamin pill and fruits and juices. Somehow she managed to buy the vitamins for me, and when she could afford it she bought canned grapefruit juice. Living in North Dakota, the growing season during which we ate anything fresh was short. The rest of the year we ate home-canned fruit and vegetables which had little or no nutrition.

This was before mass refrigeration and supermarket fresh produce. This was a time when most families in the US ate a meal of meat, potatoes, highly cooked vegetables, white bread, maybe a gelatin salad and/or a dessert. They did what they knew and thought was right, just as you and I do what we know until we learn a better way.

It's been a challenge to manage my damaged body, which has knocked on death's door several times. Learning how my body functions was the first step. Once I understood what the body needs, it was important to sort through the options.

As we have eaten denatured processed foods, disease has skyrocketed.

We were convinced the new antibiotic drugs would save the world from disease, but they too have been misused and now have added to the health problems we face. Microbes want to survive. They are mutating faster than science can create drugs to control them. What can we do? Many herbs are effective in these cases.

The purpose of vaccination across the world was to eradicate disease. It appears to have made progress in that, but with vaccinations has come a whole new set of problems of toxicity and damaged immune function. We thought we were protecting our children from communicable disease, but we had no idea that many of the ingredients in vaccines were toxic substances. Through the years children have been given an increasing number of various vaccines with little consideration given to how the onslaught of many vaccines would affect the infant or child. (58) (59)

Now we realize the effect of those vaccines may be connected with developing autoimmune disease in later life. The recent addition of the HPV (Human

44

papillomavirus) vaccine has led to terrible side effects and even death in our girls and young women. (60)

What really brought about the decline of infectious disease? Sanitation was one of the biggest factors. As sanitation improved, infectious disease became less prevalent, but vaccines were credited with the decline in infectious disease. Improved nutrition was a big factor in building a stronger immune system. A strong cellular domain will resist most infectious disease.

The Keys to Preventing Disease
1. Nutrients are the master key between you and disease.
2. Detoxification is necessary in our toxic world.
3. Changing our environment and lifestyles will be crucial to wellness.
4. Managing your emotional garbage is essential.

We need to pay attention to the weaknesses in our family health history. Diabetes was definitely a factor in mine. My mother's health history includes circulatory problems, vein replacements, and eight amputations between the ages of 82 and 96 which makes it clear I could also have genetic vein and artery weakness.

It is important for you to write up your family's health history for your own study as well as information to give your practitioners.

7 Why Do People Have Autoimmune Diseases?

I want to share another personal experience. In 2010 when I was diagnosed with sarcoidosis, an autoimmune disease, I was determined to find the cause. Conventional medicine only offered drugs, which I refused. Having studied everything I could find on sarcoidosis and autoimmune disease, one factor seemed to fit my health history. I may have an underlying infection which isstressing my immune system. I have had a lifetime of one infection after another, including strep, herpes, and Epstein-Barr virus.

I found a naturopath who guided me through thirteen intravenous hydrogen peroxide treatments, along with very strong garlic supplements and some herbal combinations. After testing, we also discovered my endocrine system was not producing adequate amounts of several hormones, for which she prescribed some natural hormones. Gradually I regained my strength and clarity.

Any auto-immune syndrome is going to need a wide-ranging, intense natural protocol to bring the immune system back into balance. A plan of management and recovery needs to be developed based on each person's individual needs.

Conventional medicine cannot handle the health issues of our time. "According to the Association of American Medical Colleges, the nation is facing a serious shortfall of primary care doctors and will be 91,500 physicians short of what it needs by 2020. That deficit could hit 130,600 by 2025, in part because Obamacare will hike the number of insured Americans seeking care and many doctors are nearing retirement age, getting into concierge medicine, or leaving the profession." (61)

With an aging population and many doctors leaving the profession, there will not be adequate doctors for our unhealthy nation. We must learn how to stay well and teach our children what their bodies need.

Degenerative disease is touching the lives of all of us. We feel helpless, as modern medicine has few answers.

There are answers. When we learn to eat from Nature, avoid toxins, and use alternatives to take care of the everyday problems, we will need to use the medical system only when we have traumas such as heart attack, stroke, or accidents.

Thomas Jefferson, whose wisdom we would do well to adopt, said, **"If people let the government decide what foods they eat and what medicines they take, their bodies will soon be in as sorry a state as are the souls of those who live under tyranny**." (62) Our government is **not** protecting us.

Disease is neither a mystery nor a roll of the dice.

We have become disconnected from our heritage and the wisdom of the ages. Instead of learning from our parents and grandparents and adding the new to the old, we have discarded the old in favor of following the media as our guide. The natural roots of health are buried deeply under the guise of "new is better". Our bodies have always needed the basic nutrients to be well, but now **we need higher quantities of these nutrients so the body can deal with the pollution and stress of modern day life.**

We are sick because we are going against the flow of Nature. We have turned our backs on the earth and the lessons that sustained our ancestors and the other species on the planet. Mark Stengler, N.D. in his book, The Natural Physician's Healing Therapies, says it so well, **"Our bodies are genetically designed to be compatible with healing substances as found in nature."** (63)

Our bodies can barely sustain life and cannot be well on the artificial or depleted foods that comprise today's diet. Our bodies cannot be well under the constant bombardment by petrochemicals, heavy metals, radiation, and electromagnetic fields in our environment. Supplementing even a good diet has become necessary for us to continually detoxify.

We can be well if we make the right choices.

8 Taking the Scare Out of Cancer

When I ask people over 50 what health issue concerns them most, it is almost universally CANCER. In discussions with people it also became apparent many people are dealing with some form of auto-immune disease. In dealing with my own auto-immune issues, I've come to believe similar causes are involved in the body becoming cancerous and fighting itself in auto-immune disease.

We are nutrient deficient and toxic.

What is your perception of cancer? Fear takes over the whole being when the doctor diagnoses the dreaded "C" word. Most of us fear being diagnosed with cancer.

Why do we fear cancer? Watching the process of cancer and the devastation caused by standard treatments has scared all of us. Having cancer is often considered a death sentence. People are told they must have chemotherapy, radiation, surgery, or a combination of those treatments or they will die. They are scared and become hopeless.

Too often I have seen intelligent people become so scared when told they had cancer that they were no longer able to think. They just froze and became so intimidated that they did whatever the doctor said without questioning the outcome.

This fear is reflected in one person's response to my discussing natural methods. "I really respect what you know about health, but I have to follow what the doctor says because he knows what to do." This comment was very frustrating to me, as it implied the power the medical community has in controlling the masses. We have been taught to do as the doctor says without evaluating it. What happened to questioning, thinking, and looking at all options, or do we believe there are no options beyond the medical protocol?

Cancer is considered the disease of the 20th century because it was hardly known until we created so many things that are altering the internal environment of the body, thus promoting the growth of disease. Free radicals are the result of the body trying to deal with antagonists such as stress, chemicals, and heavy metals. Fluoride, mercury, aluminum, pesticides, radiation, cigarette smoke, drugs, vaccines, food additives, and preservatives were just accepted as safe. Sadly, we believed that the government wouldn't let anything that could hurt us be sold. Wow! To compound the situation, our diets have been very lacking in nutrients to strengthen the body and neutralize the free radicals.

Our medical community has failed so horribly in dealing with cancer because they have frequently listened to the wrong people. Instead of understanding that the body needs nutrients to be well, they wage war on the body. The tumor is the enemy, and the patient's body is the battleground. The weapons used to attack are chemotherapy, radiation, and surgery. I know you may not want to hear it, but plain and simply cancer is big business. (64)

What is Cancer?
Basically, cancer starts when cells in a part of the body start to grow out of control. There are many kinds of cancer, but they all start because of out-of-control growth of abnormal cells called free radicals. When abnormal cancer cells multiply out of control and this unchecked growth spreads through the body, it interferes with the ability of other cells, organs, and other structures to perform their normal functions. All cancers start from a single cell that undergoes many changes.

A molecule or atom that has an unpaired electron in its outer orbit is known as a free radical. Free radicals are very unstable, highly reactive molecules. Normally free radicals are continually created in the millions in your body to carry on the metabolic activity of the body. They are essential to life as they fight infection. Our cells give a burst of free radicals to kill the germs when we become infected with bacteria, fungus, and parasites.

49

Any molecule or atom in the body can become a free radical. When it does it will try to balance itself by picking up an electron from a neighboring molecule, which in turn becomes a free radical, and the vicious cycle continues until it is checked and controlled. If it is not controlled, damage occurs in different parts of the body. (65)

As soon as free radicals are created, the body tries to control them by using antioxidant enzymes, or antioxidant nutrients such as vitamin C, vitamin E, beta carotene, and bioflavonoids from the food we eat. These antioxidants are present in plants, herbs, fruits, and vegetables and are very powerful.

When the generation of free radicals is much more than can be handled by the enzymes or anti-oxidant nutrients, then they create damage in the cell membranes. In a joint, it ultimately results in arthritis; in the lungs we have emphysema or bronchitis; in the blood vessels we have atherosclerosis or heart disease; in the stomach we have peptic ulcer; in the skin, aging and wrinkling. In each area these radicals can produce damage. In the cell nucleus, if free radicals are produced in the DNA, the DNA becomes transformed and mutated. Mutated transformed DNA will produce cancers such as leukemia, and lymphoma. <u>Many diseases such as diabetes, kidney dysfunction, liver problems, and autoimmune syndromes are triggered by the damage caused by free radicals</u>. (65)

Normally the body can handle free radicals, but if anti-oxidant enzymes or other nutrients are unavailable or inadequate, the free-radical production becomes excessive and damage will occur. (65)

What causes cells to grow out of control? Cells become cancer cells because of damage to DNA. DNA is in every cell and directs all its actions. In a normal cell, when DNA gets damaged the cell either repairs the damage or the cell dies. <u>In cancer cells the damaged DNA is not repaired and the cell doesn't die like normal cells do</u>. Instead, this cell goes on making new cells with the same damaged DNA as the first cell. People can inherit damaged DNA, but most

DNA damage is caused by mistakes that happen while the normal cell is reproducing or by some outside factor.

When a free radical isn't kept in check by the body, it tries to balance itself by picking up an electron from a neighboring molecule, which in turn becomes a free radical, and the vicious cycle continues. If not controlled, damage occurs in various parts of the body; nutrients are the control factor.(65)

It usually takes years for cancer to be serious enough for it to be diagnosed. Once cancer is diagnosed, we need to focus on helping the body control it. Often underlying emotions are feeding the cancer, and without therapy for emotional or spiritual changes, the cancer will continue to rage.

Only in understanding the process can we begin to prevent cancer or stop it. Foods and herbs provide antioxidants, but often a larger protocol is necessary. Luckily, our bodies have a host of defensive strategies for making sure damaged or mutated cells never get the chance to reproduce. But if a damaged cell does manage to get past our defenses and starts multiplying without control, it can form a mass of abnormal cells called a **tumor**.

Andreas Moritz in Cancer is not a Disease-It's a Survival Mechanism states that the body forms a tumor to collect the damaged cells to protect the vital organs. (66)

Not all tumors are dangerous. Those that arise and then go quiet are called benign, but malignant or cancerous tumors can spread into surrounding tissues, damaging nearby cells or organs. **Cancer cells can divide forever and are immortal, unless something stops them.** (67)

In many cases the cancer cells form a tumor; however, in cancers like leukemia the cancer cells involve the blood and blood-forming organs and circulate through other tissues where they grow. When cancer cells get into the bloodstream or lymph fluid they can travel to other parts of the body where they grow and form new tumors that replace normal tissue. This process is called **metastasis.**

No matter where a cancer may spread, it is always <u>named for the place where it started</u>. For example, breast cancer that has spread to the liver is still called breast cancer, not liver cancer. Likewise, prostate cancer that has spread to the bone is metastatic prostate cancer, not bone cancer. Different types of cancer can behave very differently. For example, lung cancer and breast cancer are very different diseases. They grow at different rates and respond to different specific treatments. (67)

Cancer develops in many forms in the human body:
- Carcinoma cancers affect the tissue that covers internal organs.
- Leukemia cancer grows in blood-forming tissue.
- Sarcoma cancers affect the blood vessels, bone, fat, muscle, and other connective tissues.
- Lymphoma cancer starts in the cells of the immune system and then can spread to other parts of the body.
- Melanoma is a cancer that develops in the melanocytes, the pigment cells present in the skin. It is more serious than the other forms of skin cancer because it may metastasize to other parts of the body and cause serious illness or death.

Usually a cancer cell will be extinguished by the body's natural defense system if the cells are well fed and functioning well. However, if the defense system (immune system, lymph system, liver, and elimination system) is not able to destroy and eliminate the mutant cancer cell, it will start to reproduce, often at an uncontrollable rate. It is then <u>most important</u> for us to determine <u>what is stressing the body's immune system</u>.

Often disease is blamed on genetics, which can be a factor. We can't choose our ancestry, but <u>we can choose what we eat and how we live</u>. **We need to be aware of our genetic weaknesses and live to strengthen our bodies against them**. People with an inherited weakness for cancer need to avoid chemical substances, as many are known carcinogens and nearly all are toxic to the body. Any toxicity weakens the body and takes it out of balance. They need to eat nutrient-dense food, detoxify regularly, and supplement with body building nutrients. (68)

Now that we understand cancer, we know it can be dismantled by natural means. I'm borrowing the term "dismantled" from <u>Dismantling Cancer</u> by Francisco Contreras. We can break up the cancer party in the body with the right foods, herbs, nutrients, and enzymes; detoxifying protocols; and **AVOIDING** sugar, artificial foods, chemicals, heavy metals, and toxic emotions. (69)

Let's prevent cancer, or if you already have cancer, let's dismantle it.

Start with the things you can **avoid** which are known to damage the body and/or be carcinogenic. <u>Many diseases can be prevented if we remove the cause.</u>

References for the next section are from <u>Detoxify or Die</u> (3) and <u>Natural Strategies for Cancer Patients</u>. (68) Besides the body's normal metabolism which creates free radicals the following are serious culprits:

Over-processed and created foods are not recognized by the body, thus form free radicals. Refined sugar and refined flour turn to simple sugars. **Sugar feeds cancer.** (70)

Fat – The body has always needed saturated fats. Unsaturated fat is of two types: polyunsaturated and monounsaturated. Polyunsaturated fat ultimately causes damage, as it has multiple double bonds which can become oxidized and cause an increased production of free radicals and increased incidence of colon cancer. <u>Most vegetable oils are polyunsaturated fatty acids which become very easily oxidized</u>. Hydrogenated fats are oxidized. Oxidation also occurs when foods and meats are fried or grilled. (71)

Oxidized cholesterol - Natural cholesterol is not a problem because the body needs it, but when the cholesterol has been damaged by processing foods it becomes oxidized cholesterol which forms free radicals.

Alcohol consumption is a major producer of free radicals.

It damages the liver causing cirrhosis, damages the heart causing myocardiopathy, and damages the brain.

Smoking causes susceptibility to strokes and cancer of the colon. Smoking creates free radicals that damage the lungs, so almost every smoker gets bronchitis and emphysema, if not cancer.

Sodas and other colored drinks with artificial ingredients are all toxic to the body.

Mental distress is directly linked to over production of free radicals. When somebody is angry or has anxiety, tension, or stress the body creates chemicals (cortisone and catecholamines) which react with different organs and cells, creating free radicals.

Food preservatives and additives create free radicals in the body.

Pesticides kill pests by creating free radicals, and if you consume pesticides in your food or breathe them, you will be damaged by those free radicals also. That damage may be cumulative.

Environmental pollution - All the exhaust fumes coming from cars, buses, trucks, planes, factories, and other enterprises cause a lot of pollution, creating free radicals which damage our lungs and other body systems.

Sunlight - We need sunlight for survival, but overexposure causes free radicals and skin damage.

Chemotherapy and radiation treatment for cancer kill tumor cells by producing too many free radicals. Their effects are toxic because they also damage normal cells.

Chemicals in products in the workplace, home, yard, cleaning supplies, and personal products can be damaging to the body and create free radicals.

Radiation - In recent years we are learning about the damage which is being subtly caused by various forms of radiation, whether from x-rays, EMFs from electronics, or nuclear accidents, which are damaging to our cells. (3)(68)

Be aware of what is going on in your body.

Constipation is a big clue. Everyone should have two or three soft, easy bowel movements a day. By failing to evacuate when the urge comes we allow toxic material to sit in the colon, where it putrefies and toxins can be reabsorbed through the intestinal wall into the blood stream. Eating foods with adequate fiber, enzymes and prebiotics will encourage the growth of friendly bacteria necessary for the intestines to function properly.

When we eat natural, unprocessed food we usually get adequate fiber. Eating several prunes each day along with lots of raw fruits and vegetables will usually keep you moving. If not, try an herb called cascara sagrada. Follow label instructions.

Inflammation: Chronic inflammation can be caused by poor diet, infection, lifestyle, or environmental stresses on your body. Believe it or not, elevations in blood sugar can generate free radicals which stimulate inflammation.

Infection: Often you just don't feel good! Maybe the glands in your neck hurt a bit, or your throat is slightly swollen, and you are really tired. Underlying infection is thought to be a cause of many autoimmune syndromes, cancer, and even cardiovascular disease. Every time our bodies have to deal with a microbe the immune system becomes somewhat jeopardized. Remnants of viruses, bacteria, and fungus seem to remain in the body even when we think we are "cured" or well. As soon as the body is compromised by extremes of temperature, not enough sleep, stress, or trauma, dormant microbes may become active or even mutate into a different form and become active. (72)

Allergies: In my early twenties I discovered quite by accident that eating grapefruit was causing my migraines. Be a sleuth and pay attention to what you have eaten, drunk or done before you noticed symptoms.

Stress damages the immune system: A healthy immune system is critical in dealing with free radicals and the development of any disease.

Cancer cells have a very interesting characteristic: **They create their own blood supply through a process called angiogenisis**. Tumors rely heavily on an uninterrupted blood supply; if there is deprivation of that blood supply cancerous cells will die. Thus, if we can stop the blood supply, we starve the cells. (73)

Many of antioxident foods are also anti-angiogenetic. Since testing these foods for anti-angiogenetic characteristics is quite new, I expect research will find many more natural, organic foods in this category. Here are a few:

Apples	Lavender	Pumpkin
Artichokes	Lemons	Red grape
Blackberries	Licorice	Red wine
Blueberries	Maitake	Sea cucumber
Bok choy	Mushrooms	Strawberries
Cherries	Nutmeg	Tomatoes
Dark chocolate	Olive oil	Tuna
Garlic	Oranges	(mercury-free)
Ginseng	Parsley	Turmeric (7)
Grapefruit	Pineapple	
Kale	Pomegranate	

The first step in dealing with free radicals is to understand the role toxins of all forms play in our health and to accept the power of foods, nutrients, and herbs to detoxify the body.

To quote Patrick Holford, **"The balance between your intake of antioxidants and exposure to free radicals may literally be the balance between life and death."** (75)

We need a variety of fruits and vegetables because each has its peculiar combination of nutrients. We need more than antioxidants. We need all the nutrients discovered and undiscovered that are in whole organic foods. We need the synergy from the combination of factors found in foods that no supplement or pill can replicate.

Research is continuing to find and name new factors in foods, so let's not get caught up in single factors, but always <u>look at what the whole fruit, herb, or vegetable can provide</u>.

Antioxidants are specific nutrients that counteract the harmful effects of free radicals.

Antioxidants are defined as:
1. Molecules capable of slowing or preventing the oxidation of other molecules.
2. Substances that attack free radicals, preventing them from damaging the body.
3. Substances in food that help to protect cells against damage from free radicals. (76)

Antioxidants neutralize free radicals by donating one of their own electrons, ending the "electron-stealing" reaction. The antioxidant nutrients themselves don't become free radicals by donating an electron because they are stable in either form. They act as scavengers, helping to prevent cell and tissue damage that could lead to cellular damage and disease. (76)

Known antioxidants include alpha-lipoic acid, vitamin C, vitamin E, selenium, flavonoids, enzymes, coenzyme Q10, glutathione, melatonin, methionine, superoxide dismutase (SOD), vitamin A, and carotenoids.

Glutathione, considered the master antioxidant, is a key player in both detoxifying and disease prevention. It replenishes and recycles spent antioxidants for more activity to protect cells from oxidative damage. Don't confuse oxidation or oxidative damage with oxygenation. Oxygenation is part of a healthy cell's function to properly metabolize cellular activity and growth while creating energy. Sufficient antioxidants prevent cellular damage. (76) (77)

Factors involved with glutathione production include:
- <u>Silymarin</u>, found in the herb, milk thistle, helps protect the liver and enhances glutathione production in the body.
- <u>Cumin</u> has the ability to increase glutathione tissue levels.

- Asparagus is a natural source of glutathione, plus a source of selenium, which supports production and recycling of glutathione.
- Artichokes contain the same chemicals as milk thistle, helping increase the production of glutathione and liver enzymes diminished by EMF exposure.
- Fruits and vegetables high in vitamin C help stimulate glutathione production in the body, while working to bind heavy metals for safe elimination.
- Cabbage family veggies—broccoli, Brussels sprouts, cauliflower, collards, and kale—enhance glutathione conjugation, where the liver converts fat-soluble toxins into water-soluble substances that can be passed out of the body through the urine.
- Sulfur-containing veggies like garlic and onions help trigger glutathione and SOD. (77) (78)
- Magnesium plays a critical role in glutathione levels. Magnesium deficiency causes an accumulation of oxidative products in the heart, liver, kidneys, skeletal muscle tissues and in red bloods cells. Magnesium is a crucial factor in the natural self-cleaning and detoxification in the body. (79)

Specific antioxidants found in plants include:

Alpha lipoic acid	Iodine
Anthocyananins	Lutein
Astaxanthin	Lycopene
Catechin	Proanthorcyanadins
Cinnamic acid	Pterostilbene
Ellegic acid	Quercetin
Epigallocatechin	Resveratrol
Hesperitin	Zeaxanthin (76)(77)

One of the groups of vegetables with **significant antioxidant levels** is cruciferous vegetables such as bok choy, broccoli, Brussels sprouts, cabbage, cauliflower, horseradish, kale, kohlrabi, mustard, radish, rutabaga, turnip, and watercress, which are rich sources of glucosinolates, precursors of isothiocyanates. Naturally-occurring isothiocyanates and their metabolites have been found to inhibit the development of chemically-induced cancers of the lung, liver, esophagus, stomach, small intestine, colon, and breasts in a variety of animal models. (80)

A natural compound, diindolylmethane (DIM), found in vegetables like broccoli, cabbage, turnips and mustard greens, can not only prevent cancer but may be able stop it as well. (80)

Lycopene is a special case. Scientists have significant research that supports the role of lycopene in human health, specifically in the prevention of cancers of the prostate, pancreas, stomach, breast, cervix and lung, as well as in the prevention of cardiovascular disease, cataracts, and age-related macular degeneration (a chronic eye condition in which light-sensing cells in the center of the retina stop functioning). Lycopene is thought to have prostate-protective effects and suppresses the growth of tumors. Lycopene is found in tomatoes, guava, apricots, watermelon, papaya, and pink grapefruit. Lycopene is unusual because it is more active in cooked tomatoes than in raw. Studies suggest eating cooked tomatoes along with a source of fat such as olive oil, cheese, or meat, which may improve lycopene absorption. (81)

The ORAC (Oxygen Radical Absorbance Capacity) unit, ORAC value, or "ORAC score" is a method of measuring the antioxidant levels in foods. There are many sources attempting to rate the value of antioxidant foods and they all differ slightly. The lists below are from various sources and are not in order of specific ORAC value. Consuming a variety of fruits, vegetables, and herbs (and chocolate) will provide many antioxidants which can neutralize and stop free radicals before they do damage. (82)

Herbs and spices high in antioxidants:

Allspice	Cilantro	Garlic
Angelica root	Cinnamon	Ginger root
Basil	Cloves ground	Gingko biloba
Black pepper	Cumin seed	Green/white tea
Cayenne fruit	Dill weed	Hyssop
Chamomile	Echinacea flowers	Lemon balm

Marjoram
Mustard seed
Nutmeg
Onion
Oregano
Paprika
Parsley

Peppermint
Periwinkle
Purslane
Rhodiola rosa
Rosemary
Sage
Savory

St. John's Wort
Sweet Annie
Thyme
Turmeric root
Valerian root (83)

Fruits: (berries are highest)

Acai berries
Apples
Avocados
Blackberries
Blueberries
Cherries
Chokeberries
Cranberries
Elderberries

Goji berries
Gooseberries
Grapefruit, pink
Kiwi fruit
Plums
Pomegranates
Prunes
Pumpkin
Raisins

Raspberries
  (black & red)
Red grapes
Rose hips
Seabuckthorn
  berries
Strawberries

High antioxidant vegetables:

Alfalfa sprouts
Arugula
Artichoke
  hearts
Asparagus
Beans (red,
  pinto)
Beets
Broccoli
Brussels
  sprouts

Cabbage
Cauliflower
Corn
Dried beans
Eggplant
Green peas
Kale
Leaf lettuce
Onion
Raw garlic

Red bell
  pepper
Red pepper
Russet potato
Spinach
Summer
  squash
Sweet potato
Turnips
Watercress
(84) (85) (86)

Antioxidants have only been studied for the last decade, so I'm sure there are many other natural foods that could be on these lists. All fruits, herbs, and vegetables are loaded with important nutrients besides antioxidants and the many nutrients that haven't been discovered yet, so eat a variety every day.

Do you know about plant sterols? They are plant fats, also known as phytosterols, which provide a whole array of actions in the body such as:

- decreasing both the level of cortisol in the blood and the factors that induce inflammation such as tissue damage, muscular aches, and stiffness
- reducing bowel diseases
- combating allergic reactions by decreasing the specific immune factor (Interleukin 4) that stimulates the allergic response
- enhancing the function of T-cells that attack cancer cells

The immune-modulating effect of plant sterols can be important for alleviating certain autoimmune diseases. Plant sterols are found in a variety of seeds, nuts, some grains and vegetables. (87)

Let's continue looking in depth at some other vegetables. This will emphasize the power of vegetables and herbs to lower the risk of cancer and other chronic disease and support the body when fighting disease.

I don't believe any one food or herb can cure cancer. It makes sense that using a variety of these nutrient dense foods and herbs may give the cells what they need.

Beets - Danica Collins in the *Underground Health Reporter* writes, "**Raw beet juice is astonishingly effective treatment for leukemia and other cancers."** The crimson color of the beet comes from *betacyanins*, natural compounds that happen to be extremely powerful cancer-fighting agents. Beets also contain the amino acid, *betaine*, packed with anti-cancer properties and unique phytochemicals called *betalains*. Danica goes on to say, "Betanin, one of the most researched betalains found in beets, has significant anti-inflammatory, antioxidant, and detoxifying effects." (88)

From the Whole Foods website by the George Mateljan Foundation we read, "In recent lab studies on human tumor cells, betanin pigments from beets have been shown to lessen tumor cell growth through a number of mechanisms, including inhibition of pro-inflammatory enzymes (specifically, cyclooxygenase enzymes). The tumor cell types tested in these studies include tumor cells from colon, stomach, nerve, lung, breast, prostate and testicular tissue." (89)

Asparagus: Below are some interesting stories of people who have had success treating cancer by eating asparagus. These are quoted from the website *http://www.goodhealthwellnessblog.com/210/asparagus-cures-cancer/*.

- A man with an almost hopeless case of Hodgkin's disease (cancer of the lymph glands) was completely incapacitated. Within 1 year of starting the asparagus therapy, his doctors were unable to detect any signs of cancer.
- A successful businessman, 68 years old, suffered from cancer of the bladder for 16 years. After years of medical treatments, including radiation, without improvement, he began taking asparagus. Within 3 months, examinations revealed that his bladder tumor had disappeared and that his kidneys were normal.
- On March 5th 1971, a man who had lung cancer was put on the operating table where they found lung cancer so widely spread that it was inoperable. The surgeon sewed him up and declared his case hopeless. On April 5th he heard about asparagus therapy and immediately started taking it. By August, X-ray pictures revealed that all signs of the cancer had disappeared. He is now back at his regular business routine. (90)

Why could asparagus be effective for prevention and healing? When tested asparagus contained the highest level of glutathione, the most potent antixoxidant, and contains a good supply of protein called histones, which are believed to be active in controlling cell growth. (90)

Each person has specific needs, which emphasizes the importance of individualizing routines.

Wheatgrass - <u>Did you know wheatgrass is one of the most alkaline foods known to mankind</u>? Combating acidity with alkaline foods will contribute to over-all wellness. Wheatgrass is a great source of chlorophyll, which has almost the same molecular structure as hemoglobin, so when we drink wheatgrass juice it increases hemoglobin production. Hemoglobin is the protein molecule in red blood cells that carries oxygen from the lungs to the body's tissues and returns carbon dioxide from the tissues back to the lungs. Cancer doesn't like oxygen. Wheatgrass is also a source of selenium and laetrile, which both have anticancer factors.(92)

Remember the importance of eating fruits, vegetables, and herbs grown without chemical pesticides

It is important our fruits and vegetables are free of pesticides and other toxins. The Environmental Working Group tests vegetables and fruits for pesticide and other chemical residue. <u>"The Dirty Dozen" below are the most contaminated.</u> If at all possible buy these organic or from a responsible local producer. (93) Use vegetable washes on ALL produce.

Dirty Dozen Plus as of 2015   Buy these organic

Apples	Cucumbers
Peaches	Cherry tomatoes
Nectarines	Snap peas (imported)
Strawberries	Potatoes (white)
Grapes	Hot Peppers
Celery	Kale
Spinach	Collards
Bell peppers	

Clean 15 Lowest in Pesticide

Asparagus	Eggplant	Papayas
Avocados	Grapefruit	Pineapples
Cabbage	Kiwi fruit	Sweet corn
Cauliflower	Mangos	Sweet peas
Cantaloupe	Onions	Sweet potatoes

"A small amount of sweet corn, papaya and summer squash sold in the United States is produced from GE seedstock. Buy organic varieties of these crops if you want to avoid GE produce."Environmental Working Group (94)

Unfortunately, most supermarket produce has been grown on huge farms where the soils are depleted of micronutrients and chemical fertilizers and pesticides are used. We need our produce to be free of chemicals. Studies have shown organically grown food has a higher nutrient content. Becoming "certified organic" is a long, expensive process, so also consider looking for local producers who may not use chemicals but haven't gone through the certification process. (95)

After much study and observation, I believe that most cancers can be stopped or brought into remission naturally if the person is willing to work with a good holistic doctor or alternative practitioner and follow a plan. There are many choices of healing options for cancer, but we need to be willing to **change** our lifestyles and follow some unconventional protocols. An eye-opening book on Cancer is <u>Knockout</u> by Suzanne Somers, Crown Publishers, 2009.

<u>If cancer is growing rapidly in the body, it takes drastic changes to stop it</u>. Everyone who is diagnosed with cancer needs to understand what cancer is and how it develops. Often a patient will try one or two anti-cancer herbs or supplements or a magic juice, but won't follow a cleansing routine and diet protocol. It isn't enough, they succumb to cancer, and the people around them feel natural things don't work. **Cancer needs to be stopped and the garbage cleaned out of the body using drastic cleansing measures.** An herb or two won't touch it. The cancer needs to be "dismantled". (69)

Unfortunately, most practitioners in conventional medicine are not oriented to a holistic philosophy which believes the body will usually heal itself if given what it needs. Statistics show that drugs (chemotherapy), radiation, and surgery don't always extend life beyond a short time, if at all, and usually impair the quality of life and hasten death due to the harshness of the treatment. Cancer is Big Business. (96)

A course of treatment with one cancer drug costs $93,000 but extends life by only about four months. Another cancer drug costs $120,000 to maybe give patients an extra 3.5 months. (97)

In November of 1977 Dr. Ralph Moss was fired from a distinguished cancer center for telling the public the truth about an alternative cancer treatment that was being tested. Dr. Moss in his book, Questioning Chemotherapy, documents the ineffectiveness of chemotherapy in treating most cancers. (98)

Within the last couple of years we have a new potential risk, the HPV vaccine, being forced on our young people. Parents are being coerced to have their girls and boys receive the HPV vaccine with little information of the possible dangers. The HPV vaccine is designed to prevent human papillomavirus (HPV), one of the causes of cervical cancer. From what I've read we need to question its safety, effectiveness, and certainly the side effects it is causing. (99)

Adverse reactions to the HPV vaccine include moodiness, hormonal imbalance, severe bleeding, paralysis, Bell's Palsy, Guillian-Barre' syndrome, and seizures. We are now hearing the sad results of the HPV vaccine. What's really frightening is we have no idea what the long term effects will be from the HPV vaccine. If you want statistics see the Vaccine Adverse Event Reporting System (VAERS). Was there any reliable research ensuring the safety of this vaccine or that it would even be effective? (99) (100)

There are many good protocols which integrative and alternative practitioners will help you use to dismantle cancer. Too often people are looking for a magic bullet cure for cancer and other disease. **There is no one magic juice, pill, or potion that will cure your cancer. This is your life, so do what you need to do to get well.** Don't fall for the hype that a single thing can cure cancer, not one juice or one food or one herb.

Cancer is healed only from the inside out. It will be a process of NUTRIFYING AND DETOXIFYING. Research or have someone help you research whatever you choose to dismantle your cancer. When your body has reached the point that cancer is detectable, you need a varied protocol to eliminate the cancer. Get your head in a positive place, find the best practitioners, and expect to get well as you work through the process.

The cancer protocol will depend on the individual's overall condition, age, or type of cancer

Cancer is not a mysterious disease that suddenly attacks you out of the blue. It has definite causes you may be able to correct if your body has enough time and energy. The person needs to *take action* to change the internal environment to one that creates health, not cancer, while at the same time attacking cancerous cells and tumors.

Unfortunately, conventional medicine attacks cancer by adding more toxins to the body.

Most types of radiation do not attack cancer cells specifically, and therefore cause injury to normal tissues surrounding the tumor. How can one justify beaming radiation, which we know causes cancer, at the body to cure cancer? Seems medieval to me! Burning the body may have all sorts of side effects, from injuring tissue that may become infected, to heart attacks, to new cancer cells being created by the radiation. Do your research if you are considering radiation therapy. (101)

Philip Day tells us in Cancer: Why We're Still Dying to Know the Truth, "In a survey of 79 oncologists from McGill University Cancer Center in Canada, 64 said they would not consent to treatment with Cisplatin, a common chemotherapy drug, while 58 oncologists said they would reject all the current trials being carried out by their establishment. Why? Because of the ineffectiveness of chemotherapy and its unacceptable degree of toxicity." (102)

Dealing with Cancer

Weight loss is part of the cancer process, as the cancer cells demand so much fuel that they deplete the supply for other tissues. Often cancer patients are told to eat high calorie foods so they don't lose weight. Do the medical people giving this advice not understand nutrition and how cancer survives?

Cancer thrives on sugar. The body needs only foods that are nutrient dense with no refined sugars, white or refined flour, or products made from these. Avoid hydrogenated fats. Eat only foods with good fats, especially essential fatty acids as found in fish oil, krill oil, flaxseed, and many other seeds and nuts. The diet needs to be high in antioxidant foods, and good protein is essential for maintaining and rebuilding cells, which is especially crucial in cancer patients. Avoid microwaved foods and drinks and avoid other forms of radiation. (103)

Cancer is complicated, yet understanding it becomes simpler if we understand our bodies.

If I found I had an overgrowth of cancer cells, I would find the best natural practitioner to help me sort through the many natural treatments for cancer. I would use various strategies beginning with cutting all sugars, eating lots of vegetables and herbs, and getting my head straight. I am in charge of my body.

There are many great herbal protocols to use to help the body dismantle the cancer. Herbs can assist the immune system in resisting any foreign agents that enter the body.

Garlic is the number one anti-bacterial, anti-viral, anti-fungal, and anti-parasitical herb. If something in the body needs killing, garlic is the herb for the job. Dr Richard Schulze, master herbalist and successful natural healer, strongly advocates the liberal use of garlic to aid and strengthen the body. (104)

Artemesia annua (often called Sweet Annie or sweet wormwood) has been used for years to combat malaria. After much study the active ingredient, artemisinin, has also been found to have anti-cancer properties.It was found to be capable of **selectively killing cancer cells while leaving the normal cells untouched or unharmed.** Research scientists from the University of California, found that artemisinin can stop the proliferation of prostate cancer cells by arresting the cell cycle at a certain point. They also found artemisinin could arrest the cell cycle of breast cancer cells, thus disrupting their responsiveness to estrogen. Scientists involved in these studies further said that many cancer patients who have tried artemisinin for cancer treatment have seen their situation improved and stabilized. (105)

According to studies that were published in the journal, *Life Sciences,* "Artemesinin, a derivative of the wormwood plant used in Chinese Medicine, can kill 98% of breast cancer cells in less than 16 hours. The herb used alone caused a 28% reduction in breast cancer cells, but when paired with iron, sweet wormwood was able to eradicate cancer almost entirely. What's more, normal cells were not negatively affected in the experiment by this treatment." (106)

Pacific yew (Taxus brevifolia) has been used as medicine by Native Americans and has been found to be effective against certain types of cancer. The drug, Taxol, was formulated from the constituents in Pacific yew. (107) The anticancer effects of Pacific yew are due to many constituents, including taxanes, flavonoids, and lignans." (108) I have personally used yew products from www.Bighornbotanicals.com.

Turmeric seems to be rising as the real star, with many properties to assist the body in controlling free radicals and preventing disease. Most of the hype has been about curcumin, the most studied constituent of turmeric, but I believe we should use herbs in the complete form. I would use a combination of curcumin and whole turmermic.

"In the August 15, 2005, issue of the journal *Cancer*, MD Anderson researchers reported that curcumin blocks a key biological pathway needed for development of melanoma and other cancers. They demonstrated that curcumin stops laboratory strains of melanoma from proliferating and forces the cancer cells to self-destruct. It does this by shutting down a powerful protein (NF-kB) that is known to promote an abnormal inflammatory response that leads to a variety of disorders, including arthritis and cancer. Also, dramatic results from MD Anderson Laboratory studies led to two ongoing Phase I human clinical trials, testing the ability of curcumin powder to retard growth of pancreatic cancer and multiple myeloma." (109)

Dr. Joseph Mercola wrote, "Curcumin - One of the Most Powerful Cancer Gene Regulators." He says, "It's now becoming more widely accepted that cancer is not pre-programmed into your genes, but rather it's the environment of your body that regulates your genetic expression that can trigger cancer to occur. Adverse epigenetic influences that can damage or mutate DNA and alter genetic expression, allowing cancer to proliferate, include:
- Nutritional deficiencies
- Hormonal imbalances
- Chronic stress
- Toxins and pollution
- Chronic inflammation
- Chronic infections
- Free radical damage
- Infectious toxic by-products
- Thoughts and emotional conflicts" (110)

Researchers have found that curcumin can affect more than 100 different pathways once it gets into the cell. More specifically, curcumin has been found to:
- decrease inflammation
- inhibit the proliferation of tumor cells
- help your body destroy mutated cancer cells so they cannot spread throughout your body
- inhibit the transformation of cells from normal to tumor
- inhibit the synthesis of a protein thought to be instrumental in tumor formation

- help prevent the development of additional blood supply necessary for cancer cell growth (angiogenesis) (110)

There are many herbal combinations that have been used for cancer. Often an herbalist will create formulas for cancer based on the person's needs. Essiac Tea is probably the best known combination that you can purchase. A good source for accurate information on Essiac is www.RENECAISSETEA.COM.

Hydrogen Peroxide Therapy

I remember being curious when someone said, "The most overlooked solution to all manner of illness and disease is perhaps the simplest." All pathogens, viruses, and parasites are anaerobic meaning they thrive in the **absence of oxygen,** but cannot survive with an abundance of oxygen. Even cancer cells cannot exist in oxygen. They depend on fermenting glucose to survive and multiply. (111)

I have used intravenous hydrogen peroxide treatments administered by a doctor with great success against underlying infections which weaken my immune system.

Research medicinal mushrooms for cancer.
"Medicinal mushrooms like reishi, maitake can help fight cancer"
http://www.naturalnews.com/027308_mushrooms_cancer_medicinal.html#ixzz3myJVKopR
"Chaga mushroom health benefit, review of effect on immune system and cancer" Ray Sahelian MD.
http://www.raysahelian.com/chaga.html

Rife technology is electro frequency medicine.
http://www.cancerresearchuk.org/about-cancer

I find the baking soda protocol of Dr. Simoncini intriguing. His website explains the process at
http://www.curenaturalicancro.com/therapy-simoncini.html

More information about **Dr. Simoncini's** protocol is at
https://www.cancertutor.com/simoncini/

There are many cancer treatments used around the world that are not available in the US. **I would research everything to find what might work for my situation**.

Websites with more information on healing cancer:
http://www.cancertutor.com/
http://www.healingcancernaturally.com/
http://www.cancersupportivecare.com/herbalmedicine.html
http://www.cancer-info.com/cmnherbs.htm
http://www.cancure.org/choiceoftherapy.htm

Sometimes in 3rd and 4th stage cancer the person needs to be in a constantly controlled environment for the body to get the attention it needs. I feel the following are several good cancer centers.

Cancer Centers which use basically holistic methods:

- **Bio-Med Center** (The Hoxsey Clinic) in Tijuana, Baja California, Mexico.
  http://www.cancure.org/hoxsey_clinic.htm
- **Gerson Institute** http://www.gerson.org/
- **Hippocrates Health Institute**
  http://www.healingcancer.info/resources/clinics/hippocrates
- **Rubio Cancer Center** http://rubiocancercenter.com/
- **Oasis of Hope**, Francisco Contreras, MD
  http://www.oasisofhope.com/

Great books on cancer:
- Dismantling Cancer by Francisco Contreras, MD, Jorge Barrosos-Aranda, MD, & Danel E. Kennedy
- How to Fight Cancer and Win by William Fischer
- Natural Strategies for Cancer Patients by Russell Blaylock
- Knockout by Suzanne Somers
- The Prevention of All Cancers by Hulda Clark
- Cancer Is Not a Disease—It's a Survival Mechanism by Andreas Moritz
- The Gerson Therapy by C. Gerson & Norman Walker

9 Basic Priorities for Survival

When we are sick our bodies are not getting what is needed for vital health.

The following are the basic considerations for health:
- Genetics: We need to know the history of our ancestors.
- Oxygen: What are you breathing?
- The role of water: The real staff of life.
- Potassium/Salt balance
- pH, the acid/alkaline balance: What is yours?
- Sunlight: Sunshine is crucial to health.
- Everything you consume by mouth affects your health.
- Eating a constant supply of the basic building materials for cellular growth, maintenance, and repair.
- Physical environment: Everything that touches your inside or outside affects your health.
- The mental, emotional, and spiritual climate of your life: We must find balance.

1. Genetics – Many believe we are the result of all our ancestors' thoughts and what they ate, breathed, and experienced. Some believe we carry the imprint of all the diseases our ancestors experienced.

Inherited genes play a fundamental role in health and disease. Genes are tiny molecules that contain the biological instruction that direct the functions of all cells in your body.

It was thought for many years that we had no control over our inherited genes; however, more recent research has found that these genes are flexible. Genes do not function by themselves but are dependent on the nutrients they receive. (112)

Knowing that we have some control over our genetic inheritance is comforting, especially when parents or grandparents have died of a major disease such as cancer or heart attack.

When you keep your body properly nourished with the nutrients it needs while getting adequate sunshine, sleep, and water and protecting it from physical, emotional, and environmental pollutants, you may never realize any disease from the weaknesses in genes you carry and you may endow genetically stronger characteristics to your children.

The health of the parents at the time of conception and the health of the mother during pregnancy are critical to the development of the fetus. However, the genes are continually affected by the nutrients or lack of nutrients consumed, the environment, and the lifestyle of each infant as it develops through childhood and adulthood.

Dr. F. Batmanghelidg in his book, Your Body's Many Cries for Water, says, "In their order of importance oxygen, water, salt and potassium rank as the primary elements for the survival of the human body."

2. Oxygen - We are not getting as much oxygen as our ancestors. Why?

- We have much lowered atmospheric oxygen caused by over 200,000 environmental pollutants dumped into our air over the last 50 years. Some major cities have as little as 17% oxygen. (113) At 7% life ceases to exist for humans.
- Pollution of oceans, lakes, and rivers has destroyed much of the oxygen-producing sea plankton and algae.
- Destruction of the rain forests across the planet has greatly contributed to the earth's oxygen decrease.
- Depletion of vegetation, which is being replaced by asphalt and concrete, has reduced oxygen sources.
- People are more sedentary, thus breathe more shallowly, decreasing the oxygen supply to the bloodstream.
- Poor dietary habits fill the body with toxins and acids which interfere with cellular metabolism. (113)

How can we increase oxygenation of blood and cells?
- Exercise regularly using all parts of your body.
- Learn deep breathing techniques; use those lungs.

- Drink green juices and eat green foods, which are high in chlorophyll and will build the blood and transport more oxygen to the cells.
- Use reflexology, massage, acupuncture, or acupressure to stimulate blood flow and circulation.
- Use aromatherapy (baths or diffuser) to help carry oxygen deep into the lungs.
- Use a negative-ion or zone air purifier in your home and workplace.
- Have a doctor do ozone or hydrogen peroxide therapy (113)

3. The Role of Water - My attitude about water has totally changed since I read <u>Your Body's Many Cries for Water</u> by F. Batmanghelidj and listened to his tape series. As I experimented with his ideas, I realized he has discovered something simple and basic that affects our day to day health. Most of us live in a condition of dehydration without realizing it. Often simply drinking adequate pure water can make significant changes in your life, such as lowering blood pressure, relieving headache, aiding digestion, and much more. (114)

The human body is composed of 25 percent solid matter and 75 percent water. The brain is thought to be about 85 percent water, so about 20 percent of the water circulating in the body is allotted to the brain. In 24 hours the body recycles 40,000 glasses of water and needs to replace 6-8 glasses of water which are lost each day during routine functions. (114)

The body needs water to function. Most other liquids contain water, but they also contain dehydrating agents which pull more water from the reserves in the body to clear the dissolved agents, thus leaving the body more dehydrated. In the past we were not taught to understand the role water plays in our health. (114)

Reasons the Body Needs Water:

Survival: Without water nothing lives. Shortage of water means some cells will die and others live in a state of dehydration or partial dysfunction.

Energy source: Water generates electrical and magnetic energy at the cellular level. Water is necessary for production of electrical energy for all brain functions, especially thinking, which is an energy-consuming activity. Adequate water will often lessen the effects of ADD (attention deficit disorder) and other neurological conditions. (114)

Oxygen: Water transports oxygen to every cell and takes away the waste gases.

Body's adhesive: Water is the bonding adhesive in the cells. Water prevents DNA damage and is essential in repair. Adequate water keeps the skin smooth, gives luster to the eyes, and helps maintain vision.

Transport system: Water is used for transporting all substances within the body. If water intake is insufficient, all body fluids become very concentrated, sluggish, and toxic, which overtaxes the elimination organs, often resulting in re-absorption of toxins. Adequate water decreases the depositing of toxic sediments in the tissue spaces, joints, liver, kidneys, brain, and other organs.

Blood: Water dilutes the blood, keeping the viscosity at a healthy level and lessening the chance of clots and clogging of the arteries. Water normalizes the blood-manufacturing system in the bone marrow.

Digestive Solvent: Water is the main solvent for all foods, vitamins, and minerals. Water energizes food and food particles for digestion. It is needed to break down food into small particles for their eventual metabolism. Water will increase the rate of absorption of essential substances in food. Water clears the toxic waste from different body parts, transporting them to the liver and kidneys for disposal. Drinking a glass or two of water will often alleviate GERD or other indigestion issues.

Lubricant: Water is the best lubricating laxative for proper emptying of the bowel. Water is the main lubricant in the joint spaces and thus may prevent arthritis and back pain. Water is used in the spinal discs to make them shock-absorbing water cushions.

Pain: Water can often relieve headache and premenstrual or other pain with no injurious side effects.

Immune Function: Adequate water increases the efficiency of the immune system, thus guarding against infection and cellular destruction.

Pregnancy: Pregnant women need to provide water for the fetus and themselves. There is so much happening to the woman's body; it needs water to keep all systems functioning. Morning sickness is one of the signs of dehydration. (114) (115) (116)

According to web.md, "Many prescription and nonprescription medicines can cause dehydration. A few examples are antihistamines, blood pressure medicines, chemotherapy, diuretics, and laxatives. (117) If the body receives adequate water daily, all systems will function much more efficiently, creating a healthier body with less fatigue and more normal sleep rhythms. Drinking a couple of glasses of water will often relieve stress, fatigue, malaise, anxiety, or depression. (116)

Dr. Batmanghelidj's research reveals the body needs half its body weight in ounces or a minimum of two quarts of water per day for all bodily functions. It is recommended to drink eight ounce portions spaced out throughout the day rather than just sipping. Drink 8 ounces half an hour before each meal to activate enzyme production, drink water with meals to help transport the food and instigate hydrolysis, and drink 8 ounces about 2½ hours after eating to complete digestion. Otherwise drink when thirsty. If you have not been a water drinker, increase your consumption of water gradually, so as not to overtax the kidneys. Urine production should increase in proportion to increased water consumption. Salt intake must be increased when water intake is increased. (114)

DRINK THE PUREST WATER POSSIBLE!

4. Salt/Potassium Balance - For years we have been hearing we must eat a salt-free diet in order to control our blood pressure. It is true that people who eat processed and fast foods are consuming too much salt compared to their potassium intake. But some people have taken the no-salt suggestion to extreme and are not getting enough salt. I know just such a case, in which a lady was taking Spironolactone, a potassium-sparing diuretic, and digitalis, which is known to raise serum potassium levels, and she also insisted on NO SALT in her food. She ended up in the hospital on an intravenous sodium and magnesium drip. It is very important to monitor the potassium/salt balance. (116) (118)

For years salt has been considered the enemy, but things are changing. Recently medical research is finding that salt may not be as big a factor in high blood pressure as previously thought. Studies involving 6,250 subjects, as reported in the *American Journal of Hypertension,* found no strong evidence that cutting salt intake reduces the risk for heart attacks, strokes, or death in people with normal or high blood pressure. (118)

When we eat natural foods the balance of minerals stays intact, but most processed foods are very high in sodium and low in potassium. If you eat mostly processed foods then you may be overloading the body with sodium and need to change your diet to include more natural potassium-rich foods.

Dr. Batmanghelidj explains many roles salt plays in the body:
- Salt extracts excess acidity from the cells in the body, especially the brain.
- Salt is vital in balancing the sugar level in the blood.
- Salt is necessary for the generation of hydro-electrical energy at the cell membrane.
- Salt is vital for nerve cell communication.
- Salt is processed all the time that the brain cells function.
- Salt is vital for the absorption of food particles through the intestinal tract.
- Salt is necessary for the clearance of mucus and sticky phlegm from the body.
- Salt is vital in cleaning up inflammation and congestion from the sinuses and throat.

- Salt is a strong natural antihistamine.
- Salt is needed for the prevention of muscle cramps.
- Salt is needed to prevent excess saliva production.
- Salt is vital in the formation of bone in combination with several other minerals. (119)

Potassium

Potassium hasn't received much press, so most of us don't realize how important it is to the functioning of our bodies. Many of us are potassium deficient. A few of the basic functions of potassium are:

- Promoting a healthy nervous system and muscular contraction and relaxation
- Working with sodium to maintain fluid balance in the body
- Enabling nutrients to move into and waste to move out of cells through the membranes
- Facilitating chemical reactions within the cells
- Regulating the heart beat, stabilizing blood pressure, and preventing strokes
- Helping in the secretion of insulin for control of blood sugar
- Working with magnesium to help prevent kidney stones
- Promotinghormone secretion (120) (121)

Signs of potassium deficiency include (121) (122)

Salt retention	Nausea and vomiting
Rapid irregular heartbeat	Nervousness
Swollen abdomen	Insomnia
Low blood pressure	Diarrhea
Muscle cramps	Periodic headaches
Muscle fatigue, weakness	Constipation
Fatigue	High cholesterol levels
Mental confusion	Glucose intolerance
Irritability	Impaired growth
Abnormally dry skin	Edema
Insatiable thirst	Sensation of pins and
Chills	needles, especially in
Depression	feet and ankles

Potassium deficiency may cause heart problems.

How much potassium do we need? In 2004, the Food and Nutrition Board of the Institute of Medicine established that an adequate intake of potassium ranges from 400 mg daily for an infant from 0 to 6 months, to 3,800 mg for children ages 4-8 and 4,700 mg for adults. (123)

According to a 1985 article in *The New England Journal of Medicine* entitled "Paleolithic Nutrition," "Our ancient ancestors got about 11,000 mg of potassium a day, and about 700 mg of sodium. This equates to nearly 16 times more potassium than sodium. Compare that to the Standard American Diet where daily potassium consumption averages about 2,500 mg (remember the RDA is 4,700 mg/day), along with 3,600 mg of sodium. As mentioned earlier, if you eat a diet of processed foods, you can be virtually guaranteed your potassium-sodium ratio is upside-down." (124)

Nutritionists realize there are many factors which affect the need for potassium, so an individual's appropriate dose may be lower or higher. Some factors that increase potassium deficiency include severe vomiting or diarrhea, tobacco and caffeine use, alcoholism, kidney disorders, abuse of laxatives, over-consumption of licorice, eating heavily salted foods, use of potassium-wasting drugs such as diuretics, magnesium depletion, and stress. (113)

Most foods in their natural form are sources of potassium. The dark greens are all good sources of most nutrients, including potassium. You will find a chart with the potassium values of foods later in the book.

5. What is pH?

Thanks to a wonderful little book entitled The Battle for Health Is Over pH, by Gary Tunsky, I now understand the importance of pH balance in the body. I refer to his book often.

The pH indicates the alkaline/acid balance of the body. The regulatory control for all the cellular processes and cellular communication is the pH. pH is tested on a scale of 1 to 14, with the healthiest range being 7.2 to 7.5. The body functions best when slightly alkaline. When the level goes below 7.0, it indicates an acidic state in which acid wastes are not being properly eliminated and the body is becoming clogged.

All the cells, organs, and systems communicate and work together. The function and regulation of the organ systems: respiration, digestion, metabolism, neurotransmitter release, immunity, and hormone release depend on balanced pH. **Unbalanced pH sets the stage for disease**. (113)

In the late 19th century two famous scientists arrived at different theories on the origin of disease. Louis Pasteur believed in the "germ theory," that all infectious and contagious disease is caused by germs, while Antoine Bechamp believed the condition of the cellular terrain was the basis for disease. He believed germs don't cause disease, but develop in response to the acidic condition of the cellular environment.

Bechamp was a brilliant scientist, but Pasteur had political connections and wealthy associates who saw how they could use Pasteur's "germ theory" to create a business to manage sickness. Thus, the basis for the curriculum of conventional medicine was born, in which the emphasis is on killing bacteria, virus, fungus, or tumors. What is very significant is that Pasteur, on his deathbed, admitted that "germs are nothing and cellular terrain is everything," but he was ignored by the business world, which was interested in making money, not building health. (113)

Dr. Robert O. Young says in The pH Miracle, "Overacidification of body fluids and tissues underlies all disease". It is only when the body is acidic that it is vulnerable to germs. When there is a healthy balance of acid/alkaline germs can't get a foothold." (125)

It is believed that virtually all degenerative diseases, including cancer, heart disease, arthritis, osteoporosis, kidney and gall stones, and tooth decay, are associated with excess acidity in the body. Some researchers believe that cancer cannot exist in an alkaline environment. The body has a homeostatic mechanism that maintains a constant pH of 7.4 in the blood; however, this mechanism works by depositing and withdrawing acid and alkaline minerals from other locations, including the bones, soft tissues, body fluids and saliva. Therefore, the pH of these other tissues can fluctuate greatly. The pH of saliva offers a window through which you can see the overall pH balance in your body. (126)

If over-acidification underlies all disease, we can attempt to control our cellular terrain and thus create an atmosphere in the body which is not easily invaded by germs. In whatever health situation you face you can monitor your progress toward a proper acid/alkaline balance by testing your saliva pH. (126)

The abbreviation pH stands for the power of hydrogen. A simple strip of litmus paper will measure your pH, which is the concentration of positively-charged hydrogen ions in your body. Ions make up the electrical "juice" or current your body uses to communicate. The more positively-charged hydrogen ions present, the more acidity is present. (113)

Saliva testing for pH is very simple. pH test strips (litmus strips) should be available at your health food store or pharmacy. Test before you eat or drink anything except water in the morning or wait at least 2 hours after eating. Fill your mouth with saliva and then swallow it. Do this again to help ensure that the saliva is clean. After the third time, spit some saliva onto the litmus paper. The litmus paper should turn blue, which indicates that your saliva is slightly alkaline at a healthy pH of 7.4. If it is not blue, compare the color with the chart that comes with the pH paper. (113)

What causes over-acidification? Our modern lifestyle with hours spent in traffic, financial stress, relationship stresses, an acidic fast-food diet, lack of pure water, low oxygen from lack of deep breathing, lack of exercise, and toxic environments all create acid (low pH). (126)

The body is amazing as it constantly tries to balance pH, but we need to give it the right fuel and conditions to help it keep in balance.

Sunshine and Vitamin D

We have become so afraid of the sun that we are not getting the vitamin D we need. Now the medical establishment has decided we need to take vitamin D supplements.

Our ancestors lived and worked in the sun, thus getting the sunshine the body needed naturally. In our modern world we have created unnatural conditions. Some people spend most of their daylight hours in buildings without windows, so they are rarely in a naturally lighted environment. A <u>minimum</u> of 20 to 30 minutes daily exposure to sun is needed to produce the needed vitamin D the body needs. In the northern latitudes the sun is weak during the winter, so supplementing with vitamin D is necessary. People with dark skin pigmentation may need 20 to 30 times as much exposure to sunlight as fair-skinned people to generate the same amount of vitamin D. That may be why prostate cancer is epidemic among black men. (127)

To make matters worse, we slather ourselves with sunscreens supposedly to avoid cancer, only to discover that <u>sunscreens with a protection factor of eight or greater will block the UV rays that produce vitamin D</u>. (127)

Until recently we have not understood the role vitamin D plays in our health. It is fat-soluble and found in few foods, so our supply is mostly produced in the body after exposure to the ultraviolet rays from the sun. The <u>only food sources</u> of vitamin D are eggs, wild salmon, mackerel, herring, sardines, shrimp, fortified milk and other fortified beverages, cod liver oil, dried mushrooms, and the liver of most animals. (128)

Vitamin D is technically not a vitamin but a prohormone that goes through several changes before it is activated in the body by the kidneys and liver to be used for various functions. Having kidney disease or liver damage can greatly impair your body's ability to activate circulating vitamin D. (128)

Traditionally, specific nutrients have been connected with preventing a specific disease, such as vitamin D preventing rickets or vitamin C preventing scurvy. Research in recent years has found that the body uses nutrients in combination for many body functions. Vitamin D works in concert with a number of other vitamins, minerals and hormones to promote bone mineralization. Without vitamin D and other nutrients, bones can become thin, brittle, or misshapen. There is an alarming rise in osteomalacia, osteoporosis, and other degenerative bone diseases which may be partially due to vitamin D deficiency. (129)

In order for the body to utilize Vitamin D the co-factors need to be available. <u>Magnesium</u> is the most important of these co-factors while zinc, vitamin K2, boron and Vitamin A are also necessary. It is possible that raising vitamin D levels could contribute to a magnesium deficiency, so a proper balance needs to be determined and maintained. Together Vitamin D and all the co-factors can prevent the buildup of calcium deposits in arteries and in other parts of the body. (129)

Vitamin D plays an important role in the maintenance of several organ systems, bone formation and mineralization, and the control of calcium and phosphorus metabolism. Vitamin D also performs anti-tumor functions and is vital for the maintenance of the blood/brain barrier. (128)

Deficiency of vitamin D is implicated in many diseases.

- The Vitamin D Council's current research has "implicated vitamin D deficiency as a major factor in the pathology of at least 17 varieties of cancer as well as heart disease, stroke, hypertension, autoimmune diseases, diabetes, depression, chronic pain, osteoarthritis, osteoporosis, muscle weakness, muscle wasting, birth defects, periodontal disease, and more." (133)

- Vitamin D deficiency has been associated with insulin deficiency and insulin resistance. It may be a factor in the development of type 1 diabetes in children. Insulin resistance has been found to be a factor in cancer as well as heart disease, and people in northern latitudes have increased rates of heart attack in the winter. (127)
- Some autoimmune disorders, such as rheumatoid arthritis, multiple sclerosis, Crohn's disease, and thyroiditus, have been linked with low levels of Vitamin D. (132)
- Vitamin D deficiency has been found in patients with depression, chronic pain, osteoarthritis, muscle weakness, muscle wasting, birth defects, and periodontal disease. (134)
- Vitamin D deficiency is indicated in SAD (seasonal affective disorder), which occurs in people living in upper latitudes who suffer from depression and related symptoms. (135)
- Research is making the connection between vitamin D levels and infectious diseases. Dr. Michael F. Holick, Ph.D, M.D., author of The UV Advantage, says, "It has long been recognized that patients with tuberculous do better when treated with vitamin D or exposed to sunlight. It was recently recognized that the immune cell known as the macrophage needs vitamin D in order to produce a peptide which is responsible for killing infectious agents such as tuberculosis." It has been speculated that one of the reasons that influenza occurs in the wintertime in temperate climates is that the sun's rays aren't strong enough to produce vitamin D on the skin, resulting in vitamin D insufficiency which may promote and enhance the activity of the influenza virus. (136)
- Scientists from the Department of International Health, Immunology and Microbiology at the University of Copenhagen have discovered Vitamin D is crucial to activating our immune defenses and that without sufficient intake of the vitamin, the killer cells

of the immune system, or T cells, will not be able to react to fight off serious infections in the body. (137)

- We are afraid of the sun for fear of cancer, but more and more research indicates that it may be deficiency, not an excess, of full-spectrum sunlight that is linked to melanoma. We need to understand that there is a difference between the common, easily cured basal-cell cancer, which may or may not be caused by sunlight exposure, and more serious malignant melanoma, which researchers are now saying is NOT necessarily caused by the sun. (138)

What is a safe dosage when supplementing vitamin D? Have your vitamin D and calcium levels tested to determine if you need to supplement, and if so, how much. Your health practitioner will help you decide if supplementing is necessary in your case.

The sunscreen controversy:
Despite the availability and use of sunscreens, skin cancer has risen during the past two decades. Immediately one has to question the value of sunscreens. Until recently most of the ingredients in sunscreens were not safety tested or safety approved by the FDA. The latest case studies show that sun- screens may actually be causing skin cancer. (139)

Sunscreens may contribute to skin cancer in two ways:
1. Sunscreen blocks vitamin D production, a nutrient the body needs to prevent cancer.
2. Many sunscreen products contain cancer-causing chemicals that are absorbed through the skin and enter the bloodstream, where they cause severe DNA damage leading to cancer. (140)

Sunscreens are changing, and some of the really toxic ingredients are no longer used. Check the Environmental Working Group site for the latest information on safe sunscreen ingredients. (141)

Many sunscreens often contain zinc oxide and titanium dioxide, which until recently were thought to be no threat because of the size of the particles not allowing penetration below the surface skin. However, to make the sunscreens more invisible they are now using nanopartical zinc oxide and titanium dioxide, which may penetrate deeper. There are studies being done to determine whether nanopartical zinc oxide and titanium dioxide will damage the skin cells. Watch for the results.

We now realize skin cancer, like any cancer, is linked to nutritional deficiencies. What your body needs most for protection from the sun or toxic substances are a wide array of nutrients for cell reproduction and repair, especially the antioxidants which we discussed earlier in the book.

Sunscreens and lotions whose ingredients include antioxidants used externally may be helpful in reducing free radical damage, but more importantly we need to eat those foods which are high in antioxidants so the skin will be healthy. Eating a diet rich in antioxidants and supplementing regularly, not just when you want to be in the sun, is important for good health. Some doctors are suggesting supplementing with 1,000 mcg of folic acid per day, and more if you spend a good amount of time in the sun or have a family history of skin cancer. (142)

We need sunshine on our skin, so try to get 15 or 20 minutes in the sun daily and without sunscreen. Take a short walk in the sun on your lunch break or whenever you can catch a few minutes, though when you need to be in the sun for long periods of time wear a hat, sunglasses, and lightweight protective clothing. If you wish to offer your body to the sun, safer sunning products are now on the shelves of your health food store. Read the ingredients.

**We each have a different genetic make up, so some skin types are much more sensitive than others and may need higher amounts of various nutrients and more protection to prevent damage.

10 Understanding Your Marvelous Body

Life begins in cells, which form organs, which form systems, which all work together to create an amazing body. All of this activity **depends on the nutrients** which you supply to your body every day.

In order to understand your health you need a basic understanding of the physiology and anatomy of the body. Understanding the functioning of each body system helps you realize the significance of symptoms.

It all begins with embryonic stem cells that can divide and differentiate into diverse specialized cell types and can self-renew to produce more stem cells. Adult stem cells are produced in the bone marrow and travel throughout the body repairing damaged tissues. Nutrients are required by the body to support the function of producing stem cells. (143)

All blood cells, both red and white, begin as stem cells in your bone marrow. These undifferentiated cells begin to assume individual characteristics and become either red cells (the oxygen carriers) or white cells (the cells of the immune system).

All cells in the body have receptor sites on their surfaces to receive chemical messages from hormones.

There are ten major systems in our bodies:

Circulatory system: heart, lungs, red and white blood cells, platelets, blood vessels, and the lymphatic system.

It functions to transport blood and oxygen from the lungs to the various tissues of the body via arteries and transports the waste products via veins back through the system to the elimination organs.

The lymphatic system is actually an extension of the circulatory system. It consists of bone marrow, tonsils, thymus gland, spleen, adenoids, appendix, lymph nodes, lymphatic vessels, lymph, and Peyer's patches in the small intestine.

The lymphatic system is the body's network of organs,

ducts, and tissues that filter and drain the spaces between the cells, removing the waste products, toxins, and other tissue debris. Through a one-way system of vessels lymph flows throughout the lymph nodes, where macrophages filter out the material the body doesn't need or want, and the cleaned fluid is returned to the blood. Without this recirculation of fluids to the cardiovascular system, massive swelling or edema would take place. If waste is not removed from tissues, the immune system must continually attack waste products, toxins, viruses, and bacteria lodged in the tissues.

Lymph nodes, primarily clustered in the neck, armpits, and pelvic area, are the system's battle stations against infection. Lymph nodes are connected to one another by lymphatic vessels. It is in the nodes and other secondary organs that white blood cells engulf and destroy debris to prevent them from reentering the bloodstream.

The lymph system has no pump like the circulatory system, and it has only one-way valves, which depend mainly on the movement of skeletal muscles to squeeze fluid through them. The materials are moved through the vessels by pressure exerted through physical movement such as exercise, muscular activity, breathing, and the intestines. (144)

The lymphatic system plays an important part in immunity, as it provides a continuous cleansing of the tissues at the cellular level. Almost every health crisis in my history could be traced back to the lymph system. Unlike many systems in the body, the lymph system functions or malfunctions very quietly and without much fuss, so it takes much longer to get our attention, unlike indigestion or a broken bone. When it finally breaks down, the body is usually in crisis. (144)

Dr. Joseph Mercola says, "Vaccines clog our lymphatic system and lymph nodes with large protein molecules which have not been adequately broken down by our digestive processes, since vaccines by-pass digestion with injections." (145)

Immune system: bone marrow, thymus gland, spleen, lymph nodes; 60-70% of the immune system is located in the gut

Jon Barron of The Baseline of Health Foundation wrote a paper that helped me finally understand the amazing immune system. He explains that the immune system plays two vital roles in your body.

1. It responds to foreign organisms that gain access to your body by producing antibodies and stimulating specialized cells that destroy the organisms or neutralize their toxic byproducts. It defends against foreign invaders, including germs, viruses, bacteria, fungi, and parasites.

2. It stands guard over the cells of your body to ensure they do not become abnormal or degenerate. Normally, your body produces anywhere from 100 to 10,000 abnormal cells a day as part of the normal metabolic processes, or as the result of exposure to environmental toxins or nutritional deficiencies. If your immune system is functioning properly, it can identify each and every one of those cells and eliminate them before they can do any harm. Not only is your immune system capable of identifying every single cell in your body and recognizing those that are friendly and belonging to your "self," it is also capable of singling out and identifying every single foreign invader ranging from bacteria and viruses to fungi and parasites, and knows to treat them as "non-self." (146)

Out of the trillions of cells in your body, your immune system can tell <u>when a single cell has mutated and become cancerous</u> and, in many cases, moves in to destroy it before it can do any harm. In fact, it does this thousands of times a day. If you want to learn more, visit: http://www.jonbarron.org/immunity/anatomy-physiology-immune-system-antibodies

Whether flu virus, food poison, carcinogen, or cancer cell, it is attacked as a foreign body by the immune system. If these harmful elements are not moved out of the body, they will eventually overrun the system. Gradually the immune system will be debilitated by the mounting poisons and aberrant cells until such disease-causing agents manifest as a major illness. (147)

Sixty to seventy percent of the immune system is located in the digestive system, mostly in the small intestine. If the intestinal walls are damaged nutrients are not properly absorbed, and often undigested particles pass through, which can cause many different maladies. (146)

Maintaining the balance of good bacteria to bad bacteria is crucial to a healthy intestinal tract. Most of us have damaged intestinal walls. The connection between poor flora in the gut and autism, autoimmune syndromes, and many other health issues has been verified by recent research. (147)

Digestive system: salivary glands, mouth, pharynx and esophagus, stomach, small intestine, large intestine, gall bladder, and liver. The small intestine provides us with most of the activity of the immune system.

The digestive process starts in the mouth, where food is chewed and saliva starts to break the food into smaller pieces. These smaller fragments of food travel down the esophagus, where a ring-shaped muscle called the lower esophageal sphincter, a valve, opens to allow food to enter the stomach and closes to keep the food in the stomach. Constriction of the stomach wall helps the food to be mixed with acidic gastric juices and enzymes.

The partially-digested mixture, called chyme, becomes quite liquid so it can move into the small intestine, which has three segments: duodenum, jejunum, and ileum. In the duodenum enzymes are released by the pancreas and bile from the gall bladder to continue the process, called peristalsis, which is the action of moving and mixing the food and digestive secretions. As the mixture enters the jejunum and then the ileum, nutrients are absorbed through finger-like projections on the intestinal wall called villi into the bloodstream to be carried throughout the body. The health of the intestinal tract is very dependent

90

on good bacteria, or "flora." Eating prebiotic foods and supplementing with probiotics is often necessary, especially if you have ingested antibiotics in any manner. Remember, unless we eat only grass-fed, free range meat and organic produce we are getting antibiotics every day in our foods. Antibiotics are even being found in our water supplies, so we are all being affected.

After nutrients have been absorbed, the remaining water, bacteria, and fiber pass into the large intestine, or colon. About 2/3 of this slurry is composed of water, undigested fiber, and food products. The other 1/3 is living and dead bacteria, viruses, yeast, parasites, hormones, toxins, etc. (Note: A well-formed stool should look like a brown banana.) This toxic mixture needs to be eliminated a couple of times a day to avoid putrification and reabsorption of the toxins.

The entire length of the digestive tract is coated with a bacterial layer on the surface of the gut epithelium which provides a natural barrier against invaders, undigested food, toxins, and parasites. If something has compromised this protective layer several things can happen.
- The gut can become permeated and leak undigested food into the bloodstream.
- Toxins from the body can leak into the gut.
- Foods will not be properly digested or broken down.
- Nutrients will not be properly absorbed into the bloodstream.
- Synthesis of nutrients won't happen without adequate flora.
- Pathogenic bacteria can grow unheeded.
- Energy for the gut is produced by the good bacteria, so the gut becomes malnourished. (148)
- To summarize simply, food enters your mouth, where it is acted upon by saliva. Next your stomach receives chewed food and mixes it with digestive juices (acids and enzymes) to help break down the food. This mixture slides into the small intestine, where friendly bacteria are added to further digest the food. The

resulting nutrients are absorbed through the walls into your bloodstream. The remaining matter flows into the colon, which removes water and salts from the food and supplies many more friendly bacteria to break down any undigested materials for elimination.

The liver is the largest solid organ and the largest gland in the body. The liver is actually two different types of gland. It is a secretory gland, because it has a specialized structure that is designed to allow it to make and secrete bile into the bile ducts. It also is an endocrine gland, since it makes, and secretes directly into the blood, chemicals that affect other organs in the body. Bile is a fluid that both aids in digestion and absorption of fats as well as carries waste products into the intestine. (149)

The liver has a multitude of important and complex functions. Some of these functions are to:
- Manufacture or synthesize proteins, including albumin, to help maintain the volume of blood and blood clotting factors
- Synthesize, store, and process (metabolize) fats, including fatty acids (used for energy) and cholesterol
- Metabolize and store carbohydrates, which are used as the source for the sugar (glucose) in blood that red blood cells and the brain use
- Form and secrete bile that contains bile acids to aid in the intestinal absorption (taking in) of fats and the fat-soluble vitamins A, D, E, and K
- Eliminate, by metabolizing and/or secreting, the potentially harmful biochemical products produced by the body, such as bilirubin from the breakdown of old red blood cells and ammonia from the breakdown of proteins
- Detoxify, by metabolizing and/or secreting, drugs, alcohol, and environmental toxins

The liver and gall bladder work as part of the digestive process. The liver secretes bile, a watery mixture containing bicarbonate ions to neutralize the acidic chyme arriving from the stomach and bile salts to emulsify fats in the first stage of their breakdown. Bile is transferred through the hepatic duct from the liver to the gall bladder to be stored in between meals. During digestion bile is excreted along the bile duct from the gall bladder into the duodenum (the first part of the small intestine). (149)

The endocrine system: hypothalamus, pituitary gland, thyroid and parathyroid glands, adrenal gland, pineal gland, reproductive glands and gonads, and pancreas.

The endocrine system is in charge of body processes that happen slowly. The glands of the endocrine system and the hormones they release influence almost every cell, organ, and function of our bodies. Hormones are the chemical messengers that transfer information and instructions from one set of cells to another. Each hormone affects only the cells that are genetically programmed to receive and respond to its message. They regulate tissue function, metabolism, mood, growth and development, sexual function, and the reproductive processes.

The tiny hypothalamus is really king of the endocrine system. The hypothalamus isa collection of specialized cells located in the lower central part of the brain. It is the primary link between the endocrine and nervous systems. Nerve cells in the hypothalamus control the pituitary gland by producing chemicals that either stimulate or suppress hormone secretions from the pituitary. The pituitary gland, which is about the size of a pea, and located at the base of the brain just beneath the hypothalamus, is considered the "master gland" because it makes hormones that control several other endocrine glands. However, if the hypothalamus is not functioning properly the pituitary gland is compromised. (150)

The nervous system and the endocrine system work together to help the body function properly. The nervous system controls the faster processes like breathing and body movement. We will discuss later how excitotoxins can affect the hypothalamus and thus our health.

Nervous System: The central nervous system consists of the brain and the spinal cord, while the peripheral nervous system consists of all the neurons of the body except those found in the brain and spinal cord. Different parts of the brain control different functions of the body through a specialized network of neurons. Its proper functioning depends on the coordination between the central and the peripheral nervous systems. The eyes, ears, tongue, and nose are considered part of the nervous system. (151)

Urinary System: two kidneys, two ureters, bladder, and urethra.

The urinary system removes waste products from your blood and helps maintain the proper balance of salts and water in your body. The kidneys and ureters constitute the upper urinary system, and the bladder and urethra make up the lower urinary tract. Your kidneys filter the blood and create urine to carry away the waste. Urine is a mixture of water, salts, and urea (a waste product produced from protein metabolism). It leaves the kidneys via the ureters, the muscular tubes that deliver urine to the bladder, then the urine is eliminated from the bladder. (152)

Respiratory system: nose, larynx, trachea, bronchi, lungs, and also uses the diaphragm and other muscles.

The respiratory system delivers the oxygen within the human body. Breathing starts at the nose and mouth. You inhale air into your nose or mouth, and it travels down the back of your throat and into your windpipe, or trachea. Your trachea then divides into air passages called bronchial tubes. As the bronchial tubes pass through the lungs, they divide into smaller air passages called bronchioles. The bronchioles end in tiny balloon-like air sacs called alveoli. The alveoli are surrounded by a mesh of tiny blood vessels called capillaries. Oxygen from the inhaled air passes through the alveoli walls and into the blood. After absorbing oxygen, the blood leaves the lungs and is carried to your heart. Your heart then pumps it through your body to provide oxygen to the cells of your tissues and organs.

As the cells use the oxygen, carbon dioxide is produced and absorbed into the blood. Your blood then carries the carbon dioxide back to your lungs through the capillaries, where it is removed from the body when you exhale. (153)

Skeletal System: all of the bones in the body and the tissues such as tendons, ligaments and cartilage that connect them. Your teeth are also considered part of your skeletal system, but they are not counted as bones.

The skeleton basically has three jobs:

- To provide support for our body. Without your skeleton your body would collapse into a heap.
- To help protect your internal organs and fragile body tissues. The brain, eyes, heart, lungs, and spinal cord are all protected by your skeleton. Your cranium (skull) protects your brain and eyes, the ribs protect your heart and lungs, and your vertebrae (spine, backbones) protect your spinal cord.
- Bones provide the structure for muscles to attach so our bodies are able to move. Tendons are tough inelastic bands that attach muscle to bone. Ligaments are stretchy bands of tissues that hold bones to bones.

The human skeleton is more than just bones, vertebrae, and joints. It is an active organ that is constantly linked to our brain, our muscles, and our fatty tissue. **Stem cells**, the body's most important cells, are formed in the bones of the skeleton, which is also home to hormones that control the body's blood sugar and obesity by sending signals to other organs. (154)

Muscular System: skeletal, smooth, and cardiac muscles. There are over 600 muscles that provide the forces that enable the body to move. The muscles give your body shape and hold the other systems in the body together. The cardiac muscles in the heart relax and contract to pump the blood through the heart and throughout the body. (155)

Reproductive System: <u>Female</u>: vagina, uterus, ovaries, fallopian tubes.

<u>Male</u>: penis, testicles, vas deferens, prostate.

A great website for explaining the reproductive system is: http://kidshealth.org/parent/general/body_basics/female_reproductive_system.html#

11 Your Spine, the Column of Life

It was quite a revelation to discover that my teeth and my spine could be affecting my internal health. Once again, we need to look at the body holistically, understanding how everything is interconnected.

Most of us have had our falls, traumas, and accidents which have left damage in our structural systems. I have used chiropractors and other body work practitioners for years to keep the energy flowing efficiently through my body. Even babies can benefit from body and energy work.

Gray's Anatomy 29th Edition tells us, "The nervous system controls and coordinates all organs and structure of the human body." It is through the spinal column that the spinal cord passes which connects the brain to all parts of the body. There are thirty-two pairs of spinal nerves that pass from the spinal cord through small openings between the vertebrae to various parts of the body. It makes sense then that misalignment of spinal vertebrae and discs may cause irritation or blockage to the nervous system which could affect the structure, organs, and functions of the body. (162)

The simplest explanation of chiropractic care is a quote from www.echiropractic.net: "A subluxation (a.k.a. Vertebral Subluxation) is when one or more of the bones of your spine (vertebrae) move out of position and create pressure on, or irritate spinal nerves. Spinal nerves are the nerves that come out from between each of the bones in your spine. This pressure or irritation on the nerves then causes those nerves to malfunction and interfere with the signals traveling over those nerves." (163)

"How does this affect you? Your nervous system controls and coordinates <u>all</u> the functions of your body. If anything interferes with the signals traveling over nerves, parts of your body will not get the proper nerve messages and will not be able to function at 100% of their innate abilities. In other words, some part of your body will not be working properly.

It is the responsibility of the Doctor of Chiropractic to locate subluxations and reduce or correct them. This is done through a series of chiropractic adjustments specifically designed to correct the vertebral subluxations in your spine." (164)

12 Your Teeth Affect Your Health

Most biological dentists acknowledge findings that each tooth relates to a nerve and a meridian which is connected to an organ of the body. Infection in that tooth can affect the related organ. I experienced that when I had a root canal in which the infection was buried for several years. I finally had the tooth extracted and now have no more problems. There is now also specific evidence that periodontal disease can cause heart problems. (156)

To view an amazing interactive chart go to http://naturaldentistry.us/holistic-dentistry/meridian-tooth-chart-from-encinitas-dentist/

The renowned German physician Dr. Reinhard Voll "estimated that nearly 80% of all illness is related entirely or partially to problems in the mouth. The reason the teeth are such a threat to health is that, in addition to their connection to every organ and gland in the body, they can harbor infections without symptoms. There's no pain or discomfort. Yet, there may be chronic infection eroding the body's immune response and wearing out the immune system. This infection is very difficult to detect. Few people today have escaped the problems of dental cavities and gum infection. About 98% of Americans have some areas of diseased gum tissue in their mouths; over half of these are also experiencing a progressive bone loss." Fortunately, cavities and pyorrhea (gum disease

and bone loss) are both 100% preventable and reversible."
(157)

Fluoride is still being used in dentistry, in dental
products, and in water supplies. We know fluoride is a
very toxic substance that is related to many health issues,
but the politics behind the continuation runs very deep. I
recommend the website of Fluoride Action Network,
www.FlourideAlert.org, for a wealth of information on the
dangers of fluoride. Paul Connett, PhD, the executive
director and researcher has said, "The teeth are windows
to what's happening in the bones." Since his research has
connected fluoride with bone cancer in young males, we
need to take note of the fluorosis which is found on the
teeth of many young people as an indicator of other health
problems. As Dr. Connett says, "We need a national
campaign to end fluoridation and minimize fluoride
exposure." That will entail all of us becoming involved in
the issue in every state. (158)

One of the two biggest issues connected with the teeth and
health is amalgam fillings. A controversy has been raging
for many years over the safety of amalgam fillings, which
contain mercury and other metals. The FDA says, "Dental
amalgam contains elemental mercury. It releases low
levels of mercury in the form of a vapor that can be
inhaled and absorbed by the lungs. High levels of
mercury vapor exposure are associated with adverse
effects in the brain and the kidneys." (159)

This toxicity is connected to many health problems
including autism, fatigue, Parkinson's, Multiple Sclerosis,
ALS, Alzheimer's disease, immune dysfunctions,
schizophrenia, hormone disruption, bone and muscular
issues, colitis, and many unnamed syndromes that people
have experienced. (160) For more information read *Dental
Truth*, a newsletter published by DAMS, Intl. or call 1-800-
311-6265.

Norway was the first to ban the use of mercury in all
products in 2008, including dental materials. Sweden and
Denmark followed in the same year. France's 40,000
dentists use mercury amalgams less and less, while

Germany, Spain, and Austria have restrictions or guidelines on amalgams in place. (161) The dangers of mercury are discussed in various sections of this book.

Finding a biological dentist was the best dental decision I ever made. I can trust her to do the safest procedures and use the least toxic products. Since you know the facts, when you visit the dentist:

- If your dentist suggests internal fluoride tablets for your children or oral treatments, you will be able to make better decisions. You decide if you want your children to have any kind of fluoride treatments.
- If x-rays are required, ask for minimal x-rays and ask to wear a lead collar to protect your thyroid when they are taking dental x-rays.
- If they want to do varnishes or protective coatings, ask what the ingredients are and decide if the value outweighs the dangers.
- If you need fillings ask what your options are. After what you have read I assume you don't want amalgam fillings. Ask if they give the composite compatibility test to find what composite would be best for you.
- If the dentist feels you need a root canal, do as much study as you can to see if there are other options.
- If you have an extraction, consider asking the dentist to provide infrared treatment and/or magnets to assist healing.

Advocate locally and nationally to have fluoride removed from municipal water systems and the practice of dentistry.

How to find a biological dentist:
- Call DAMS, Intl. at 1-800-311-6265.
- American Academy of Biological Dentistry Tel: (813) 659-5385.
- The Holistic Dental Association (HDA) offers a biological dentist list for US for $2.50 and stamped self-addressed envelope sent to: P.O. Box 5007, Durango Colorado 81301 Tel / Fax (970) 259-1091.
- E-mail: hdd@frontier.net or online at http://www.holisticdental.org

13 The Body is More than Parts

The body, mind and spirit need to be in balance for there to be wellness.

Our health can be measured by our **Vital Force**, which is a term that is used by herbalists, homeopaths, and many other natural practitioners. The Chinese call this invisible force "*qi*," while the Ayurvedic tradition calls it "*prana*". Vital Forcecan be defined as an invisible, dynamic, automatic power which preserves the life in a living being. It is the energy which performs all the phenomenon of health and disease of the material body. It maintains the balance between mind and body. It protects the body from injurious or harmful influences to which the body is constantly exposed, such as bacteria, viruses, and toxic substances found in our food, water, and atmosphere.

Health is when the Vital Force is in a normal state, or in other words, when a person is balanced. Disease is when the Vital Force is deranged or disturbed.

DISEASE IS THE BODY OUT OF BALANCE

We often call the body a "machine," and in some ways it is, but it is so much more.

If something is wrong with my car, the mechanic often jerks out the defective part and replaces it with a new one. It is easy and complete.

To some extent modern medicine can now replace parts, too. Joint replacements are becoming very common and are quite successful in most cases. However, organ transplants such as liver and heart transplants require the use of massive amounts of drugs to avoid rejection and infection.

The human body is a complex being of intricate cells. Those cells are interconnected by blood vessels and nerves orchestrated by a magnificent brain. The human body has a vital force.

Could the transplants have been avoided if we had known all the factors to keep us healthy?

100

The interesting thing about comparing our bodies to cars is that <u>we often take much better care of our cars than we do our bodies</u>. Do you put cola or sugar in your gas tank? Of course not, because cola and sugar are not fuel for an automobile. Far fetched? Is it any different than putting cola, sugar, aspartame, monosodium glutamate, and drugs in our bodies? NO! **Putting non-foods or adulterated foods in our bodies is just as detrimental to humans as putting cola or sugar in the gas tank of your car.**

Natural, organic foods will give us what we need for health and vitality.

<u>Drugs and created ingredients are NOT in our food chain!</u>

I need to share a story about a friend's eighty-year old mother who went in for a routine physical. She was in good health and wasn't taking any medications. After the exam, the doctor said she had no problems but sat down to write a prescription. The woman asked why he was writing a prescription if there was nothing wrong with her. He replied, "Everyone your age needs to take this drug because their bones wouldn't be strong without it." She was confused because he had just said she was in good health. To make it even more ludicrous, since when are our bones dependent on drugs? It is nutrients that build and maintain bone.

I find it very interesting that doctors and others have come to believe that people need drugs to maintain health. Something has gone awry in our thinking. How do they think people lived to be over eighty in the past when there were no synthetic drugs?

Another story I love is about a very spritely man I met in a craft store. He said proudly, "I'm 92 years old and until a few months ago had never taken a drug. I went for a physical and the doctor said my cholesterol was high so gave me a statin drug. After a couple of weeks I started feeling weak, and my muscles didn't seem to work. I stopped the drug and now I'm fine again."

101

Drugs are <u>NOT in our food chain</u>, thus cannot replace nutrition. Drugs <u>should be used in trauma and critical situations</u> and only rarely on an everyday basis. When you have an ailment for which the doctor wants to prescribe a drug, consider if there are other less toxic options which will remedy the problem.

Surgery is a major trauma to the body. Those are not spare parts to be discarded, by the way; we need those organs. When we start cutting out organs we break the synergy of the whole. Each part is connected and affected by the others. Yes, there are times when surgery may be necessary. I resent having had parts removed through surgery because my doctors didn't understand the value of detoxifying and using nutrition and herbs to build the body. Now I deal with scar tissue and damaged nerves from those surgeries. Conventional medicine threw out natural remedies that had worked for centuries when they discovered drugs and technology.

So many middle-aged people tell me they have various digestive problems. When I ask a few questions, I find many have had their gall bladders removed because they had problems and the doctor said they didn't need a gall bladder anyway.

You need your gall bladder. <u>It is NOT a spare part.</u> Your liver produces bile, which emulsifies fats for improved fat digestion. The liver sends bile to the gall bladder to be stored until it is needed for digestion. When the gall bladder is removed, the liver stores the bile, which impacts the liver.

14 Health Begins Before Conception

The health of a person actually begins before conception. Scientists have discovered that a mother's <u>health and nutrition during pre-conception and pregnancy</u> have a great effect on the health of the infant and patterns of disease in their childhood. The best time to begin prevention of disease in the child is many months before conception. It takes three months for sperm to mature and a month for an egg to mature. <u>The health of both partners determines the health of fetus.</u> (165)

As a former school teacher I saw an increasing number of children with various neurological and behavioral problems. Society has labeled these kids as having hyperactivity syndrome, ADD, ADHD, Autism, or Aspberger's Disease Syndrome, but the causes may be very similar—poor nutrition and toxicity from many sources. It is heartbreaking to see and feel the agony of the child who is out of control and to see the pain and frustration of the entire family.

Today, we are realizing that autism and so many of the other neurological malfunctions in children may be preventable and that chemicals and vaccines may be dangerous. We blindly accepted that our government agencies and medical people would not allow harmful things. We were so wrong.

<u>The health of both parents prior to conception is very important</u>. Both partners need to correct the following before becoming pregnant:

- <u>Toxicity</u> in either prospective parent from chemicals, heavy metals, vaccinations, drugs, alcohol, and smoking. Heavy metals toxicity, especially mercury and aluminum, are indicated in neurological problems. (166)
- <u>Nutrient deficiency</u> (especially vitamin D) in parents prohibits them from producing healthy sperm and eggs. Also, B vitamins are crucial to the development of a healthy fetus.

- Damage to the immune systems of parents caused by vaccinations which may be genetically passed the fetus. (167)
- Lack of a healthy gut where the immune system resides.
- Emotional environment of the parents. (166)
- Fungal, bacterial, and viral infections that could be transferred to the fetus and enter a baby's brain. (167)

Everything that happens to a pregnant woman happens to her fetus.

What can the mother-to-be do?

Drink adequate purified water. Drink half your body weight in ounces or a minimum of two quarts per day of pure water. It is also important that there is some salt in your diet. Avoid all sodas, fruit drinks, and anything else that has non-food ingredients, artificial sweeteners, artificial colors, or preservatives. Drinking adequate water helps the detoxification and elimination of the cellular wastes of mother and fetus. Drinking adequate water will often eliminate morning sickness. (168)

Maximize nutrition. Eating good organic food and supplementing with food-grade vitamins and minerals will give the baby a better chance of being born with a strong immune system and without defects.

It is very important for the pregnant woman to consume adequate nutrients and calories for herself and the fetus and avoid fast food and processed food with additives. The **brain and nervous system of a fetus use more than half the available nutrients** supplied during development in the womb. The nutrients will go to the fetus first and may leave the mother deficient and vulnerable. Severe nutritional deficiencies can cause birth abnormalities.

Note: It is important for the pregnant woman to consult a **holistic practitioner** who understands nutrition. Consuming synthetic supplements may not provide the nutrients necessary for the health of fetus and mother.

IMPORTANT Factors for the pregnant woman:

1. The non-fat philosophy is very dangerous, both in pregnancy and for everyone else. The fetus and a growing child need fats, which include saturated fats; so does the mother. (169)

2. Essential Fatty Acids—Omega 3, 6, and 9: Our modern diet has created an improper balance of essential fatty acids. Many people are consuming few foods that are rich in Omega-3s and many foods high in Omega-6s. A diet of fast or otherwise processed foods provides more Omega-6s than Omega-3s. A <u>proper balance of essential fatty acids is crucial in the development of the brain and nervous system of the fetus as well as in protecting the mother</u>. DHA, an Omega-3 fatty acid, can prevent many premature deliveries, protects the baby from brain injuries, and can maximize intelligence in the child. Omega-3 fats are also very useful in treating the depression that may accompany pregnancy. (170)

Cold water fish were once considered a healthy source of animal protein, vitamin A and Omega 3s. That has changed in the last decade, as testing for mercury and other pollutants has found <u>most fish to be too contaminated to be safe to eat</u>. In addition, farmed fish are usually extremely polluted from the conditions in which they are raised.

Studies recommend taking a fish oil supplement (from uncontaminated sources) which is high in Omega 3, DHA and EPA. Avoid using high Omega 6 sunflower, corn, soy, and safflower, which may also be contaminated with pesticides and/or may be GMO, and products made with these oils. Canola oil has a balanced Omega 6 to Omega 3 ratio, but is usually genetically modified and has been refined with toxic substances. (171)

Acceptable fats include high quality extra-virgin olive oil, coconut oil, avocados, and organic butter. Grass-fed beef and free range poultry, bison, ostrich, and wild game are high in Omega 3 and good choices as well.

There are a few good plant sources of Omega 3, such as spirulina, purslane, flaxseed, chia seed, and walnuts, but there are no plants that provide significant DHA and EPA.

Omega-9 is found in: olive oil, black olives, walnuts, avocados, almonds, hemp, cashews, macadamia nuts, peanuts, pistachios, sesame oil, pecans, and hazelnuts.

3. The bad guys: Trans fats are damaged fats produced when oils are processed at high temperatures, often using chemical solvents, and then hydrogenated. The altered fat is damaging to the body. We need to **avoid all hydrogenated or partially hydrogenated fats (trans-fats)**. That includes most margarine, hydrogenated peanut butter, solid white shortening used in baking, and partially hydrogenated oils such as corn, soy, safflower, and sunflower oils, and ALL bakery products made with these fats. (172)

Do include medium-chain fatty acids "MCFAs" such as coconut oil, real butter, and whole dairy products

4. Multi-vitamin/mineral supplements: Nutritionists and research supports the need to take a good **natural** vitamin/mineral supplement to meet the body's needs in our modern world. The pregnant woman needs a plan designed to meet her individual needs. It is best to consult with a nutritionist or other natural practitioner who will test you before setting up a nutritional plan to ensure you are getting adequate nutrients, including trace minerals and antioxidants. Your body's needs for vitamins and minerals change during pregnancy. Vitamin C is especially important to strengthen the integrity of your vascular system and to support the immune system. Vitamin E is an antioxidant, helps alleviate fatigue, and helps prevent miscarriage in pregnant women. (173)

It is important to remember that nutrients in your body work in synergy. Any time we supplement with only one or two nutrients and the diet is deficient in other nutrients, imbalances or even toxicity may occur. For example, some authorities recommend no more than 5,000 units of Vitamin A in supplement form per day during pregnancy. When supplementing with a multivitamin/mineral supplement and eating a variety of fruits and vegetables each day, hopefully the pregnant woman will be getting adequate vitamin A.

In my second pregnancy, I was taking the pre-natal supplement prescribed by my doctor and still broke five bones in my foot by merely stepping on the edge of a manhole cover. Looking back, I'm sure I was very deficient in magnesium and trace minerals, so the calcium I was consuming was not absorbed. <u>We weren't told that magnesium and vitamin D are always needed when we supplement with calcium</u>. Doctors are rarely knowledgeable about nutrition beyond the RDAs, which are <u>not adequate</u> in today's world. The calcium to magnesium ratio is still not understood by many doctors. The fetus will remain alkaline until birth and will often deplete the mother's minerals in the process. <u>Magnesium</u> is especially important for many processes in the mother as well as development of the fetus. (174) You will find charts indicating the foods with high levels of magnesium, calcium, and potassium in Part B of this book.

5. B vitamins, especially folic acid (folate): If a woman of childbearing age is always taking a good multi-vitamin that incorporates a B-complex which has at least 400 mcg of folic-acid, her body will be better prepared for pregnancy. It is recommended that every woman of childbearing age understand that a lack of folic acid in the early stages of pregnancy can cause a variety of serious birth defects. The effect of this ignorance is that your baby may be born with spina bifida (split/open spine), microcephaly (small head), or anencephaly (rudimentary or no head. Doctors usually recommend 800 mcg of folic acid daily. (175)

<u>Folate</u> is the natural form found in food, and <u>folic acid</u> is the synthetic form found in supplements. <u>It is very important to never take an isolated supplement, so start by making sure your multiple vitamin/mineral supplement has at least 25 mg of the B-complex.</u> This will ensure you are getting some folic acid and the other B

vitamins. Then if needed, you can take additional folic acid supplement during pregnancy. Supplementing with folic acid and not receiving enough of the other B vitamins can lead to a serious B12 deficiency. (175)

The best food sources of folate are: organic calf's liver, avocados, Brussels sprouts, spinach and other dark greens, parsley, asparagus, green peas and split peas, broccoli, cauliflower, beets, parsnips, sweet potatoes, chickpeas, orange fall squash, and cooked dried beans and lentils. (176)

Eat vegetables raw whenever possible. Nutrients are quickly lost in cooking. If you need them cooked, lightly steam or stir-fry them. Many cereal products are enriched with folic acid, so read the labels on breads, cereals, flours, cornmeal, pastas, rice, and processed foods to see what your daily consumption of folic acid actually is.

Certain drugs can lower a woman's folic acid levels and increase the risk of birth defects, should she become pregnant. Visit with your physician about the drugs you are taking or ask for a list of drugs associated with birth defects. (177)

Homocysteine levels tend to rise in pregnancy. High levels of homocysteine are indicated in cardiovascular disease and many other health issues. It's been found that pregnant women with higher levels of homocysteine are at greater risk of having babies with neural tube defects (myelomeningocele) and other congenital abnormalities, as well as greater risk of pre-eclampsia. (178) Increased intake of folate along with betaine, B6, B12, and vitamin C have been found to lower homocysteine levels.

6. Vitamin D/Sunshine: The importance of getting regular **sunshine** during pregnancy cannot be overstressed. If the woman is getting enough **vitamin D**, the infant will be stronger. I'm not recommending anyone bake for hours in the heat of the day, but she should try to get at least 15 minutes of sunshine each day on her face, arms, or whatever she is willing to bare. Ask your doctor about taking cod liver oil or supplementing with

D3. <u>Adequate vitamin D is crucial for a healthy fetus</u>. Most Americans are deficient in vitamin D, which is crucial for almost all bodily functions. (179)

7. Probiotics: It has been found that pregnancy alters gut bacteria. Taking a mixed probiotic supplement will keep the intestinal tract healthy, which is important for the proper absorption of nutrients, for preventing yeast infection, and for a strong immune system. Eating plain yogurt with several cultures (add fruit and stevia if you like) or taking a probiotic supplement works well. Avoid sugared or artificially sweetened yogurt, especially the new highly advertised probiotic foods, which are often full of sugar and unhealthful ingredients.

Eating cultured or fermented vegetables is also a great way to keep intestinal bacteria balanced. (180)

<u>Exercise</u>: Walking and getting other regular exercise will help the pregnant woman feel better, help maintain a healthy weight, and make delivery easier. If she has a sedentary job, getting up and walking a few minutes every hour is very important for mother's circulatory and lymph systems, and she should take longer walks whenever possible. Usually she can continue with her regular activities unless her physician recommends changes.

<u>Safeguard the fetus</u>: One of the great tragedies of our time is how the toxins in our lives are affecting the pregnant mom and the fetus. Of great concern is guarding as best we can against the causes of autism and other neurological disorders. There is no way everything that is listed can be avoided, but be aware of what can be avoided so you can make healthy choices.

Major areas now under study, as related to childhood autism, include:

1. infant and childhood immunizations (179)
2. toxic environmental chemicals (181)
3. commercial food processing and excitotoxins (182)
4. the overuse of antibiotics (183)

Recently research has questioned several specific factors that may be involved in the development of autism:

- **Mercury toxicity** mostly from vaccinations. **The mercury in vaccines is in the form of thimerosal, which is 50 times more toxic than plain old mercury.** (184) (185)
- **MSG** that is highly reactive in the human brain and other organs. (182)
- **Drugs** like Augmentin, which some sources report has been implicated in autism. (183)
- **MMR vaccinations**. "CDC research scientist comes forward, anonymously, comes clean, tells Dr. Brian Hooker that the CDC has known about the MMR vaccine connection to autism for at least 11 years." (184)
- **A damaged small intestine** which is deficient in good bacteria can be the basis of a compromised immune system. (185)
- **Nutritional deficiencies** resulting from lack of understanding that the body needs all nutrients in balance for the growth of the fetus and health of the mother.
- **Toxic internal environment in the body,** which can be inherited or obtained from foods and drinks or from chemicals in products used on the child or in its surroundings. (185)

Guidelines for a healthy pregnancy and baby:

Avoid mercury and vaccines during pregnancy, which includes avoiding flu shots. Many vaccines still contain mercury and other ingredients which could affect your baby. Studies have linked mercury in vaccines with autism, other neurological disorders, and death in children. As early as February 9, 2004, the National Autism Association issued a press release that reported on one of the larger studies under review based on the Centers for Disease Control's Vaccine Safety Datalink. Under independent investigation, the association reported, of the CDC's data, <u>children were found to be 27 times more likely to develop autism after exposure to three</u>

thimerosal-containing vaccines (TCVs) than those who received thimerosal-free versions. Consider this evidence before getting a flu shot or having other vaccinations. (186) (187)

The Agency for Toxic Substance and Disease Registration says, "Very young children are more sensitive to mercury than adults. Mercury in the mother's body passes to the fetus and may accumulate there." (188) Mercury can also be passed to a nursing infant through breast milk; however, the benefits of breast feeding may be greater than the possible adverse effects of mercury in breast milk. Mercury's harmful effects can cause brain damage, mental retardation, lack of coordination, blindness, seizures, and inability to speak. Children poisoned by mercury may develop problems with their nervous and digestive systems and have kidney damage. (188)

Besides the mercury in vaccines, other sources of mercury are:
- Eating fish or shellfish contaminated with methylmercury
- Breathing vapors in air from spills, incinerators, and industries that burn mercury-containing fuels
- Release of mercury from dental work (amalgam fillings) and medical treatments
- Breathing contaminated workplace air or skin contact during use in the workplace (dental, health services, chemical, and other industries that use mercury) (188)

**Note: If you are planning to get pregnant and have amalgam fillings in your mouth, you may want to have them properly removed before you become pregnant and also thoroughly detoxify your body to remove the mercury from your system. Call DAMS, Intl. at 1-800-311-6265 to find a qualified biological dentist to remove the mercury so it does not affect your baby or your health. It is not recommended to have amalgam fillings removed if you are already pregnant as the toxins given off in the removal may damage the fetus.

Avoid excitotoxins such aspartame, MSG, food colorings, nitrates, nitrites, and other preservatives. According to

111

Dr. Russell Blaylock, "the infant's brain is four times more sensitive to excitotxoins than is the adult brain." (182) Excess glutamate has been shown to cause significant impairment of brain development in babies and can lead to mental retardation. (182)

According to some sources, Aspartame, when ingested during pregnancy, can damage the brain of the fetus as well as cause other birth defects. The potential damage includes parts of the brain involved in complex learning as well as the hypothalamus, which is the hormonal control center. Hormonal problems may not be seen until after the child reaches puberty. (182)

Avoid refined sugar, high fructose corn syrup, and white flour products, which are sources of highly refined carbohydrates. They have little or no nutritional value and lead to sugar sensitivity in the fetus.

Avoid drinking alcohol and using recreational drugs. Alcohol and drugs damage the fetus

Avoid or curtail caffeine intake. Substitute with herbal teas.

Avoid processed food of all kinds, as it is dead and will not support the nutritional needs of the fetus or the mother and is usually filled with preservatives. Eat organic food raw or freshly prepared. (177)

Avoid drinking sodas, which take the place of drinking water and have many toxic factors: (189)

- Carbonation: Any drink with fizz, including sparkling water, has been subjected to carbon dioxide gas under pressure. Carbon dioxide is a waste product given off by the body, so by drinking anything with CO2 you are adding waste to your body.

- Phosphoric acid-caused acidification: Most sodas have a very low pH of 2, which creates an acidic environment in the body. The normal pH balance of the body is 7-7.3. The acids in soda demineralize the bones and teeth.

- Sweeteners: Sodas are sweetened with sugar, high fructose corn syrup, sucralose (Splenda), or artificial sweeteners such as aspartame, a neurotoxin. They may all be deleterious to your health.

- Artificial coloring, which usually comes from coal tars or other chemicals.
- Caffeine, which taxes the liver
- Containers such as an aluminum can, which gives you a dose of toxic aluminum, or a plastic bottle, for a dose of toxic Bisphenol-A (BPA).

Rethink soy: There is much controversy about soy, but more and more research has found that soy products should be avoided during pregnancy. The phytoestrogens in soy are potent hormonal influences and can adversely affect the health of infants. (190)

Daniel Doerge and Daniel Sheehan in "The Guardian" indicated research that isoflavones in soy products consumed during pregnancy could be a risk factor for abnormal brain and reproductive tract development. (191)

Avoid microwaved food as much as possible and avoid being a near a microwave when you are pregnant. There are many studies which alert us to the dangers to our health as a result of eating microwaved food. Some conclusions of the Swiss, Russian, and German scientific clinical studies are found in "Ten Reasons to Throw Out Your Microwave Oven" at: http://humansarefree.com/2013/09/ten-reasons-to-throw-out-your-microwave.html. For example:

- Continually eating food processed from a microwave oven causes long term to permanent brain damage by "shorting out" electrical impulses in the brain (de-polarizing or de-magnetizing the brain tissue).
- The human body cannot metabolize (break down) the unknown by-products created in microwaved food.
- Male and female hormone production is shut down and/or altered by continually eating microwaved foods.
- The effects of microwaved food by-products are residual (long term to permanent) within the human body.

113

- Minerals, vitamins, and other nutrients are reduced or altered when food is microwaved. Instead of nutritious food, the body absorbs altered compounds that cannot be broken down. The minerals in vegetables are altered and become free radicals when cooked in microwave ovens.
- Microwaved foods are being studied as a cause of stomach and intestinal cancerous growths (tumors). This may explain the rapidly increasing rate of colon cancer in America.
- The prolonged eating of microwaved foods causes cancerous cells to increase in human blood.
- Continual ingestion of microwaved food causes immune system deficiencies through lymph gland and blood serum alterations.
- Eating microwaved food causes loss of memory and concentration, emotional instability, and a decrease of intelligence. (192) (193)

In addition, carcinogenic **phthalates** are formed when microwaving foods in plastic containers or covered with plastic wrap. (154)

Besides the above reasons, microwaves should <u>never</u> be used to heat a baby's bottle or food. The food or liquid may become internally too hot and severely burn the baby. (193)

<u>Avoid exposure to chemicals and other toxins.</u> We have heard the dangers of fluoride in water, but there are more chemicals to consider.

1. A Norwegian study of 141,000 births over a three-year period found the risk of birth defects increased 14 percent in areas with chlorinated water. Scientists have already found an association between chlorine and an increased risk of bowel, kidney, and bladder cancer, but it is the first time a link has been verified with higher levels of spina bifida. (196)

2. <u>Avoid exposure to chemicals in personal products, household cleansers, laundry products, yard products, and chemicals in the workplace.</u> For example, damage

114

from two commonly used chemicals, an insecticide called methoxychlor and a fungicide called vinclozolin, are known to cause infertility in the male offspring of pregnant animals. (194)

Paul Turek, a male infertility specialist at the University of California at San Francisco says, "Everyone agrees that exposure of the fetus at a certain critical time can cause malformed organs and birth defects. But no one ever imagined this might persist at some level for three more generations." (194)

PFOA (pentadecafluorooctanoic acid), more commonly known as Teflon, was found in a risk assessment by the U.S. Environmental Protection Agency to increase developmental and reproductive risks to humans. PFOA is found in many areas of our lives. It is used as a stain repellent in clothes and furniture, in food packaging and cosmetics, and is most commonly found in Teflon coatings on cooking pans. (197)

3. Avoid phthalates, chemicals commonly used in plastics and personal products such as flexible food storage containers, water bottles, hair spray, insect repellent, nail polish, and moisturizers. It leaches out into the environment. We breathe it, ingest it, and absorb it through our skin. The effects of phthalates on the endocrine system, particularly during pregnancy, breastfeeding, and childhood can be very serious. (198)

"Phthalate exposure has been linked to malformed sex organs in male lab animals, but recently there is a human study linking mothers exposed to phthalates to genital birth defects in male infants." (199)

Phthalates have been associated with:
- Increase in testicular cancer
- Declining sperm rates
- Early puberty
- Increased sexual deformities

There is so much information on phthalates and other chemicals that I can't begin to cover it, so I recommend you go to www.Mercola.com and search "phthalates".

Another great website is http://www.bodyburden.org/ with information from the Human Toxome Project by Environmental Working Group, which has information on many chemicals and heavy metals that are toxic to the body and especially the fetus. (199)

It was previously thought the placenta shielded cord blood and the developing baby from most chemicals and pollutants in the environment. A most disturbing study about chemicals found in the umbilical cords of newborns has proven otherwise. We now know that at the critical time when organs, vessels, membranes, and systems are knit together from single cells to finished form in a span of weeks, the umbilical cord carries not only the building blocks of life, but also a steady stream of industrial chemicals, pollutants, and pesticides that cross the placenta as readily as residues from cigarettes and alcohol. (200)

The Environmental Working Group commissioned five laboratories to examine the umbilical cord blood of 10 babies and found more than 200 chemicals in each newborn.

The 10 children in this study were chosen randomly, from among 2004's summer season of live births from mothers in Red Cross Volunteer national cord blood collection program. They were not chosen because their parents work in the chemical industry or because they were known to bear problems from chemical exposures in the womb. Nevertheless, each baby was born polluted with a broad array of contaminants. (201)

The cords were tested for only 413 of the over 75,000 chemicals the US manufactures or imports. In this study 287 out of the 413 chemicals were found in the umbilical cords of newborns. Most of the chemicals found were industrial pollutants, so it does not give us any idea of the contamination by the pollutants in our personal environments. (201)

4. Avoid drugs: *The Indian Journal of Pharmaceutical*

Sciences says, "In general, drugs unless absolutely
necessary should not be used during pregnancy because
drugs taken by a pregnant woman can reach the fetus and
harm it by crossing the placenta, the same route taken by
oxygen and nutrients, which are needed for the growth
and development of fetus."
https://www.ncbi.nlm.nih.gov/pmc/articles/PMC2810038/

NSAIDs (Nonsteroidal anti-inflammatory drugs): "Pregnant
women who use (NSAIDs) and aspirin increase their risk of
miscarriage by 80 percent." (202)

Antibiotics: The use of antibiotics should be kept to a
minimum during pregnancy. Researchers have found the
babies of mothers who were treated with antibiotics during
pregnancy were often resistant to an antibiotic. This
could be serious if the baby develops a bacterial infection
in those first weeks. (203) Another reason for avoiding
antibiotics if possible, is that yeast infection often follows
antibiotic use and could be passed to the fetus. (203)

Antidepressants: I recommend researching the use of
antidepressants during pregnancy discussing it with your
doctor or pharmacist. Some Internet sites to read include:
"Should You Use Antidepressants During Pregnancy?"
American Journal of Obstetrics and Gynecology, March,
2003 at www.Mercola.com, and "Antidepressant in
Pregnancy Not a Great Idea," *New England Journal of
Medicine,* April 11, 2002 at www.Mercola.com

Other things to consider
1) Avoid extreme emotional and physical stress. A happy
   mom will usually have a happy baby.
2) EMF's: Avoid electric blankets or electric heating pads
   during conception or pregnancy as the EMF's may be a
   factor in premature births. We are learning about the
   dangers of radiation from cell phones, so keep it
   away from the fetus. (204)
3) Get plenty of rest and enjoy the pregnancy.

**Remember, whatever affects a pregnant woman's body
affects the fetus.**

Morning Sickness: One of the discomforts of pregnancy

is often morning sickness. Morning sickness can indicate a lack of nutrients the baby needs to develop or insufficient water intake. Dr. F.Batmanghelidj says, "Morning sickness of the mother is a thirst signal of both the fetus and the mother." (205) Ginger tea may be helpful in relieving symptoms of morning sickness.

Red raspberry leaf tea is an excellent herbal food for expectant mothers. (Don't confuse herbal raspberry leaf tea with the many flavored black teas on the market.) Start with one cup a day.

- Raspberry leaves contains a high level of cellulose, vitamins A, B, and C, calcium, magnesium, potassium, and phosphorus, and are rich in citrate of iron which is an astringent and contractive agent for the reproductive area. It strengthens the uterine walls and eases the pain of childbirth.
- Red raspberry tea helps alleviate nausea during pregnancy.
- Red raspberry leaves stimulate, tone, and regulate.
http://www.pregnancy.com.au/resources/topics-of-interest/pregnancy/raspberry-leaf.shtml

To prepare tea, measure 1 teaspoon of leaves per cup of boiling water. Let it steep for 15 to 20 minutes. The tea may be drunk hot or cold. (206) Herbs for a Healthy Pregnancy by Penelope Ody is a good book.

Besides the references already discussed, I'd like to recommend the following reading:
- La Leche League International, at http://www.lalecheleague.org/.
- Having a Baby, Naturally, by Peggy O'Mara
- *Mothering: the Magazine of Natural Family Living,* www.mothering.com

15 Nutrify Your Cells

There is much discussion lately about genes and DNA. The DNA in your genes is the entire set of instructions which guides the behavior of every cell in the body. I knew that but didn't realize the specificity of nutrients needed to run the process until I read <u>Feed Your Genes Right</u> by Jack Challem. (207)

The human body is amazing! It consists of approximately 70 million cells. Inside the nucleus of each cell are twenty-three pairs of chromosomes, which are divided into approximately 30,000 genes. Each of these genes contains two strands of DNA which contain the instructions for making a specific protein or enzyme.

In order for the genes to be healthy and functional, their DNA must be fed the proper nutrients, such as certain B vitamins. DNA needs selenium and zinc for specific tasks. Each nutrient has a specific task for the body to be able to make or repair specific cells. Nutrients are needed by the DNA to produce energy for the body to function, to make and repair DNA, as well as to protect DNA from damage.

To quote Jack Challem, "Your genes are always responding to what you eat, to your emotions, your stresses, your experiences and to the nutritional microenvironment within each of your body's cells." (207)

PART B: FOODS TO NUTRIFY

1. Getting off the Diet Roller Coaster

In these times when obesity has become a big issue, you may wonder why the topic of weight control is not listed in the Table of Contents. When you understand what your body needs and what your body will not tolerate you will be on the path to your perfect weight.

A major factor in our battle with the bulge is that we are consuming products which not only are not only nutrient deficient but also add empty calories and toxic substances, causing us to be bloated and look fat. A huge business has developed around dieting. You will be healthier mentally and physically if you forget "dieting" and embrace eating well.

False Fat: Toxicity may be making you feel and look fat. Most of us have never considered that some of our weight might be toxins created in our bodies by an allergic reaction to certain foods or combination of foods. To quote Dr. Elson Haas from The False Fat Diet, "You're not nearly as overweight as you may think. Much of your weight isn't even fat. It's false fat, the bloating and swelling caused by allergy-like food reaction and you can shed it almost immediately. As your false fat fades, so will your food cravings and certain metabolic disorders (such as hormone imbalances." (1)

Food sensitivities, intolerances, and allergies are more common than people realize. Many people are aware that eating certain foods makes them uncomfortable, but often there is no overt symptom that the body is reacting to a food, so we don't connect a particular food with a chronic health problem.

According to WebMD, "A food allergy is an immune system response. It occurs when the body mistakes an ingredient in food--usually a protein--as harmful and creates a defense system (antibodies) to fight it. Food allergy symptoms develop when the antibodies are battling the 'invading' food. The most common food allergies are peanuts, tree nuts (such as walnuts, pecans and almonds), fish, and shellfish, milk, eggs, soy, and wheat." (2)

Food allergies are an immune response which can be triggered by even a small amount of the food and occur every time the food is consumed. Food allergies can cause or aggravate an enormous variety of symptoms including upset stomach, gastroenteritis, runny nose, fever, dark circles under the eyes, headaches, shock, edema or swelling, anxiety, ulcers, joint pain, rashes, diarrhea, constipation, low stomach acid, acne, sore throat, depression, colic, insomnia, hoarseness, delusions, ringing in the ears, dizziness, addictions, memory loss, bronchitis, chronic fatigue, hay fever, hyperactivity, bowel disease, iron deficiency anemia due to blood loss, malabsorption, myalgia, and failure to thrive. Food allergies can be life threatening! (3)

Food intolerance is a digestive system response which occurs when something in a food irritates a person's digestive system or when a person is unable to properly digest or break down, the food. Intolerance to lactose, which is found in milk and other dairy products, is the most common food intolerance. (3)

There are many differentphilosophies telling us what we should eat, which is very confusing. We don't know who or what to believe. Few people fit exactly into any of the plans that are touted as the "best." Your needs are not exactly like anyone else's needs. People who sell materials and supplements for a specific philosophy are sure they are right. Use these philosophies ONLY as general guidelines to find what works best for you.

Vegetarianism: There are many health advocates who feel everyone would be healthier on a vegetarian diet. Contrary to what we are often told by vegetarian advocates, man in ancient times was not a vegetarian. I found it very interesting when studying ancient people in many of the European countries to discover that they ate a variety of foods in season with meat and fish being the constant in many cultures. They ate what was available in their surroundings or they moved following the food source until some groups settled and became farmers. (4)

From my observation, many vegetarians don't eat enough vegetables and fruits; insteadthey load up on pastas, rice, breads, dairy products, and combination dishes. Often they are not really health conscious--they just don't eat meat.Even for those whose blood and metabolic type lean toward less meat, there are dangers of nutrient deficiency if one is not very careful. The most discussed deficiency in vegetarian diets is vitamin B12. All bodies need all the vitamins, minerals, and amino acids indicated earlier. (5)

Another factor is a lack of carnosine in the vegetarian diet. Carnosine is actually two amino acids, L-histadine and alanine, linked. It is a dipeptide that acts as a very powerful antioxidant. Most importantly, it prevents glycoselation, which is one of the main factors in aging, inflammation, and free radicals. Glycoselation is a process in which sugar molecules attach to protein molecules, which impairs the normal function of the protein. (5) (6)

All nutrients work together, and a deficiency of just one nutrient can cause malfunctioning.

The need for protein: We are finding many people, especially children, teens, and the elderly, aren't getting enough protein. While waiting in a chiropractor's office, I was pleased to hear the chiropractor telling his elderly patients to make sure they ate saturated fats and protein, preferably meat, at every meal. He emphasized that proteins provide the building blocks needed for growth, maintenance and repair of the body. It was a good reminder, as people seem to forget that the real purpose of eating is to provide fuel and nutrients to keep our bodies healthy and repaired. The body does not store protein, so we need to provide it daily.

I find the study of man's path to survive on the planet fascinating. In the 1920s and 30s Dr. Weston Price, the dentist/anthropologist who studied people across the globe, was one of the first to realize a link between modern eating habits and chronic degenerative disease. He found that primitive cultures, when they ate the nature-based diet of their ancestors, were healthy and vigorous. When they started to eat food of the civilized world their health deteriorated quickly. (7)

It is very interesting to note that indigenous cultures living in very different environments and eating very different foods were healthy and nearly free of disease until explorers brought infectious disease and different foods to them. The Eskimos, for example, had excellent immunity and cardiovascular health thriving on large quantities of fat and several pounds of meat a day. In comparison, the aboriginals in the Australian Outback were fit and strong on a diet of insects, beetles, grubs, berries, and occasionally meat from kangaroo or wallaby. The Scottish, Welsh, Celtic, and Irish diet was high in fatty fish, whereas the Italians lived quite well on fish, pasta, garlic, olive oil, vegetables, and wine. (7)

Through the ages cultures intermixed, and people moved to new locations with different foods available. Today most people in the US are a mixture of several cultures. Knowing our blood, body, and metabolic types can give us some diet and lifestyle guidelines.

The work of Loren Cordain, Ph.D. in The Paleo Diet continues to explain the importance of the diet ofancestry as to the diet and lifestyle we individually need. At one time our ancestors were all hunter/gatherers, and that is the origin of our nutritional needs. Animal foods dominated their diet, and they ate whatever wild fruits, vegetables, roots, and seeds were available, which set the pattern for what our bodies need today.(8)

Dr. Peters J. D'Adamo says in Eat Right 4 Your Type Encyclopedia, "As humans migrated and were forced to adapt their diets to local conditions, the new diets provoked changes in their digestive tracts and immune systems, necessary for them to first survive and later thrive in their new habitats. Different foods metabolized in a unique manner by each ABO blood group probably resulted in that blood group achieving a certain level of susceptibility (good or bad) to the endemic bacteria, viruses and parasites of the area." (9)

"Variations, strengths and weaknesses of each blood group can be seen as part of humanity's continual process of acclimating to different environmental challenges. Most of these challenges have involved the digestive and immune systems. It is interesting to note that virtually all the major infectious diseases that ran so rampant throughout our pre-antibiotic history have preferences for one ABO blood group or another." (9)

The O gene blood group was the first of which anthropologists have found evidence. They were the hunters and gatherers and thought to have first originated in eastern Africa. It is thought that the interactions that occurred between early man and his environment as he moved out of his original habitat caused the mutating of the original O blood type gene to A, B, and AB types. Today the percentages of the world's population are approximately O (40-45%) and A (35-40%) versus much lower rates of groups B (4-11%) and AB (0-2%). (10)

I have found that planning my eating around the concepts of the Paleo and Blood-Type philosophies works for me. The Paleo philosophy is basic to mankind, but following the more specific guidelines for my O blood type makes a difference for me. When I follow the plan, I feel light and energetic, but when I eat things that are to be avoided, I don't feel as well. You decide what works for you.

For more in depth information on blood types please read Eat Right 4 Your Type by Dr. Peter J. D'Adamo or go to http://www.dadamo.com/

Your metabolic type is another factor which has evolved through the years.Some people are fast oxidizers, and some are slow oxidizers. To discover more about your individual needs you may want to read The Metabolic Typing Diet by William Wolcott and Trish FaheyThey believe the body functions in such a way that "the efficiency of any system is dependent upon the efficiency of each of its organs and glands, each of which in turn is

124

dependent upon the efficiency of its cells. The cells in turn are dependent upon their capacity for energy production in order to carry out their assigned roles."(11)

Wolcott has taken the research on individuality and created a metabolic typing system which can be used by everyone. You can take the Metabolic Test in his book, The Metabolic Typing Diet, or if you want specifics you can find tests online: www.MetabolicTypingOnline.com.

I personally found that knowing I was an O blood type and a Protein metabolic type helped me to understand the food choices and activities that were best for me. Dr. Joseph Mercola has taken this philosophy a step further and calls it the Nutritional Type. http://products.mercola.com/nutritional-typing/.

Another philosophy to explore is Dr. Abravanel's Body Type System, which you can find at http://www.bodytypes.com/.

Food Combining Principles for Digestion is another philosophy that makes sense to me. It is understood that the human stomach digests food at varying rates by using different enzymes. There are many versions of this philosophy, so I will give you my short version.

- Proteins (especially meats) and starches should not be eaten at the same meal, as they neutralize each other and prevent proper digestion of either food.
- Greens and non-starchy vegetables can be eaten with proteins or starches.
- Eat no fruits with other foods at a meal. Tomatoes are an exception.
- **Never eat fruit or dessert after a meal** as it becomes trapped in your stomach with all the other food, where it starts to rot as it's not being chemically digested there. **Eat fruit 30-60 minutes before dinner or alone during the day as a snack.**
- Melon does eaten with other foods does not digest well and can cause problems. (12)

I know people who have found great intestinal relief through food combining. I really believe we should never eat fruit or dessert after a meal. Allow a couple of hours for your other food to have digested. To learn more about food combining see: http://www.trueactivist.com/6-food-combining-rules-for-optimal-digestion/

Obesity May Actually Be Malnutrition!

Obese people seem always to be hungry. They eat and drink often, sometimes constantly, but never feel satisfied. They seem to be constantly craving something.

The body is crying for nutrients. It is screaming, "Feed me what I need!"

How can you get fat if you are malnourished? Most of the processed food we eat doesn't nourish the body; it barely keeps us alive and deposits what the cells can't use as fat or false fat. In 1993-4 when I was very sick and started to detoxify, I lost fifty-five pounds. Since I wasn't obese, it is quite likely most of those pounds were "false fat" caused by the storage of toxins which included cellular waste, prescription drug residue, Candida die-off, heavy metals, and petrochemicals that my body had not been eliminating.

Many obese people are actually starving for nutrients!

Drinking diet sodas containing aspartame can actually cause many toxic reactions. Dr. Richard Wurtman demonstrated that aspartame inhibits the carbohydrate induced synthesis of serotonin (Congressional Record – Senate 1985a, P. S 5511). "Serotonin is an important component of the feedback system that helps limit one's consumption of carbohydrate to appropriate levels by blunting the carbohydrate craving."(13)

We have followed the wrong drummers, the food manufacturers and marketers, who wanted to make money without regard for the actual needs of the body. We were told that processed food is nutritious because it is "enriched." Processing takes out most of the natural nutrients (many which have not even been discovered or named), and adds a few synthetic vitamins or minerals to make us believe the product is nutritious. There is a danger in eating a variety of processed foods that are enriched, as in some cases we may be actually getting too much of a synthetic vitamin or an isolated poorly assimilated form of a mineral. Such is the case with men eating several products enriched with iron. Men require less iron and may be getting too much of the wrong form of iron in enriched products. (14)

The key is to discover what your body needs and can tolerate. When you eat foods to fuel your cells and avoid foods that work against you, you will usually find:

- your metabolism balances and you will no longer crave certain foods
- you are feeling emotionally more balanced
- you have more energy
- chronic complaints start to lessen and often disappear
- your weight will balance to what is right for you

We should consume only that which will fuel all the cells in the body.

2. Adulterated Foods and Additives to Avoid

When you buy food, are you thinking about how this will enhance your health or the health of your family? Often we eat because we are hungry, need energy, or have cravings with little thought as to how what we eat affects our bodies. Many of the products we consume contain few if any nutrients and may contain ingredients that actually harm the body. Researchers are beginning to agree much of modern disease is caused by metabolic disrupters found in many "food products" we eat. (15)

Learning what ingredients are metabolic disrupters and then reading labels will give you an indication as to what a product really is. Manufacturers are not always required to list all ingredients, and may have included hidden ingredients which sound OK but really aren't. For example, a packaged muffin mix says it has blueberry bits, which sounds nutritious. But are they really bits of blueberries or an imitation made from a <u>combination of corn syrup solids with artificial blue and green food colorings derived from coal tar</u>? There are so many deceptions in our processed food that I will only mention a few to give you a start. Do your research to make informed decisions. I personally choose to avoid processed foods.

EXCITOTOXINS

"Excitotoxin" is a relatively new term to reference several created toxins that bind to certain receptors on the cells. They may cause neuronal cell death and may be involved in brain damage associated with strokes and many other conditions. Excitotoxins are chemicals that cause a brain cell to become "overexcited" and fire uncontrollably. <u>Monosodium glutamate and aspartame are two of the most common and potentially dangerous excitotoxins.</u> (16)

Professor John Olney of Washington University in St. Louis found that not only did MSG destroy the nerve cells in the inner layers of an animal's retina, but MSG also was toxic to the brain. Free glutamic acid **(MSG) mostly from food sources, can get into the brain, injuring and**

sometimes killing neurons. In animal studies specialized cells in the **hypothalamus**, the critical area of the brain, were destroyed after a single dose of MSG. (17)

The hypothalamus regulates the autonomic nervous system which is involved with:
- contraction of smooth muscle
- cardiac muscle
- secretions of glands
- feelings of rage and aggression
- regulating body temperature
- regulating food intake and thirst
- maintaining wake and sleep patterns (16)

A few symptoms of MSG reaction:
- headache (migraine type)
- flushing of face
- hyperactivity
- distortions of vision
- rapid, irregular heartbeat
- abdominal cramping, bloating
- sweating
- facial pressure or tightness
- numbness, tingling
- loss of consciousness
- chest pain
- nausea
- weakness
- extreme tiredness
- skin rashes
- distortions of vision
- asthma attacks
- severe depression
- insomnia (16)

MSG (monosodium glutamate):
Early in the 1900s Japanese cooks learned that adding kombu to bland foods improved the taste. Dr. Kikunae Ikeda, a chemist, was able to isolate the chemical that was responsible for the taste-enhancing powers as glutamate. By 1909 Dr. Ikeda and a friend had formed a company to manufacture monosodium glutamate. During WWII,

servicemen became aware that Japanese rations tasted much better than American, which led American food processors to explore what was making the difference. Soon American food processors were adding large amounts to their foods. (18)

All pregnant women should be warned about potential dangers to the fetus from **excitotoxins.** Again we are reminded how important the diet of the pregnant woman is. Often infants and young children are given commercial baby food which may contain significant amounts of MSG. Through Dr. Olney's work pure MSG has been removed from baby food, but some food manufacturers are still using an "even more dangerous product, hydrolyzed vegetable protein, which contains three known excitotoxins and has added MSG." Read those labels. Usually baby food purchased at a health food store will be less likely to contain excitotoxins. (18)

MSG is added to most soups, chips, fast foods, frozen foods, ready-made dinners, processed meats, and canned goods. The food industry can create a tasteless, inferior product and, by adding MSG, make it taste great. Often MSG and related toxins are added to foods in disguised forms. For example, among the food manufacturers' favorite disguises are: hydrolyzed vegetable protein (HVP), vegetable protein, "natural flavorings," spices, autolyzed yeast, caseinate, meat tenderizer, flavor enhancers, yeast extract, chicken and beef broths. Foods often contain from 12 per cent to 40 per cent MSG. (17)

I've learned that taking 100 mg of Vitamin B 6 when I feel I'm having an MSG reaction is a fast antidote for this vicious migraine-type headache and other symptoms. I've also discovered that taking potassium and magnesium supplements and the homeopathic remedy Kali Phosphoricum will ease the symptoms. I don't have scientific reasoning for these, but I know they help me.

Excitotoxins may play a major role in the massive behavioral problems in kids such as Attention Deficit Disease. Too often these kids are put on Ritalin and other drugs when changing their diets to avoid additives may alleviate the situation. (17)

Alzheimers Disease (AD) has risen greatly in the last forty years. Many feel chemical toxins in our foods and environment including excitotoxins such as MSG contribute to the damage to the brain in people with Alzheimer's. Experiments have been done where AD like symptoms have been produced in the laboratory from MSG. (19)

When I'm reading labels or asking a waitperson if there is MSG in something on the menu, the response is often, "I'm glad I don't have to worry about eating MSG." I always tell him/her that MSG is affecting everyone in different ways and with varying intensity, depending on the body's ability to detoxify it.

A story comes to mind. I was in the Twin Cities of Minnesota for a national conference. After a long day of organizing a friend and I went to an upscale chain restaurant and had a tasty dinner. Too tasty I thought as I was eating it. About an hour later while we were shopping for supplies for the conference, my friend said, "I feel like I'm going to have a stroke." Her vision was distorted, and she felt sick all over. I knew what it was because I was starting to have my own reaction. That tasty food was heavily laced with MSG. Neither of us felt very well for the start of the conference the next morning. At that time I had not learned the natural antidotes, so we just suffered through it. Even when I take the antidotes, though, my system is disturbed for at least 12 hours; we can't assess the cumulative damage.

I doubt that anyone is truly immune to the dangers of excitotoxins. Every time we consume foods containing them, they are damaging cells in our bodies which will eventually manifest in symptoms.

Why is MSG or any form of processed free glutamic acid still used in our food products when we have so much evidence that it is damaging to the body?

MSG is added to food for the **addictive effect it has on the human body**. In his book, The Slow Poisoning of America, University of Waterloo research assistant John Erb called MSG an *addictive substance*, like a drug that is slipped into the food to get you hooked. He said it is no secret that the preservative has addictive properties, and that is exactly why manufacturers use it. Processed free glutamic acid is cheap, and since its neurotoxic nerve stimulation enhances so wonderfully the flavor of basically bland and tasteless foods, manufacturers are eager to go on using it. (20)

Many of the symptoms of discomfort in our lives can be eliminated by avoiding foods and drinks that contain MSG and its many other names.

Consider some common sources of MSG:
Low-fat and no-fat milk products often contain milk solids that contain MSG, and many dairy products also contain carrageenan, guar gum, and/or locust bean gum. Protein powders often contain processed free glutamic acid (MSG). Individual amino acids are not always listed on labels of protein powders. (21)

When a product has been hydrolyzed, it will usually have free glutamic acid, such as hydrolyzed soy protein, hydrolyzed wheat protein, hydrolyzed pea protein, hydrolyzed whey protein, hydrolyzed, corn protein. If a tomato, for example, were whole, it would be identified as a tomato. Calling an ingredient tomato protein indicates that the tomato has been hydrolyzed, at least in part, and that processed free glutamic acid (MSG) is present. (22)

MSG reactions have been reported from soaps, shampoos, hair conditioners, and cosmetics, where MSG is hidden in ingredients with names that include the words hydrolyzed, amino acids, and/or protein. Sun block creams and insect repellents may also contain MSG. Drinks, candy, and chewing gum are potential sources of hidden MSG and/or aspartame, neotame, and AminoSweet (the new name for aspartame). Binders and fillers for medications, nutrients, supplements, and some fluids administered intravenously in hospitals may contain MSG. (23)

According to the manufacturer, Varivax–Merck, chicken pox vaccine (Varicella Virus Live) contains L-monosodium glutamate and hydrolyzed gelatin, both of which contain processed free glutamic acid (MSG), which causes brain lesions in young laboratory animals and endocrine disturbances like obesity and reproductive disorders later in life. It would appear that most, if not all, live virus vaccines contain some ingredient(s) that contains MSG. (24)

Reactions to MSG are dose-related, which means some people react to even very small amounts. MSG-induced reactions may occur immediately after ingestion or after as much as 48 hours later. The time lapse between ingestion and reaction is typically the same each time for a particular individual who ingests an amount of MSG that exceeds his or her individual tolerance level. We know some people get reactions after eating the food with monosodium glutamate—reactions that include migraine headaches, upset stomach, fuzzy thinking, diarrhea, heart irregularities, asthma, and/or mood swings.(25)

Remember: By food industry definition, all MSG is "naturally occurring". **"Natural" doesn't mean safe.** Natural only means that the ingredient started out in nature. So did arsenic. (25)

The following ingredients are suspected of containing or creating sufficient processed free glutamic acid to serve as MSG-reaction triggers in HIGHLY SENSITIVE people:
- Corn starch
- Corn syrup
- Modified food starch
- Lipolyzed butter fat
- Dextrose
- Rice syrup
- Brown rice syrup
- Milk powder
- Reduced fat milk (skim; 1%; 2%)
- Most "low fat" or "no fat"
- Anything "enriched"
- Anything "Vitamin enriched"

More sources for information on MSG:
http://www.msgmyth.com/
http://www.truthinlabeling.org/adversereactions.html
Excitotoxins --The Taste That Kills by Dr. Russell
Blaylock, MD
Battling the MSG Myth by Debby Anglesey
In Bad Taste: The MSG Symptom Complex by George R.
Schwartz & Kathleen A. Schwartz

Adulterated Foods and Additives to Avoid

http://www.truthinlabeling.org/MSG

Ingredients that <u>always</u> contain processed free glutamic acid:	Ingredients that <u>often</u> contain or produce processed free glutamic acid:
Glutamic acid (E 620)[2], Glutamate (E 620) Monosodium glutamate (E 621) Monopotassium glutamate (E 622) Calcium glutamate (E 623) Monoammonium glutamate (E 624) Magnesium glutamate (E 625) Natrium glutamate Yeast extract Anything "hydrolyzed" Any "hydrolyzed protein" Calcium caseinate Sodium caseinate Yeast food, Yeast nutrient Autolyzed yeast Gelatin Textured protein Soy protein soy protein concentrate Soy protein isolate Whey protein whey protein concentrate Whey protein isolate Anything "...protein" Vetsin Ajinomoto	Carrageenan (E 407) Bouillon and broth Stock Any "flavors" or "flavoring" Maltodextrin Citric acid, Citrate (E 330) Anything "ultra-pasteurized" Barley malt Pectin (E 440) Protease Anything "enzyme modified" Anything containing "enzymes" Malt extract Soy sauce Soy sauce extract Anything "protein fortified" Anything "fermented" Seasonings (1) Glutamic acid found **in unadulterated protein** does not cause adverse reactions. To cause adverse reactions, the glutamic acid must have been processed/manufactured or come from protein that has been fermented. (2) E numbers are used in Europe in place of food additive names

ASPARTAME: (artificial sweetener found under the names of Equal or Nutri-Sweet) is an excitotoxin. Aspartic acid, found in neotame, aspartame (NutraSweet), and AminoSweet, ordinarily causes MSG type reactions in MSG-sensitive people. (26)

Aspartame is found in some medications, including children's medications. For questions about the ingredients in pharmaceuticals, check with your pharmacist and/or read the product inserts for the names of "other" or "inert" ingredients.

Aspartame accounts for over 75 percent of the adverse reactions to food additives reported to the FDA. Many of these reactions are very serious, including seizures and death. (26)

Aspartame consists of several factors:

1. Aspartic Acid (40 percent of Aspartame) and **glutamate** act as neurotransmitters in the brain by facilitating the transmission of information from neuron to neuron. Too much aspartate or glutamate in the brain kills certain neurons by allowing the influx of too much calcium into the cells. This influx <u>triggers excessive amounts of free radicals, which kill the cells</u>. The neural cell damage that can be caused by excessive aspartate and glutamate is why they are referred to as "excitotoxins." They "excite" or stimulate the neural cells to death. (26)

2. Methanol (aka wood alcohol) (10 percent of aspartame): Methanol/wood alcohol is a deadly poison. Free methanol is created from aspartame when it is heated to above 86 Fahrenheit (30 Centigrade). This would occur when an aspartame-containing product is improperly stored or when it is heated (e.g., as part of a "food" product such as Jello).Methanol breaks down into formic acid and formaldehyde in the body. Formaldehyde is a deadly neurotoxin. (27)

3. Phenylalanine (50 percent of aspartame): Even a single use of aspartame raises the blood phenylalanine levels. In his testimony before the U.S. Congress, Dr.

Louis J. Elsas showed that high blood phenylalanine can be concentrated in parts of the brain and is especially dangerous for infants and fetuses. Blood phenylalanine levels build up in the brain, specifically the hypothalamus, medulla oblongata, and corpus striatum. (27) Dr. Blaylock points out that excessive buildup of phenylalanine in the brain can cause schizophrenia or make one more susceptible to seizures. (27)

4. Diketopiperazine (DKP): DKP is a byproduct of aspartame metabolism. DKP has been implicated in the occurrence of brain tumors. (27)

Excitotoxins are negatively impacting the health of our nation, especially our children, but the food industry just keeps manufacturing products that contain them. It's estimated that aspartame is in over 5,000 products and MSG under its various names is found in nearly all processed foods.

Russell Blaylock, MD, in the summary of his book, Excitotoxins: The Taste that Kills, says "Today, virtually all of the neurodegenerative disease are now considered to be intimately related to the excitotoxic process. Seizures, headaches, strokes, brain injury, subarachnoid hemorrhage, and developmental brain disorders are all intimately related to excitotoxins." (28)

Evidence is gathering that excitotoxins aggravate or even precipitate many of the neurodegenerative brain diseases of our time, among them Parkinsons' disease, Alzheimer's disease, ALS, and others. Recognizing the dangers to the unborn child and to infants should make people work for the production of these products to be discontinued, but it has not. Dr. John Olney, a neuroscientist who did research for years on the effects of excitotoxins said, "The amount of MSG in a single bowl of commercially available soup is probably enough to cause blood glutamate levels to rise higher in a human child than levels that predictably cause brain damage in immature animals." Dr. Blaylock says, "A child's brain is four times more sensitive to these toxins than is the brain of an adult." (29)

Over 460,000 people per year are now dying of a disorder called <u>sudden cardiac death</u> according to CDC statistics. (30)

Dr. Blaylock also reports, "Numerous glutamate receptors have been found within the heart's electrical conduction system, as well as heart muscle. When an excess of food-borne excitotoxins, such as MSG, hydrolyzed protein, soy protein isolate and concentrate, natural flavoring, sodium caseinate and aspartate from aspartame, are consumed, these glutamatereceptors are over stimulated, producing cardiac arrhythmias."(31)

Researchers at the University of Liverpool examined the toxic effects on nerve cells in the laboratory when a combination of four common food additives - aspartame, monosodium glutamate (MSG) and the artificial colorings Brilliant Blue and Quinoline Yellow were used. The research team reported that when mouse nerve cells were exposed to MSG and Brilliant Blue or aspartame and Quinoline Yellow in laboratory conditions, combined in concentrations that theoretically reflect the compound that enters the bloodstream after a typical children's snack and drink, the <u>additives stopped the nerve cells growing and interfered with proper signaling systems</u>. The mixtures of the additives had a much more potent effect on nerve cells than each additive on its own. (32)

Aspartame is being called the "saddest joke on the American consumer" because aspartame-sweetened sodas are marketed as "diet" soft drinks. The truth is that **aspartame suppresses the production of serotonin**. Reduced serotonin leads to carb/sugar binging and cravings causing people to eat and drink more, thus gaining weight. (26)

<u>Some of the common early symptoms of aspartame poisoning:</u>
Headaches, nausea, vertigo, insomnia, numbness, blurred vision, blindness and other eye problems, memory loss, slurred speech, depression, personality changes, hyperactivity, stomach disorders, seizures, skin lesions, rashes, anxiety attacks, muscle cramping and joint pain,

loss of energy, symptoms mimicking heart attacks, hearing loss and ear ringing, and loss or change of taste. (33)

One federal (United States) report lists 92 symptoms triggered by Aspartame, including symptoms of multiple sclerosis and systemic lupus, four types of seizures, sexual dysfunction, coma, and death. Millions of individuals are now apparently suffering from "Aspartame Disease." (33)

The quickest way to understand aspartame is to watch the documentary, "Sweet Misery: a Poisoned World" by Cori Brackett, Sound and Fury Productions. If you buy a copy and share it with your friends and colleagues, you could make a difference in the health of everyone who watches it. "Sweet Misery" is available online from several sources.

Dr. Joseph Mercola says,"Diet products containing the chemical sweetener aspartame can have multiple neurotoxic, metabolic, allergenic, fetal and carcinogenic effects." Dr. Joseph Mercola has collected great information on his website: www.Mercola.com (Search Aspartame for great articles.)

Avoid consuming aspartame while flying. The methanol in aspartame can lead to oxygen deprivation, and at high altitudes this can lead to dizziness, sudden memory loss, loss of vision, and even convulsions. (34)

Aspartame literally stimulates brain neurons to death and depletes insulin, inducing hypoglycemia and seizures. Further, the phenylalanine in aspartame drops the brain's seizure threshold, depletes serotonin, and can trigger panic attacks, paranoia, manic depression, rage, and suicidal tendencies. (34)

An article in Flying Safety warns that "People have suffered aspartame related disorders with doses as small as that carried in a single stick of chewing gum. This could mean a pilot who drinks diet sodas or coffee laced with aspartame is more susceptible to flicker vertigo or to flicker induced epileptic activity." That would mean any pilot who consumes aspartame is a potential victim for

<u>sudden memory loss, dizziness, gradual loss of vision or epileptic seizure.</u> (34)The health conditions and death of several commercial and military pilots have been connected with aspartame use. One airline pilot who sipped Equal-laced coffee on long flights, suddenly developed atrial fibrillation. A second pilot and heavy aspartame user died in flight. A third pilot, who was also an aspartame user, sustained a grand mal seizure, was grounded, developed a brain tumor, and died. (34)

Everyone really needs to understand how food additives are affecting their health.

I can't begin to devote the pages needed to cover the subject of excitotoxins and other additives adequately, so I hope you will access some of the suggested reading below.
<u>The Crazy Makers</u> by Carol Simontacchi
<u>Excitotoxins: the Taste that Kills</u> by Russell L. Blaylock, M.D.
http://www.aspartamesafety.com/Transcript3.htm
http://www.nutrition4health.org/NOHAnews/NNW95Exci toxins.htm

BEWARE OF OTHER ADDITIVES:
The Environmental Working Group's Dirty Dozen list of food additives includes:
1.   Nitrites and nitrates
2.   Potassium bromate
3.   Propyl paraben
4.   Butylated hydroxyanisole (BHA)
5.   Butylated hydroxytoluene (BHT)
6.   Propyl gallate
7.   Theobromine
8.   Secret flavor ingredients
9.   Artificial colors
10. Diacetyl
11. Phosphate-based food additives (Watch List)
12. Aluminum-based additives (Watch List) (35)

Sodium nitrite and sodium nitrate
Nitrate becomes a health hazard because of its conversion to nitrite. Once ingested, conversion of nitrate to nitrite

takes place in the saliva of people of all age groups, and in the gastrointestinal tract of infants. Infants convert approximately double, or 10 percent of ingested nitrate to nitrite, compared to 5 percent conversion in older children and adults. (36)

Nitrite changes the normal form of hemoglobin, which carries oxygen in the blood to the rest of the body, into a form called methemoglobin that <u>cannot carry oxygen</u>. High enough concentrations of nitrate such as in drinking water can result in a temporary blood disorder in infants called methemoglobinemia, commonly called "blue baby syndrome." In severe, untreated cases, brain damage and eventually death can result from suffocation due to lack of oxygen. Early symptoms of methemoglobinemia can include irritability, lack of energy, headache, dizziness, vomiting, diarrhea, labored breathing, and a blue-gray or pale purple coloration to areas around the eyes, mouth, lips, hands and feet. (37)

<u>Infants up to six months of age are considered to be the most sensitive population.</u> Not only do they convert a greater percentage of nitrate to nitrite, their hemoglobin is more easily converted to methemoglobin and they have less of the enzyme that changes methemoglobin back to its oxygen-carrying form. <u>Pregnant women are more sensitive to the effects of nitrate due to a natural increase in methemoglobin levels in blood during the later stage of pregnancy beginning around the 30th week</u>. (37) (38)

It is believed that after nitrate is converted to nitrite in the body, it can react with certain amine-containing substances found in food to form nitrosamines, which are known to be potent cancer causing chemicals. <u>Nitrosamine formation is inhibited by antioxidants that may be present in food such as vitamin C and vitamin E</u>. (39)

Even though it is known nitrates and nitrites are precursors to highly carcinogenic nitrosamines, potent cancer-causing chemicals such as nitrate and nitrite are still in breakfast sausage, hot dogs, jerky, bacon, lunch meat, and even meats in canned soup products.

141

Processed meat consumption results in as much as a 67% increase in pancreatic cancer risk. (38)

It is true that many vegetables, particularly spinach, celery, beets, lettuce, and root vegetables, contain nitrites, but these vegetables also contain the antioxidants that provide the enzyme that inhibits toxicity. (39)

Not only are nitrites and nitrates a cause for cancer, but they are also now being researched as to their role in the development of many other diseases such as Alzheimer's, autism, diabetes, MS, Parkinson's and ALS. (36)

BHA (Butylated hydroxyanisole) and BHT (butylated hydroxytoluene) are used to keep fats and oils from going rancid. They are commonly found in cereals, baked goods, chewing gum, vegetable oil, potato chips, and other packed foods to ensure freshness. These additives have been found by some studies to cause cancer in rats and are being phased out of the food industry. (35)

Propyl Gallate is a preservative used to prevent fats and oils from spoiling. It's used in such products as vegetable oil, meat products, potato chips, chicken soup base and chewing gum. It is being studied for its carcinogenic properties but seems less toxic than BHA, BHT, or nitrates. (35)

Potassium Bromate is an additive used in breads and rolls to increase the volume and produce a fine crumb structure. Although most bromate breaks down into bromide, which is harmless, the bromate that does remain causes cancer in animals. I find it interesting that bromate has been banned throughout the world, except in the United States and Japan. (35)

Artificial colors: Artificial food colorings are often made from coal tars and contain heavy metals such as lead and mercury as well as many other chemicals. These chemicals are not on the food chain of any animal. (40)

In 2010 The Center for Science in the Public Interest (CSPI) published a comprehensive report called "Food

Dyes: A Rainbow of Risks,"which details the inherent risks of different dyes used in common foods. (41)

The colors below have been found to be health hazards:

Blue #1 (Brilliant Blue)	Green #3
Blue #2 (Indigo Carm	Red #40 (Allura Red)
Red #3	Yellow #5 (Tartrazine)
Citrus Red #2	Yellow #6 (Sunset Yel)

Natural food dyes that conscientious food manufacturers are using include:

Beet juice	Paprika
Blueberry juice	Purple sweet potato
Caramel -burnt sugar	Red cabbage
Carrot juice	Saffron
Grape skin extract	Turmeric (41)
Algae	

The European Union has passed a law requiring companies to post a notice on each dyed product sold in Europe. The notice states, "May have an adverse effect on activity and attention in children."This law is expected to encourage the companies to completely eliminate them inside all of Europe. (41)

Soda Pop and Flavored Drinks
Our society seems to have a love affair with sodas. Unfortunately, most soda drinkers are not aware of the health hazards of consuming this beverage.

1. Soda pop (regardless of the kind or brand) is 100% acid forming! Most soda has a pH of 2 which is a very low pH number.**Our bodies were made to have a natural pH balance of 7.3, which is slightly alkaline.**
- A pH of 6 is ten times more acidic than a pH of 7.
- A pH of 5 is 100 times more acidic than a pH of 7.
- A pH of 4 is 1,000 times more acidic than a pH of 7.
- A pH of 3 is 10,000 times more acidic than a pH of 7.
- At a pH of 2, one can of soda is 100,000 more acidic than your natural pH level.

A pH of 2 means a person would have to drink 32 eight ounce glasses of alkaline water just to neutralize the effect of one can of soda. We have already learned that over-acidification of the body fluids and tissues is an underlying factor in all disease. (42) (43)

2. Phosphoric acid, a basic ingredient in sodas, is seriously corrosive and caustic, damaging the skeletal system and greatly upsetting the body calcium-phosphorus ratio. It is so acidic it dissolves calcium out of the bones, which plays a major role in the development of osteoporosis (a weakening of the bones and skeletal structure) which makes a person, especially a woman, very susceptible to broken bones due to the bones becoming fragile. The teeth are alkaline in nature due to calcium, the most alkalizing mineral in the body. (43)

Increased soft drink consumption may be a major factor contributing to **poor bone mineralization in children.** When phosphate levels are high and calcium levels are low, calcium is pulled out of the bones. The phosphate content of soft drinks is very high, and they contain virtually no calcium. (42)

3. Sodas can be especially hazardous for anyone over 40, because the kidneys are less able to excrete excess phosphorus, causing depletion of vital calcium. Phosphoric acid even kills brain cells and fights with hydrochloric acid (which is needed for digestion) in human stomachs rendering it ineffective. (44)

4. And what makes soda pop so effervescent in nature? It is carbon dioxide. Carbon dioxide is a natural waste product the body produces, which is released with every exhalation. So why do we put carbon dioxide back into the body via ingestion of soda pop when the body naturally expels it with every exhalation? Nature takes out the carbon dioxide and then man puts it back in. Hmm!

5. Most carbonated beverages are sweetened with HFCS (high fructose corn syrup) or artificial sweeteners whose dangers we have already explored.In a recent chemical

analysis of eleven carbonated soft drinks sweetened with high fructose corn syrup, Dr. Chi-Tang Ho and his team of researchers from Rutgers University found very high levels of reactive carbonyls. Elevated levels of reactive carbonyls are normally found in diabetics and have been linked to tissue damage and complications of diabetes. In the study they found that a single can of HCFS sweetened carbonated beverage contained five times the amount of reactive carbonyls found in the blood of a person with diabetes. Old-fashioned table sugar (sucrose), on the other hand, has no reactive carbonyls. (45)

We already know the dangers of refined sugar and artificial sweeteners, so to date all sweeteners in sodas are hazardous to health.

6. Children are consuming more caffeine than most of us imagine. A 12-ounce can of cola contains about 45 milligrams of caffeine, but the amounts in more potent soft drinks can exceed 100 milligrams, almost that found in coffee. No wonder the kids are bouncing all over the classrooms of America.

7. Soft drinks have replaced milk in the diets of many American children. Although milk has its downside, it does provide protein, calcium, and other nutrients, whereas soda provides nothing healthful and has major disadvantages.

8. Some soft drinks are high in sodium, which may upset the body's sodium/potassium balance, leading to health issues such as high blood pressure. (47)

9. Sodium benzoate is a common preservative in soft drinks because it suppresses the growth of bacteria and fungi under the acidic conditions found in carbonated beverages. There seem to be several issues concerning sodium benzoate. In the presence of citric and/or ascorbic acid, sodium benzoate breaks down into the carcinogen, benzene. Tests show a rise in hyperactivity in children consuming a product with sodium benzoate. (48)

10. The containers from which sodas are consumed are questionable. We know that any acidic food or drink in an

145

aluminum container will dissolve traces of aluminum. (49) Recently we're hearing more about the dangers of plastic bottling. Polyethylene terephthalate (PET) is used in many soft drink containers and is known to release small amounts of dimethyl terephthalate into foods or beverages. Some experts believe this compound to be carcinogenic. BPA found in plastic soda bottles is thought to be an endocrine disruptor or "gender bender". (50)

Whether you drink sodas, fruit drinks, powdered drinks, sports drinks, power drinks, or vitamin waters, you must read the label and understand it. There are often other additives in various sodas which are detrimental to health. Health food store sodas usually have fewer health destroying ingredients, but they usually contain phosphoric acid and carbon dioxide.

3. Sweeteners, Good and Bad

We've already discussed the dangers of Aspartame, so let's look at some other sweeteners.

Sucralose (Splenda): Sucralose is sometimes advertised as a natural sugar, but it is not. It is made in a laboratory from sugar (sucrose) but becomes a chlorocarbon through a chemical process in which hydroxyl groups in a sugar molecule are replaced with chlorine atoms. Chlorocarbons have long been known for causing organ, genetic, and reproductive damage. Several other toxic chemicals are also involved in the process of creating sucralose. We know chlorine is a carcinogen, so what does that tell us about sucralose? (51)

The research of sucralose in animals has revealed some very serious side effects such as:
1. Shrinking of the thymus gland (up to 40 percent shrinkage)
2. Swelling of the liver
3. Swelling and calcification of the kidneys
4. Irritated bladder
5. Atrophy of lymph follicles in the spleen and thymus
6. Reduced growth rate
7. Decreased red blood cell count
8. Extension of the pregnancy period
9. Aborted pregnancy
10. Decreased fetal body and placental weights
11. Diarrhea (52)

You can find actual complaint cases from people who suffered side effects from sucralose in products. In each case the symptoms subsided after avoiding products with sucralose. These include:
- water retention, swelling
- blurred vision
- muscles and joints ached so bad, brain was in a fog all the time
- horrible red very itchy splotchy rash
- severe headache
- flu-like symptoms

147

- tumor and seizures
- gastric distress, cramping, and diarrhea
- rash and welts,
- sad, upset, angry
- light headed, drop in blood pressure (53)

Saccharin: The little pink packets of Sweet and Low are still in restaurants, and it is still available on the grocery shelf, even after it was thought to be a carcinogen back in the 70s and warning labels were required. In 2001 the warning labels were removed from the saccharin products, so we now assume they are safe. However, according to Science in the Public Interest, a committee of non-governmental scientists, the National Toxicology Program's Board of Scientific Counselors, reviewed saccharin data and concluded in <u>1997 that saccharin should still be considered a cancer risk.</u> Saccharin is sold as: Sweet Twin, Sweet'N Low, and Necta Sweet. (54)

Acesulfame-K (sold as Sunette or Sweet One):
Acesulfame-K is an artificial sweetener that's about 200 times sweeter than sugar. It's used in baked goods, chewing gum, gelatin desserts and soft drink. The testing has been inconclusive that Acesulfame-K breaks down into acetoacetamide, which has been found to affect the thyroid in rats, rabbits and dogs. In tests it caused cancer in animals. (55)

Refined sugar: I've discovered most people don't want to hear how damaging sugar is to their health because people love and crave the taste. They are addicted. Dr. Abram Hoffer, father of orthomolecular medicine and vitamin therapy for schizophrenia, is convinced that "Sugar is an addiction far stronger than what we see with heroin." He goes on to say that "It is the basic addictive substance from which all other addictions flow." (56)

Studies are showing that not only can a diet rich in sugar boost the risk of type 2 diabetes and contribute to obesity, but also it may lead to colon cancer. (57)

Sugar is so damaging that Nancy Appleton has listed over a hundred reasons not to use sugar. I'll give you a few to make my point. To see the whole list, "143 Reasons Why Sugar Is Ruining Your Health," go to http://www.nancyappleton.com/ or read <u>Lick the Sugar Habit</u> by Nancy Appleton. (58)

1. Sugar reduces the effectiveness of white blood cells, which are responsible for destroying germs in the body. So even in small amounts, sugar negatively affects the body's ability to fight off infection.
2. Sugar can cause cancer. It also helps the cancer cells progress by meeting the cancer cell's energy needs. Sugar (glucose) is cancer's fuel or food. Regular cells use oxygen for energy through normal respiration.
3. Sugar can weaken the eyes and cause cataracts.
4. Sugar can raise homocysteine levels in the blood stream, thus increasing inflammation in the body.
5. Sugar can contribute to metabolic syndrome.
6. Sugar suppresses the immune system, which is our main defense against disease.
7. Sugar upsets the mineral relationships in the body and can cause mineral deficiencies.
8. Sugar can cause hyperactivity, anxiety, difficulty concentrating, and crankiness in children.
9. Sugar can increase your blood pressure and contribute to heart disease.
10. Sugar contributes to obesity, which is becoming a great health threat to many people.

In the 1930s, Dr. Weston A. Price travelled around the world examining the teeth and skulls of every primitive race he could find – American Indians, Swiss Alps villagers, Eskimos, aborigines, Scottish primitives, Fiji islanders, and more. Price's conclusions are not subject to debate—in instance after instance, when a people were exposed to western foods such as white sugar and white flour, within a very few years, they experienced rates of tooth decay, tuberculosis and arthritis equal to the "civilized" nations. Price found that as long as a group of people could remain isolated and eat their 'primitive' simple foods, the rates of tooth decay and degenerative disease were practically zero. You can read more about

149

Dr. Price's discoveries see his book, <u>Nutrition and Physical Degeneration.</u>

One of the most informative articles I've found is "Sugar: The Sweet Thief of Life," found at http://www.thedoctorwithin.com/sugar. A great book is <u>Sugar Blues,</u> by William Dufty.

White flour and products made with refined white flour are high on the glycemic index (GI), meaning they cause a quick rise in blood sugar levels. A steady intake of high GI foods causes a gradual insensitivity to insulin, which can lead to Type 2 diabetes, weight gain, and other health issues. See more on grains in the *Carbohydrate* section.

High fructose corn syrup (HFCS) was introduced into the American food supply in the 1970s and 80s as a cheap replacement for sugar.

HFCS is processed from <u>hydrolyzed</u> corn starch, so <u>it's not natural</u>. During processing it is subjected to three separate enzymatic processes: first a bacteria, then a fungus, and finally a chemical. From the Westin A. Price website we learn most HFCS is made from genetically modified corn and then it is processed with genetically modified enzymes. (59)

The result is a product high in fructose. Since fructose does <u>not</u> stimulate the release of insulin, we were told for many years that using HFCS was good for diabetics. I found that is not true. Insulin is a naturally-occurring hormone that helps to metabolize our foods by pushing carbohydrates into our muscle cells to be used as energy and allows carbohydrates to be stored in the liver for later use. It also stimulates production of another hormone, leptin, which helps to regulate our storage of body fat and increases our metabolism when needed. These two hormones are important in regulating our body fat. (60)

Most sugars like sucrose, with the help of insulin, can be processed by every cell in the human body, but <u>fructose must be metabolized by the liver</u>. The liver is already very busy doing all the normal bodily functions. The chemicals, heavy metals, and drugs which assault our bodies must be processed by the liver, and then we are ask the liver to work overtime to process a diet heavy in fructose. The livers of the rats on the high fructose diet looked like the livers of alcoholics, plugged with fat and cirrhotic. (59)

Metabolic syndrome is a cluster of conditions that occur together—increased blood pressure, elevated insulin levels, excess body fat around the waist, or abnormal cholesterol levels. Just one of these increases your risk of serious disease, but the combination of factors in metabolic syndrome greatly increases your risk of a cardiovascular event. (62)

The rise in obesity in the US parallels the increased use of HFCS in the food and drink industry. Studies show that obesity leads to many other conditions such as diabetes. The occurrence of new cases of type-2 diabetes has doubled over the past three decades, according to a report in the American Heart Association's journal, *Circulation*, June 2006. The percentage of overweight children in the United States has tripled since 1980. The epidemic of type 2 diabetes cases across the nation is likely to lead to a substantially higher incidence of strokes among middle-aged adults and newly diagnosed diabetics. (59)(60)

Researchers have found that men who consume very high levels of fructose elevated their triglyceride level by 32 percent. **As a trygliceride enters our blood stream, it makes our cells resistant to insulin, making our body's fat burning and storage system even more sluggish.** (63) The body metabolizes high fructose corn syrup differently than sugar. It blunts the body's ability to recognize when it is full and increases a person's appetite. (59)

So what are **triglycerides** and why is their level important? When we eat, the body uses the calories it needs for quick energy and extra calories are turned into triglycerides and stored in fat cells to be used later. **If you regularly eat or drink more calories than you burn,**

you may have high triglycerides which can translate to higher cardiovascular risk. (64)

There is considerable research connecting HFCS with the rise of Type II Diabetes and related complications. Researchers at Rutgers University, in a chemical analysis of eleven carbonated soft drinks sweetened with high fructose corn syrup (HFCS), found very high levels of reactive carbonyls. Elevated levels of reactive carbonyls have been found in the blood of people with diabetes and have been linked to tissue damage and complications of diabetes. (65)

Agave syrup is the latest sweetener to hit the media. Agave is a highly processed and concentrated fructose sugar. The hype tells us because it is low on the "glycemic index" and doesn't spike your blood sugar, it is good for diabetics. That is NOT true. It is important to understand fructose does not increase insulin levels, which is not necessarily good because it does radically increase insulin resistance, which is far more dangerous. It's normal for your insulin levels to rise and fall, but it is dangerous when these insulin levels remain elevated, which is what insulin resistance causes. (66)

The Good Sweet Alternatives

Raw Honey:
Honey is essentially a highly concentrated water solution of many sugars. (67) These sugars do not all need to be broken down by the digestive process, so honey is quickly absorbed into the bloodstream, giving a quick energy boost to the body. It contains important minerals like magnesium, potassium, calcium, sodium chlorine, sulfur, iron, phosphate, and small amounts of copper, iodine, and zinc. It also contains vitamins B1, B2, C, B6, B5, and B3, all of which change according to the qualities of the nectar and pollen. (67) (68)

Raw honey is an excellent substitute for refined sugar in our drinks and food and also has many medicinal qualities. (67)

There is more information about honey in "Superfoods".

When purchasing honey, be sure to know your source, as much of the honey on the market is altered and has additives. Often I have found that a package says "honey" on the front label, but on the ingredient panel it lists refined sugar, dextrose, sucrose, corn syrup, or artificial sweeteners and then honey is listed near the end. Ingredients are listed in the order of the percentage of quantity in the product.

Note: Honey should not be given to infants in the first year. (69)

Stevia: As a diabetic who doesn't want to use artificial sweeteners, stevia has brought "sweet" back into my life. However, I have learned not all stevia products are pure.

Stevia comes from the leaves of the stevia shrub (Stevia rebaudiana), which is native to Paraguay and has been used by people in South America for 1500 years. It's been used by the Japanese food industry since the 1970s. However, in the US, due to FDA politics, it can only be purchased in the supplement section of your health food store. The controversy over the safety of stevia in the US seems to be unwarranted, since it has been used in other countries for years. (70)

Extracts of stevia leaves have been found to be up to 300 times as sweet as cane sugar, with no calories, and it does not metabolize to glucose. In fact, it is thought to enhance the glucose tolerance of some diabetics and replaces the need to use artificial sweeteners. However, use stevia sparingly until you discover how your body reacts to it. It is a very concentrated sweetener, so start using a tiny bit. A few grains sweeten my cup of tea and not much more to whip up a bowl of cream. (70)

There are stevia products on the market that contain very little stevia and some questionable other ingredients such as a popular stevia brand, contains **erythritol,** a sugar alcohol, and natural flavors along with the stevia leaf extract. Erythritol is made by processing corn into a food grade starch which it then ferments with yeast to create glucose and is then processed further to create erythritol.

The corn most likely is genetically modified. Erythrtol is known to cause abdominal cramping and excess flatulence in some people. One stevia product contains dextrose, a starch-derived glucose, which is often extracted from corn, wheat or rice. (71)

** **Note:** I use the purest stevia I can buy. Read labels.

Sugar alcohols--good or bad? Sugar alcohol is new terminology for many of us, but sugar alcohols have been used in food products for many years. Actually, sugar alcohols are neither sugars nor alcohols. They are carbohydrates with a chemical structure that partially resembles both sugar and alcohol, but they don't contain ethanol as alcoholic beverages do. (72)

The metabolism of sugar alcohols is very different than the metabolism of regular sugars. Sugar alcohols are not completely absorbed by the body from the small intestine. Some is absorbed into the blood, but the rest passes through the small intestine and is fermented by bacteria in the large intestine. The part that is absorbed into the blood is converted to energy by processes that require little or no insulin. Because of the fermentation in the large intestine, consumption of alcohol sugars may produce abdominal gas and discomfort in some individuals. (73)

The common sugar alcohols found in food products are: sorbitol, xylitol, mannitol, glycol, glycerol, arabitol, ribitol, maltitol, maltitol syrup, lactitol, erythritol, isomalt, and hydrogenated starch hydrolysates. All forms of sugar alcohols except xylitol are six-carbon sugars, which feed dangerous bacteria and fungi. (73)

Xylitol has been depicted as a good sugar, which it is in its natural form as found in fibrous vegetables and fruit, hardwood trees like birch, and some other natural substances. It has 40% fewer calories and 75% fewer carbohydrates than sugar and is slowly absorbed and metabolized, resulting in very negligible changes in insulin. (74) **HOWEVER, most of the xylitol available is a chemically extracted sugar alcohol** the body is unable to fully digest, which causes an uproar in the digestive tract. To make matters worse, xylitol is frequently made from GMO corn and produced in China. Studies have found sugar alcohol is extremely toxic to dogs and can cause liver failure. (74) Organic chemist Shane Elison explains the production process of the sweetener in "Xylitol: Should We Stop Calling it Natural?" Quoting Elison, "Xylitol is a molecular cousin to <u>sugar</u> and is derived from the crushed fibers of sugar cane, birch wood or corn, using a **multi-step chemical reaction** that involves the use of sulfuric acid, calcium oxide, phosphoric acid and active charcoal. The end product is a bleached, powdery blend of sugar alcohols that taste sweet on the tongue but are **not absorbed by the body**. Xylitol will rip up your insides, namely the digestive tract." (75) Xylitol is considered a five-carbon sugar, which means it is antimicrobial, preventing the growth of bacteria. While sugar is acid-forming, xylitol is alkaline-enhancing. Using toothpaste and mouthwash with xylitol may benefit your mouth, gums, and teeth, but ingesting it makes me sick.

Other natural sweeteners: Blackstrap molasses, brown rice syrup, date sugar, sorghum, and natural fruit concentrates are all healthier alternatives to refined sugar or artificial sweeteners. Remember they are still sugars, though, so go lightly on them as well.

4. Understanding the Nutritional Jargon

NUTRIENTS ARE THE KEY IN PROTECTING YOU FROM DISEASE

This dictionary definition for food says it all. "Food is material, usually <u>of plant or animal origin</u> that contains or <u>consists of essential body nutrients</u>, such as carbohydrates, fats, proteins, vitamins, or minerals, and is ingested and assimilated by an organism to produce energy, stimulate growth, and maintain life."(76)

<u>The Optimum Nutrition Bible</u> by Patrick Holford was one of the main texts in my study of nutrition and so is reflected in this section. You will note along the way many other researchers and authors who have contributed to my broadening scope of foods as the basis for health. The following information on nutrients comes basically from his work.

Vitamin A is a fat-soluble vitamin. Vitamin A:
*   is needed for new cell and tissue growth.
*   is needed for healthy skin and hair
*   helps to preserve and improve your eyesight, especially night vision
*   boosts your immune function and protects against infection
*   is needed to maintain healthy bones and teeth
*   aids in preventing the formation of kidney stones
*   works as a powerful antioxidant, Vitamin A fights against oxidative stress, thus protecting us from cataracts, atherosclerosis, chronic obstructive pulmonary disease, and cancer.
*   is essential for the reproductive process for both males and females

Vitamin A is found in animal sources. The best animal sources are from grass-fed animal sources including organ meats, milk, butter, cheese, eggs, and cod liver oil. Beta carotene in plant foods is converted in the body to vitamin A. Carotenes are found in dark green and yellow vegetables and yellow fruits such as carrot juice, pumpkins, carrots, winter squash, sweet potatoes, apricots, leafy greens, broccoli, Chinese cabbage, cantaloupe, papayas, red sweet pepper, tomatoes, mangos, asparagus, watercress, and many herbs.

Vitamin B Complex is needed for almost every process in the human body, including the skin, eyes, hair, liver, and healthy muscle tone throughout the body. It is essential for the functioning of the nervous system and proper brain function. B vitamins are involved with energy production and are helpful in alleviating depression. B vitamins play a crucial role in preventing atherosclerosis.

B-1 (Thiamine) helps circulation and assists in blood formation. It is important in many processes of the gastrointestinal and nervous systems. Thiamine is needed for energy metabolism and the proper function of the nervous system. The richest sources are brown rice, egg yolks, fish, legumes, liver, peanuts, peas, pork, poultry, rice bran, wheat germ and whole grains; others include watercress, zucchini, asparagus, mushrooms, peas, greens, peppers, cabbage, cauliflower, Brussels sprouts, tomatoes, and legumes.

B-2 (Riboflavin) helps maintain your supply of other B vitamins and is critical in the production of vitamin B-3 (niacin) in the body. Riboflavin:
* helps protect cells from oxygen damage
* plays a crucial role in the body's energy production
* allows the recycling of the antioxidant glutathione to take place.

Vitamin B2 is a cofactor for the enzyme glutathione reductase that reduces the oxidized form of glutathione back to its reduced version. Food sources: asparagus, avocados, broccoli, Brusssels sprouts, bean sprouts, cabbage, currants, dandelion greens, dulse, green beans, kelp, leafy greens such as collards, mustard, turnip greens, spinach, and chard, mushrooms, pumpkin, tomatoes, watercress, wheat germ, venison, and eggs.

B3 (Niacin) (nicotinic acid and 2 other forms, niacinamide/nicotinamide and inositol hexanicotinate which have different effects from niacin) is needed for

157

energy metabolism, proper digestion, and a healthy nervous system. Researchers have recently found that <u>high doses</u> of vitamin B3 in the form of niacinamide stimulate the gene C/EBPe which enhances your white blood cells' ability to fight staph infections, regardless of antibiotic resistance. (77) Niacinamide also:

- helps lower cholesterol levels.
- helps the body process fats.
- stabilizes your blood sugar.
- supports genetic processes in your cells. (78)

<u>Food sources</u>: mushrooms, watercress, cabbage, asparagus, broccoli, pumpkin, bean sprouts, mackerel, milk, bamboo shoots, tomatoes, chicken, tuna, halibut, venison, calf's liver, and turkey.

B-5 (Pantothenic acid) functions as part of the molecule called coenzyme A that is important in cellular metabolism of carbohydrates and fats to release energy.

- It supports the adrenal glands to increase production of cortisone and other adrenal hormones to help counteract stress and enhance metabolism.
- It is also thought to help prevent aging.
- It is generally important to healthy skin and nerves.
- It may reduce potentially toxic effects of antibiotics and radiation.
- It supports the synthesis of acetylcholine, a very important neurotransmitter agent that works throughout the body in a variety of neuromuscular reactions.
- It is vital in the synthesis of fatty acids, cholesterol, steroids, and phospholipids.
- It also helps synthesize porphyrin, which is connected to hemoglobin. (79) (80)

Some vitamin B-5 is made by the bacterial flora of human intestines, but food sources are very important. <u>Food sources</u>: mushrooms, watercress, broccoli, alfalfa sprouts, green peas, tomatoes, cabbage, celery, strawberries, squash, avocados, sweet potatoes, legumes, cauliflower, molasses, organ meats, brewer's yeast, egg yolks, fish, chicken, whole grain cereals, and cheese.

158

B-6 (Pyridoxine) is a water-soluble vitamin which the body <u>cannot store</u>, which means we need a continuous supply in our diets. <u>Vitamin B-6:</u>

- helps the immune system produce antibodies needed to fight many diseases
- is used by the body in more than 100 enzymatic reactions. Enzymes are proteins that help chemical reactions take place, so vitamin B-6 is active virtually everywhere in the body. Many of the building blocks of protein, amino acids, require B6 for their synthesis, as do the nucleic acids used in the creation of our DNA. Because amino and nucleic acids are such critical parts of new cell formation, <u>vitamin B6 is essential for the formation of virtually all new cells in the body</u>.
- is needed to help break down proteins. The more protein you eat, the more vitamin B-6 you need.
- is necessary for the production of Heme, the protein center of our red blood cells, and phospholipids, cell membrane components that enable messaging between cells.
- is necessary for the breakdown of glycogen, the form in which sugar is stored in our muscle cells and liver, making vitamin B-6 a key player in athletic performance and endurance.
- plays numerous roles in our nervous system, many of which involve neurological (especially brain cell) activity.
- plays a critical role in methylation, a chemical process in which methyl groups are transferred from one molecule to another. <u>Methylation changes a potentially dangerous molecule called homocysteine into other, benign substances</u>. Since homocysteine can directly damage blood vessel walls greatly increasing the progression of atherosclerosis, high homocysteine levels are associated with a significantly increased risk for heart attack and stroke. (81)

<u>Most vegetables and fruits are sources of B-6, but those listed below have the highest level:</u> Watercress, basil, cayenne, garlic, leafy greens, cauliflower, cabbage,

159

peppers, bananas, squash, broccoli, Brussels sprouts, asparagus, onions, seeds, nuts, cod, and tuna.

B-7 (Biotin) is needed in cell growth, the production of fatty acids, and metabolism of fats and proteins.
- It plays a role in the Kreb cycle, which is the process in which energy is released from food.
- Biotin is needed for healthy hair and skin, sweat glands, nerve tissue, and bone marrow, and for assisting with muscle pain.
- Biotin not only assists in various metabolic chemical conversions, but it also helps with the transfer of carbon dioxide.
- Biotin is helpful in maintaining a steady blood sugar level.

**Note: Natural bacteria living in the small intestine in humans produce biotin. Egg whites have a chemical that binds to biotin very tightly, preventing its uptake in the body's bloodstream, <u>so eating only egg whites can adversely affect biotin in the body.</u> Also, because of the micro flora that produce biotin in the human intestines, <u>prolonged use of antibiotic medication can lower the amount of biotin within the body</u>. (82) <u>Food Sources:</u> organ meats, eggs yolks, raw cauliflower, peas, tomatoes, oysters, lettuce, grapefruit, watermelon, sweet corn, cabbage, cherries, avocado, nuts, milk, bananas, and almonds.

B-9 (Folate or folic acid) is complex in its structure, needing enzymes in the intestines to chemically alter food forms of folate in order for this vitamin to be absorbed. Even when the body is operating at full efficiency, <u>only about 50% of ingested food folate can be absorbed</u>. The daily recommended intake of folate is 400 mcg. Folate:
- promotes healthy cell and tissue development. This is especially important during periods of rapid cell division and growth such as infancy and pregnancy.
- is important for functioning of the nervous system for everyone.

- deficiencies in the mother can cause malformation of the neural tube in the fetus, resulting in spina bifida (split/open spine) or deformed head.
- may be the most important nutrient in regulating homocysteine levels in the body.
- supports red blood cell production which helps prevent anemia.
- supports cell production in your skin.
- helps prevent osteoporosis-related bone fractures.
- helps prevent dementia, including Alzheimer's disease. (83) (84)

Too little folate or disturbed folate metabolism may contribute to depression in some people.

Food sources: wheat germ, spinach, peanuts, asparagus, turnip greens, mustard greens, calf's liver, parsley, broccoli, beets, lentils, romaine lettuce, collard greens, cauliflower, barley,beef, bran, brown rice, citrus fruits, lima beans, cantaloupe, garbanzo beans, watermelon, peas, cashews, walnuts, hazelnuts, sesame seeds, sprouts, poultry, shellfish, pork, and liver from organically raised animals.

B-12 (Cyanocobalamin or methylcobalamin) is important in almost all functions of the body.

- A deficiency of either vitamin B-12 or folate can result in significantly reduced white blood cell production and abnormal white blood cell responses.
- Deficiency of B-12 and folate in pregnant women may raise the risk of spina bifida and other neural tube defects in the fetus.
- B-12 is linked to the production of acetylcholine, a neurotransmitter that assists memory and learning.
- Adequate vitamin B-12 levels in the body are needed for a properly functioning thyroid gland.
- B-12 promotes proper breakdown of sugars and starches.
- B-12 helps prevent homocysteine buildup in your blood.

- An interesting theory contends the body can make B-12 in the intestines if there are adequate good bacteria (flora).
- Studies are being done looking at low vitamin B-12 levels in people diagnosed with Alzheimer's disease.
- B-12 deficiency can cause pernicious anemia.

Many of us, especially vegetarians, are often deficient in B-12. (85)

Some symptoms of B-12 deficiency are:
- weakness and tiredness
- light-headedness, brain fog, or lack of focus
- rapid heartbeat and breathing
- pale skin
- sore tongue
- easy bruising or bleeding, including bleeding gums
- stomach upset and weight loss
- diarrhea or constipation
- tingling or numbness in fingers and toes
- difficulty walking
- mood changes or depression
- memory loss, disorientation, and dementia (86)

Food sources: calf's liver, sardines, salmon, venison, shrimp, scallops, clams, lamb, cod, halibut, beef, herring, kidney, mackerel, dark turkey meat, brewer's yeast, eggs, yogurt, and other dairy products.

Note: If you are deficient in B-12, work with your health practitioner for the best form of supplementing for you.

Choline is a nutrient that helps the body absorb and use fats, particularly those that become part of cell membranes.
- It is needed for proper transmission of nerve impulses from the brain throughout the nervous system.
- It is necessary for the proper brain function.
- It is necessary for liver and gall bladder function.

Choline is a precursor for acetylcholine, an important neurotransmitter involved in muscle control, memory, and many other functions. It's been found acetylcholine is crucial for short-term memory and is lacking in Alzheimer's patients. (87)

Food sources: lecithin, egg yolk, liver, pork, beef, fish, milk, cauliflower, spinach, lettuce, nuts, soybeans, and whole grains. The body can produce choline from lecithin.

Inositol, sometimes called **B-8**, is important in the metabolism of fat and cholesterol and helps remove fats from the liver. Inositol also:
- prevents hardening of the arteries
- is calming to the nervous system
- is vital for hair growth
- helps in treating anxiety and depression
- helps in treating skin disorders like eczema
- is beneficial in treating eye problems
- helps with respiratory distress in babies

Food sources: brewer's yeast, fruits, lecithin, legumes, meats, milk, unrefined molasses, raisins, vegetables, and whole grains. (88) (89)

Vitamin C is also known as **ascorbic acid**. Researchers are discovering increasingly diverse uses for vitamin C for the promotion of health and disease prevention. Linus Pauling is known as the father of vitamin C research. In his book, Vitamin C and the Common Cold, first published in 1970, he revealed the benefits of vitamin C in relation to colds. Vitamin C acts as a natural antihistamine, which by reducing the histamine levels of the body controls the symptoms and duration of the common cold and may decrease the risk of serious respiratory conditions like asthma.

- Vitamin C is probably best known for preventing scurvy, a disease where the body cannot create enough collagen due to a lack of vitamin C. Without enough vitamin C your body cannot manufacture the connective tissue which holds your organs and teeth in place and cushions your joints. Two amino acids, proline and lysine, are also needed to create collagen, thus preventing scurvy.

163

- As a potent antioxidant, vitamin C boosts the immune system, thus helping the body develop resistance against infectious agents and aid in wound healing.
- It scavenges harmful oxygen free radicals, thus protecting against cancer.
- Vitamin C's antioxidant characteristics are showing great power in reducing or even reversing some changes in blood vessels (atherosclerosis) that can lead to strokes and other vascular catastrophes.
- Vitamin C reduces the cellular DNA damage that is the first step in cancer initiation and also reduces the inflammatory changes that allow a malignant cell to grow into a dangerous tumor.
- Vitamin C enhances the health-promoting effects of exercise and reduces exercise-induced oxidative damage.
- Vitamin C dramatically combats the oxidative damage caused by smoking and exposure to tobacco smoke.
- As an antioxidant, vitamin C is understood to prevent the oxidation of cholesterol in the blood and thereby may reduce the possibility of heart disease and strokes.
- Vitamin C is effective against stomach disease caused by bacterium Helicobacter pylori and cuts the risk of gastric cancer it could cause.
- The human eye requires vitamin C, as it is believed to protect the lens from the damage caused by sunlight.
- Vitamin C improves iron absorption. (90) (91)

Excellent Food Sources: hot chili peppers, fresh herbs such as parsley and thyme,

bell peppers, broccoli, cauliflower, Brussels sprouts, cabbage, citrus fruits, berries (especially strawberries), kale, romaine lettuce and all dark greens, tomatoes, summer and winter squash, cranberries, cantaloupe, kiwi fruit, watermelon, and papayas. (90) (91)

Note: It is very difficult to get enough vitamin C from foods in our toxic world, so I feel it is necessary to supplement.

Vitamin D is technically not a vitamin but a prohormone that behaves like a steroid in that it binds to receptor sites and has a regulatory effect on gene expression. Vitamin D was already discussed in "Priorities".

- Vitamin D plays an important role in the maintenance of several organ systems, bone formation and mineralization, and the control of calcium and phosphorus metabolism.
- It is vital in maintaining a healthy immune system.
- Vitamin D performs anti-tumor functions and is vital for the maintenance of the blood/brain barrier.

Sunshine is still the best source, but supplementing is often needed depending on where you live and the amount of time you spend outdoors.

Food sources: eggs, dried mushrooms, herring, mackerel, salmon, herring, sardines, catfish, tuna, cod liver oil, and the liver of most animals. (92)

Vitamin E is a term that covers eight fat-soluble compounds found in nature. Four of them are called tocopherols; the other four are tocotrienols.

Vitamin E:
- is important in the formation of red blood cells and helps the body use vitamin K
- is a powerful antioxidant that protects your cells from damaging free radicals and may protect against aging, cancer, and Alzheimer's disease
- helps your cells communicate effectively
- helps boost your immune system
- plays a role in healthy skin and hair
- protects against cardiovascular disease
- prevents the formation of thick scars from wounds
- helps alleviate fatigue
- helps prevent miscarriage in pregnant women

Food sources: wheat germ, olives, seeds and nuts, tuna, sardines, and salmon are some of the best sources of vitamin E. Asparagus, green peas, carrots, spinach, turnips, broccoli, mustard and other green leafy vegetables, tomato paste and sauce, avocados, papaya, sweet potatoes, and kiwifruit are good sources.

If you are going to use vitamin E supplements, please choose only a natural form. On a supplement label, natural vitamin E is listed as d-alpha tocopherol, d-alpha tocopheryl acetate, or d-alpha tocopheryl succinate. In contrast, synthetic forms of vitamin E are labeled with a dl- prefix. (93)

Vitamin F refers to essential fatty acids, which are discussed under "Fats."

Vitamin K intake by humans comes from <u>two main sources--our diets and synthesis from intestinal bacteria</u>. Vitamin K is found in nature in two forms. K1, also called phylloquinone, is found in plants, and vitamin K2, also called menaquinone, can be synthesized by good bacteria in the intestines. Vitamin K3, menadione, is a man-made synthetic form of this vitamin. Since vitamin K is a fat-soluble vitamin, it should be consumed with a fat.

- Vitamin K plays an important role in bone health by promoting bone formation and repair.
- Adequate vitamin K levels in the diet help limit neuronal damage in the brain.
- Vitamin K is used in the body to control blood clotting. It is essential in the creation of prothrombin in the body, which is the precursor to thrombin, a very important factor in blood clotting.
- In the intestines it also assists in converting glucose to glycogen, which can then be stored in the liver.

<u>Eating a variety of green vegetables will usually provide an adequate supply of vitamin K</u>. <u>Food sources</u>: spinach, broccoli, cabbage, all leafy greens and herbs, asparagus, Brussels sprouts, scallions, tomatoes, eggs, liver, green tea, and cheese. Yogurt with active bacterial cultures and probiotics help create vitamin K in the intestines.

<u>Caution:</u> High vitamin K intake can interfere with anticoagulant medication. Remember to check with your doctor before making any diet or supplement modifications if you are on anticoagulants. (94)

Betaine, also known as trimethylglycine, is produced by the body from choline and also from the amino acid glycine. Betaine functions very closely with choline, folic acid, vitamin B12, and a form of the amino acid methionine known as S-adenosylmethionine (SAMe) in the controlling of homocysteine by converting it to methionine.

- Betaine has been found to protect liver cells from toxins.
- Betaine is being studied to prevent or stop the progression of plaque formation seen during the initial stages of Alzheimer's disease.
- Betaine is a mood modifier.
- Betaine also plays a role in the manufacture of carnitine and serves to protect the kidneys from damage. (95)

Food sources: beets, broccoli, spinach, eggs, liver, seafood and wheat.

**Note: Betaine hcl (betaine hydrochloride) is betaine with hydrochloric acid, which is used as a digestive aid supplement. (96)

Calcium is often considered the most important mineral in the body. However, studies are showing calcium needs some buddies—phosphorus, magnesium, trace minerals, and vitamin D—to be properly utilized by the body. We need calcium from birth through old age. (97) Calcium:

- helps maintain strong bones, supports nerve and muscle function, and may help maintain normal blood pressure
- aids in maintaining bone health from the fetus through aging. During infancy calcium is required for proper bone and teeth growth; during adolescence it is essential for proper development of the skeletal structure; calcium is again essential as we get older, as our bones tend to get porous and weak.
- helps cardiac muscles contract and relax properly
- helps the nervous system
- helps in maintaining healthy blood pressure
- helps prevent coloncancer (97)

Food sources: all leafy greens, broccoli, blackstrap molasses, tofu, sesame seeds, fennel, cabbage, summer squash, green beans, garlic, Brussels sprouts, celery, oranges, asparagus, leeks, crimini mushrooms, basil, thyme, dill seed, oregano, cinnamon, rosemary, cumin seeds, cloves, coriander seeds, scallops, and kelp. Fermented dairy products yogurt and kefir. (98)

Chromium works with insulin to improve the transportation of glucose out of the blood and into the cells. Chromium may:

- help to reduce the amount of sugar circulating in your blood, decreasing your risk of diabetes and metabolic syndrome
- improve your body's insulin sensitivity, helping to reduce body fat and increase muscle mass
- help to reduce the amount of bad cholesterol circulating in your blood and raise the amount of good cholesterol in your blood
- help to reduce your blood pressure (99)

Food sources: onions, tomatoes, green beans, potatoes, green pepper, grape juice, orange juice, parsnips, apples, brewer's yeast, eggs, chicken, butter, oysters, beef, turkey breast, lamb, and Swiss cheese. Food processing methods often remove the naturally occurring chromium from the foods. (99)

**Note: Consult your holistic health practitioner before using a chromium supplement.

Copper plays a role in:

- aiding critical enzymes needed for proper metabolism
- maintaining a balance with zinc in the body
- iron utilization
- development of bone and connective tissue
- the production of the skin and hair pigment called melanin
- reducing tissue damage caused by free radicals
- building healthy blood
- the formation of collagen and elastin

Copper is a cofactor for many vital enzymes, including cytochrome c-oxidase and superoxide dismutase (cofactors for this enzyme are manganese and zinc.) (100)

Food sources: calf's liver; oysters, calamari, and lobster; sesame seeds, sunflower seeds, pumpkin seeds, dried basil, cocoa, nuts, crimini mushrooms; greens (turnip, mustard, kale, Swiss chard, spinach), blackstrap molasses, summer squash, asparagus, eggplant, cashews, tomatoes, ginger root, green beans, baked potato, tempeh, sweet potato, kiwi fruit, bell peppers, winter squash, and most unprocessed foods have some copper. (101)

Iodine is an essential trace element needed for the normal growth and development. About 60% of the iodine in the body is stored in the thyroid gland. Iodine:
- is required to ensure proper development and metabolism in human beings
- influences the functioning of thyroid glands by assisting in production of hormones, which are directly responsible for controlling the basic metabolic rate. Hormones, like thyroxin and triodothyronine, influence heart rate, blood pressure, body weight and temperature.
- plays an important role in maintaining optimum energy levels of the body by ensuring optimum utilization of calories
- helps in the normal growth and maturity of reproductive organs
- is necessary in the formation of healthy and shiny skin, teeth and hair

Iodine deficiency can cause mental retardation, abnormal weight gain, goiter, coarse skin, constipation and many other symptoms. Food sources: marine plant and animals, including shellfish, white deep-water fish, and brown seaweed kelp. Garlic, lima beans, Swiss chard, summer squash, sesame seeds, soybeans, turnip greens, and spinach are rich in iodine. Using iodized salt is an option. (102)

Iron's main activity is carrying life-giving oxygen to human blood cells. Iron is required for cellular oxidation and red blood cell formation. Women of childbearing age need more iron than men. Balanced iron in the diet is:

- vital for muscle health. It is present in the muscle tissues and helps supply oxygen required for contraction of muscles.
- crucial to brain health. Iron is involved in supplying about 20% of the blood oxygen needed by the brain to function.
- an important constituent of different enzyme systems
- key in providing strength to the immune system of human body

Deficiencies in iron may contribute to fatigue, restless legs, insomnia, and amnesia.

Food sources: Iron is found in many unprocessed foods, including meats and eggs, whole grains, many herbs, leafy greens, blackstrap molasses, beets, avocados, raisins, legumes, dried apricots, prunes, pumpkin, and sesame and sunflower seeds, to name a few. (103)

**Note: There is a danger when eating enriched processed foods of consuming too much of the wrong kind of iron. If you are eating iron-enriched foods, your vitamin/mineral supplement should be "without iron." (104)

Magnesium is needed by every organ in the body, especially the skeletal system, heart, muscles, kidneys, and teeth.

- It helps regulate calcium levels, as well as levels of copper, zinc, potassium, vitamin D, and other important nutrients in the body.
- Magnesium is responsible for the correct metabolic function of over 350 enzymes in the body.
- Magnesium affects the creation of ATP (adenosine triphosphate) the energy molecules of the body, the action of the heart muscle, the proper formation of bones and teeth, relaxation of blood vessels, and the promotion of proper bowel function. (105)

Conventional medicine has not understood the significance of magnesium to health. Since 99 percent of the magnesium in our bodies is located within the cells with only 1 percent in the blood, the usual blood test is not an accurate test of magnesium levels in the tissues and organs. (106)

About two thirds of all magnesium in our body is found in our bones. Researchers have discovered, however, that bone magnesium has two very different roles to play in our health. Some of the magnesium in our bones helps give them their physical structure. Magnesium is part of the bone's crystal lattice "bone scaffolding" together with phosphorus, calcium, and trace minerals. Other amounts of magnesium are found on the surface of the bone. This surface magnesium does not appear to be involved in the bone's structure but instead acts as a storage site for magnesium which the body can draw upon in times of poor dietary supply. (107)

Low magnesium levels in the body may be the single largest cause of bone loss and make high calcium intake ineffective. Without enough magnesium, your body pulls calcium from bones and deposits the surplus calcium into arteries (causing arteriosclerosis), joints (causing arthritis), muscles (causing fibromyalgia), capillaries of the brain (causing mental function disorders), blood vessels of the arms and legs (causing cold hands and feet), bone spurs, and kidney stones. (105) Magnesium is just as important as calcium to prevent osteoporosis. Magnesium's roles in bone health are many:

- Adequate levels of magnesium are essential for the absorption and metabolism of calcium.
- Magnesium stimulates a particular hormone, calcitonin, that helps preserve bone structure and draws calcium out of the blood and soft tissues back into the bones, preventing some forms of arthritis and kidney stones.
- Magnesium suppresses another bone hormone called parathyroid, preventing it from breaking down bone.

171

- Magnesium converts vitamin D into its active form so that it can help with calcium absorption.
- Magnesium is required to activate an enzyme that is necessary to form new bone.
- Magnesium regulates active calcium transport. (105)

Magnesium deficiency can trigger the following conditions:

Anxiety attacks	Liver disease
Asthma	Metabolic
Blood clot	Syndrome
Bowel disease	Migraines
Cystitis	Musculoskelal
Diabetes	Nerveproblems
Fatigue	Osteoporosis
Heart disease	Raynaud's
Hypertension	Syndrome
Hypoglycemia	Syndrome X
Insomnia	Tooth decay
Kidney disease	

Women's issues: premenstrual syndrome, dysmenorrhea (cramping pain during menses), infertility, premature contractions, preeclampsia, and eclampsia in pregnancy.

Adequate magnesium lessens the risk of cerebral palsy and Sudden Infant Death Syndrome (SIDS). (105)

The introduction of magnesium, either by a high-magnesium diet, with green drinks, or via magnesium supplements, can help alleviate the above conditions.

Reading The Miracle of Magnesium by Carolyn Dean, MD, ND made it very clear to me how important magnesium is to our overall health and how deficient most of us are. There has been a great push for people to supplement with calcium and lately vitamin D, but few have understood the role magnesium plays in the body's use of those nutrients.

Food sources: Almost all raw vegetables, nuts, seeds, and many herbs are good sources of magnesium.

Manganese is an essential cofactor in a number of enzymes important in **energy production and antioxidant defenses.** It is used by the body as a co-factor for the antioxidant enzyme, superoxide dismutase, which helps break down potentially harmful oxygen molecules in cells. Few people have manganese deficiencies.

- Manganese helps assist iron in the oxygenation of the blood and formation of hemoglobin. Interestingly, manganese is also concentrated in tears.
- It helps form healthy bones, cartilage, tissues, and nerves.
- Manganese helps produce energy from protein and carbohydrates and is involved in the synthesis of fatty acids, which are important for a healthy nervous system, and in the production of cholesterol, which is used by the body to produce sex hormones. (108)

Food sources: dried herbs and spices such as cloves, cardamom, ground ginger, cinnamon, spearmint, parsley, bay leaf, tarragon, turmeric, coriander, chili powder, and marjoram; watercress, pineapple, okra, endive, blackberries, raspberries, lettuce, grapes, strawberries, oats, beets, celery, wheat, rice and oat bran; nuts, mussels, oysters, and clams; sunflower, sesame, and pumpkin seeds; dark cocoa powder; and soybeans. (109)

Molybdenum is a trace mineral that functions as a cofactor for a number of enzymes that catalyze important chemical transformations in the carbon, nitrogen, and sulfur cycles. Molybedenum:

- is an integral component of the enzyme sulfite oxidase, which is responsible for detoxifying sulfites. If you have ever reacted to sulfites, it may be because your molybdenum stores were insufficient to detoxify them.
- provides energy and vigor by aiding in carbohydrate and fat metabolism
- helps with alcohol detoxification and sulfur metabolism
- plays a role in the detoxification of cancer-causing chemicals
- helps prevent tooth decay

173

- promotes normal cell function
- activates the enzyme that produces uric acid, the substance that helps carry excess nitrogen out of the body when you urinate (110)

Food sources: beans, lentils, peas, grains, nuts, yeast, lentils, dark green leafy vegetables such as spinach, green cabbage, brown rice, red beans, liver and kidney (organ meats), eggs, and milk. (111)

Potassium was introduced in "Basic Priorities for Survival". Potassium is a very important component of cells and body fluids. Many people are deficient in potassium. Potassium:

- has various roles in metabolism and body functions and is essential for the proper function of all cells, tissues, and organs
- helps control heart rate and blood pressure by countering the effects of sodium
- is classified as an electrolyte, which means it can carry an electric charge in body fluids
- assists in the regulation of the acid/alkaline balance
- assists in protein synthesis from amino acids and in carbohydrate metabolism
- is necessary for the building of muscle and for normal body growth
- helps your nerves and muscles function properly (112)
- maintains normal blood pressure and helps regulate body fluids

Food sources: For a quick potassium pick-me-up try a 6 oz. glass of prune juice at 530 mg, orange juice at 345 mg, tomato juice at 400 mg, carrot juice at 345 mg, or a vegetable cocktail at 335mg, a banana at 467 mg; or a hand full of dried prunes, raisins, apricots, or dates with a few nuts and seeds. (112)

174

High Potassium Foods		Mg
Apricots, dried	10 halves	407
Artichoke hearts	1 cup	595
Avocados	3 oz.	540
Bananas	1 medium	467
Beets, cooked	1 cup	519
Beet Greens, cooked	1 cup	1,309
Black-eyed peas	1 cup	690
Broccoli	1 cup	505
Brussels Sprouts	1 cup	504
Cantaloupe	1 cup	495
Carrot juice	1 cup	689
Chicken	6 oz	440
Chick peas, cooked	1 cup	477
Cod	4 oz.	585
Collard greens, cooked	1 cup	494
Dates, dried	10	615
Figs, dried	4	542
Halibut	4 oz.	653
Jerusalem artichokes	1 cup	644
Kidney beans, cooked	1 cup	713
Lima beans, cooked	1 cup	955
Lentils, cooked	1 cup	731
Molasses	1 T	498
Orange juice	1 cup	496
Papaya	1 med	781
Parsnips	1 cup	573
Pinto beans, cooked	1 cup	800
Pork	6 oz	716
Potato, white, w/skin	1 med	1081
Prunes, dried	1 cup	828

Prune juice	1 cup	707
Pumpkin, cooked	1 cup	550
Raisins	1/2 cup	544
Salmon	4 oz.	425
Soybeans	1 cup	886
Spinach, cooked	1 cup	839
Sweet potatoes	1 cup	508
Swiss chard, cooked	1 cup	961
Tomatoes, cooked	1 cup	909
Tomato juice	1 cup	535
Trout	4 oz.	500
Tuna	4 oz.	645
Turkey	6 oz.	524
White beans, cooked	1 cup	1,189
Winter squash	1 cup	896
Yogurt, plain	1 cup	579

Medium Potassium Foods		
Almonds	2 oz.	412
Carrots, raw	1 cup	394
Celery, raw	1 cup	344
Green beans, cooked	1 cup	374
Kale, cooked	1 cup	296
Kiwifruit	1	252
Milk, nonfat	1 cup	376
Mustard greens, cooked	1 cup	283
Orange	1	237
Peanuts	2 oz.	374
Split peas	1/2 cup	355
Tomato, ripe raw	1 cup	400
Turnip greens, cooked	1 cup	292

Phosphorus is essential for many activities in the body. We don't hear much about phosphorus because deficiencies are rare. Phosphorus:

- is needed in combination with calcium, magnesium, vitamin D and trace minerals to form and maintain bones and teeth
- is required for the metabolization of fats and starches into energy
- is needed to build muscle tissue
- is a component of DNA and RNA
- helps maintain pH in body
- helps maintain regularity of the heartbeat
- aids in proper digestion of nutrients such as riboflavin and niacin.
- aids in transmission of nerve impulses
- is needed for cellular repair of burns and other wounds
- helps your kidneys effectively excrete wastes
- helps form the proteins that aid in reproduction
- is being studied for its role in blocking cancer
- is necessary for balancing hormones. (113)

Food sources: Phosphorus is found in almost all foods. Calcium and phosphorus are found naturally in dairy products.

**Note: People who eat a fast food diet and drink sodas may actually be getting too much phosphorus, which can cause an imbalance of other minerals in the body.

Selenium is an essential component of several major metabolic pathways, including thyroid hormone metabolism, antioxidant defense systems, and immune function. Selenium has been shown **to induce DNA repair and synthesis in damaged cells, to inhibit the proliferation of cancer cells, and to induce their apoptosis, the self-destruct sequence the body uses to eliminate worn out or abnormal cells.** (114)

Selenium plays a critical role in cancer prevention as a cofactor of glutathione peroxidase, which is particularly important for cancer protection. Glutathione peroxidase is one of the body's most powerful antioxidant enzymes and

176

is used in the liver to detoxify a wide range of potentially harmful molecules. When levels of glutathione peroxidase are too low, these toxic molecules are not disarmed and wreak havoc on any cells with which they come in contact, damaging their cellular DNA and promoting the development of cancer cells. (114) (115)

Selenim also works with vitamin E in numerous other vital antioxidant systems throughout the body. The powerful antioxidant actions are helpful in the prevention of heart disease and in decreasing the symptoms of asthma and the pain of inflammation in rheumatoid arthritis.

Food sources: Brazil nuts are the most concentrated source. Good sources are: mushrooms, cod, shrimp, tuna, halibut, salmon, sardines, scallops, turkey, eggs, beef, chicken, lamb, venison, garlic, mustard seeds, asparagus, barley, tofu, brown rice, oats, blackstrap molasses, broccoli, spinach, sesame seeds, and cheese. (114)

Silica may be even more important in the body than iron, though we don't hear much about it. It is necessary for many of the bodily functions and metabolic reactions.

- Silica is important in the development of the skeletal system. Without it, there are bone deformities.
- Silica restores balance between calcium and magnesium in the body.
- Silica is needed for the body to assimilate phosphorous. Phosphorous is important in building bones, repairing tissue and filtering waste.
- Silica does the job of depositing minerals into the bone and speeds healing, if there's a fracture. Silica in the diet relieves the pain of osteoporosis.
- Silica is one of the primary components of collagen, a fibrous protein that connects and supports other bodily tissues, such as skin, bone, tendons, muscles, cartilage, and also supports the internal organs. (116)

Good sources of silica are: Horesetail (eqisetum arvense), nettles, oat straw, alfalfa, and raw cacao. It is also found in asparagus, Brussels sprouts, cucumbers, beet root,

177

rhubarb, green beans, garbanzo beans, strawberries, mango, celery, leafy vegetables, apples, oranges, cherries, raisins, almonds, peanuts, raw cabbage, onions, endives, carrots, eggplants, pumpkin, celery, honey, corn, tomatoes, soybeans, and fish. (117)

Sodium has been discussed in "Priorities," as it is crucial to the existence of life.

Sulfur is usually considered to be the fourth most plentiful mineral in the body, and you cannot survive without it. (118) Sulfur is a sticky, smelly molecule, which acts like fly paper and all the bad things in the body stick onto it, including free radicals and toxins like mercury and other heavy metals.

Sulfur is needed:
- for the manufacture of many proteins, including those forming hair, muscles, and skin
- to make bile acids which aid in fat digestion and absorption
- as a constituent of bones, teeth, and collagen (the protein in connective tissue)
- as a component of insulin, which is needed to regulate blood sugar

Most of the body's sulfur is found in the sulfur-containing amino acids methionine, cystine, and cysteine. Vitamin B1, biotin, and pantothenic acid also contain small amounts of sulfur.

Most dietary sulfur is consumed in protein-rich foods such as: meat, poultry, organ meats, fish, eggs, beans, and dairy products. Egg yolks are one of the better sources of sulfur, followed by onions and garlic. Fesh, unprocessed vegetables like, cabbage, Brussels sprouts, cabbage, broccoli, cauliflower, and turnips are also sources of sulfur; grains and legumes as well as.

Vegetarians in particular may be deficient in sulfur, and should be encouraged to eat raw and slightly cooked vegetables. Sulfur works synergistically with vitamin C to build healthy cells. If supplementing sulfur, it is ideal to take it in combination with vitamin C and bioflavonoids. (118) (119)

Zinc plays a critical role in the immune system, liver, pancreas, and skin. Zinc:
- is key to proper T-cell and natural killer cell function and proper lymphocyte activity; it may be directly involved in antibody production to help you fight infection
- is involved in thousands of enzymatic reactions throughout the human body
- is a co-factor in many enzymes that regulate growth and development, sperm generation, digestion, and nucleic acid synthesis
- supports good prostate and reproductive health
- is very important for teenagers during sexual development
- may protect against the toxic effects of chemical exposures
- intensifies elimination of free radicals
- promotes central nervous system function (120)

The zinc /copper balance is important. They are usually balanced when eating unprocessed foods, but when using zinc supplements it may be necessary to add a small amount of copper, 1-2 mg daily. (121)

MIXED NUTRIENTS

	A	B	C	D	E	F	G
	FOOD	SERVING	MAGNESIUM	POTASSIUM	CALCIUM	OTHER SIGNIFICANT NUTRIENTS/VITAMINS	ORAC
2	Almonds, raw	1 oz.	76	200	75	Protein, E, monounsaturated fats	
3	Apricots, dried	1/2 cup	21	756	36	A, carotenoids	Med
4	Artichokes, globe	1 med.	50	343	25	Phytonutrients	High
5	Asparagus, cooked	1 cup	26	400	42	Folate, K, A, C, E, prebiotics, trace minerals, molybdenum	High
6	Avocado	1 med.	58	974	24	Folate, K, C, E, oleic acid, lutein	High
7	Banana	1 med.	32	467	6	B6, C, FOS, pectin	
8	Beef, lean cooked	6 oz.	32	393	27	Protein, zinc; (if grass-fed--Omega-3 and B vitamins)	
9	Beets, boiled	1 cup	39	519	N/A	Folate, anthycyanins, betacyanin	High
10	Black beans, cooked	1/2 cup	140	710	54	Protein, molybdenum, folate, prebiotics	Med
11	Blackstrap molasses	1 T.	44	512	177	Iron, copper, B-6	
12	Brazil nuts	1 oz.	107	187	45	Protein, selenium	
13	Broccoli, steamed	1 cup	39	505	62	Zeaxanthin, folate, A, C, lutein	High
14	Brown rice, cooked	1 cup	84	84	20	Selenium	
15	Brussels sprouts, steamed	1 cup	32	504	56	A, K, C, E, folate, phytonutrients	High
16	Buckwheat, cooked	1 cup	264	526	20	Flavonoids, zinc, copper	
17	Cabbage, boiled	1 cup	12	146	47	Sulforaphane & indoles, A, C, folate	Med
18	Carrots, raw	1 cup	18	394	46	A, carotenoids, K	Med
19	Cashews, raw	1 oz.	83	187	10	Protein, copper, tryptophan	
20	Cauliflower, steamed	1 cup	12	176	20	Phytonutrients, C, K, folate	Med
21	Celery, raw	1 cup	18	426	63	Folate	
22	Cherries	1 cup	15	306	18	Phytonutrients	High
23	Chia seeds	2 Tbsp.	78	140	143	Protein, Omega-3, lignins, iron, essential aminos	
24	Chicken, white meat	4 oz.	30	260	17	Protein	
25	Chickpeas, cooked	1/2 cup	96	582	98	Protein, selenium, prebiotics	
26	Chocolate, dark	1 oz (sq)	33	103	9	Polyphenols	High

180

MIXED NUTRIENTS

	A	B	C	D	E	F	G
27	Cocoa powder	1 T.	25	75	6	Polyphenols	High
28	Collard greens, steamed	1 cup	32	494	226	K, A, E folate, Omega-3, lutein, prebiotics	High
29	Corn, large ear, cooked	1 ear	31	257	5	8 amino acids, lutein, B-1, B-5, folate	Med
30	Dates, dried	1/4 cup	34	307	20	Selenium, copper, beta-carotene, lutein, zeaxanthin	Med
31	Eggplant, cooked, cubed	1 cup	11	122	6	Phytonutrients, copper, manganese, vitamin Bs	Med
32	Flaxseeds	2 Tbsp.	80	168	52	Protein, Omega-3, lignins, prebiotics	
33	Green beans, steamed	1 cup	31	374	58	Carotenoids, A, C, K, folate	
34	Green peas, steamed	1 cup	62	434	43	Lutein, zeaxanthin	Med
35	Halibut, baked/broiled	5 oz.	145	812	N/A	Protein, D, tryptophan, selenium, Omega-3	
36	Kale, steamed	1 cup	23	296	94	A, K, zeaxanthin, lutein, prebiotics	High
37	Kelp (sea vegetable)	1 oz.	174	3714	286	Iodine, amino acids, vitamins, trace minerals	
38	Kidney beans, cooked	1/2 cup	90	806	56	Protein, molybdenum, tryptophan, folate, prebiotics	Med
39	Kiwifruit	1 each	12	215	23	C, folate, E, lutein	High
40	Lima beans, cooked	1 cup	81	955	32	Protein, molybdenum, tryptophan, folate	
41	Milk, cow's, whole	1 cup	24	322	276	Protein, iodine, tryptophan, D, Bs	
42	Oatmeal, cooked	1 cup	138	362	52	Protein, Omega-3, tryptophan, K, B-1, prebiotics	
43	Pinto beans, cooked	1/2 cup	100	872	92	Protein, molybdenum, tryptophan, folate	Med
44	Potato, white w/skin	1 med.	48	1,081	26	C, copper, B6, manganese, kukoamines	High
45	Prunes, dried	1/2 cup	64	1058	72	Carotenoids, , phytonutrients, copper	High
46	Pumpkin seeds, raw	1 oz.	156	223	15	Protein, tryptophan, zinc, iron, selenium	
47	Pumpkin, cooked	1 cup	22	564	37	A, E, carotenoids, phytonutrients	Med
48	Quinoa, cooked	1/2 cup	68	180	20	E, riboflavin, zinc, iron, copper	Med
49	Raisins	3 oz.	28	644	44	Phenols, boron,	High
50	Raspberries	1 cup	27	186	31	Phytonutrients vitamins A, C, prebiotics	High
51	Salmon, baked/broiled	4 oz.	138	425	17	Protein, Omega-3	Med
52	Sesame seeds	1 Tbsp.	32	42	88	Protein, selenium	

181

MIXED NUTRIENTS

	A	B	C	D	E	F	G
53	Shrimp, steamed/boiled	4 oz.	29	119	54	Protein, selenium	
54	Soybeans, cooked	1 cup	148	885	175	Protein, molybedenum, tryptophan, Omega-3	
55	Spinach, steamed	1 cup	157	839	245	A, K, C, E folate, zeaxanthin, prebiotics	High
56	Strawberries	1 cup	19	220	23	C, iodine, phytonutrients, folate, prebiotics	High
57	Summer squash, yellow	1 cup	43	345	27	C, A, K, folate, copper	High
58	Sunflower seeds, raw	1/4 cup	74	482	40	B-1, E, folate, selenium, copper, fatty acids	
59	Sweet potatoes, cooked	1 med.	31	542	43	A, C, E niacin, B6, carotenoids	Med
60	Swiss chard, steamed	1 cup	151	961	102	A, K, C, phytonutrients	High
61	Tofu, raw	1/2 cup	68	N/S	200	Protein, tryptophan, iron, Omega-3	
62	Tomato, ripe	1 cup	20	400	12	Lycopene, C, A, K, molybdenum, folate, prebiotics	Med
63	Tuna, yellowfin	4 oz.	73	645	14	Protein, tryptophan, selenium, Bs	
64	Watermelon, diced	1 cup	15	176	15	Carotenoids, lycopene, C, A, B-6	
65	Wheat flour	1 cup	166	486	41	Protein, folate, selenium	
66	Yogurt, low fat	1 cup	40	573	447	Protein, iodine, Bs, tryptophan	

Phytonutrients/Phytochemicals

These terms are often used interchangeably to indicate biologically active substances in plants.

Antioxidants are natural compounds that protect the body from free radicals.

The antioxidant level in foods and drinks is calculated through a test tube test measuring the oxygen radical absorptive capacity (ORAC). It specifically measures both the degree to which a sample inhibits the action of an oxidizing agent and how long it takes to do so.

Researchers can't agree on the amount of antioxidants we need per day, but I'm observing that it seems to be a minimum of 5,000 ORAC units per day and up to 10,000 needed for good health. (122)

Antioxidants include:
- 4 enzymes which the body makes:
  - Superoxide dismutase (SOD)
  - Methionine reductase
  - Catalase
  - Glutathinone peroxidase (123)
- Carotenoids
- Flavonoids including bioflavonoids
- Vitamins A, C, E
- Coenzyme Q-10 (CoQ-10)
- Alpha-lipoic acid (ALA)
- Minerals – selenium and zinc
- Hormone – melatonin (124)

Specific antioxidants found in plants include:

Alpha lipoic acid	Iodide
Apigenin	Lutein
Anthocyanins	Luteolin
Astaxanthin	Lycopene
Catechin	Proanthocyanis
Ellegic acid	Pterostilbene
Epigallocatechn	Quercetin
Hesperitin	Resveratrol
	Zeaxanthin
	(124) (125)

Alpha-Lipoic Acid (ALA) is a vitamin-like compound which the body produces in small quantities. ALA is considered a **universal antioxidant because it dissolves in both water and fat.**

- ALA is able to scavenge more wayward free radical cells than most antioxidants, the majority of which tend to dissolve in either fat or water, but not both.
- It assists the B vitamins in producing energy from the proteins, carbohydrates, and fats absorbed from digested food.
- It shields the liver from potentially harmful cell changes and assists it in flushing toxins from the body. (ALA is administered in hospitals in intravenous form to treat cases of acute mushroom poisoning and for other cases of acute poisoning that affect the liver.)
- ALA has been used for decades in Europe to counter nerve damage in diabetics known as neuropathy.
- It is being studied as a supplement to improve long-term memory.
- It increases the blood flow to the nerves and improved transmission of nerve impulses.
- It increases the potency of vitamins C and E, both nutrients that protect the lens of the eye from harmful ultraviolet light. (126)

Food sources: potatoes, spinach, broccoli, other green leafy greens, organ meats, red meats, brewer's yeast, tomatoes, and Brussels sprouts. (126)

Flavonoids/Bioflavonoids There are approximately 4,000 different flavonoids, but only a portion of the known flavonoids are considered bioflavonoids. Bioflavonoids are not produced by the body; they must be ingested. They work with other antioxidants to protect the body, but their unique role is protecting vitamin C from oxidation in the body, which allows the body to reap more benefits from vitamin C. (127)

Food sources of bioflavonoids include:

apples	mangos
apricots	onions
black beans	papayas
blueberries	parsley
broccoli	pears
Brussels sprouts	raspberries
cabbage	red peppers
citrus fruits	spinach
garlic	strawberries
green tea	tomatoes (127)

Herbal sources of bioflavonoids include:

- the inner skin of citrus fruits
- buckwheat greens or sprouts are an exceptional source of bioflavonoids; grow them at home like alfalfa sprouts
- the leaves of yellow dock (Rumex crispus) or any knotweed
- the flowers and berries of the elder bush
- hawthorn berries, flowers, and leaves
- rose hips or rose blossoms
- shepherd's purse aerial parts, which are wonderful in salads
- sea buckthorn leaves and berries, rich in many nutrients needed by post-menopausal women including: bioflavonoids, carotenes (vitamin A), vitamin C, vitamin E, and the B vitamin complex, especially B6
- toadflax flowers, which can be added to salads
- white dead nettle (Lamium album), which doesn't sting, so try it in salads, or dry bunches when it's flowering and get your bioflavonoids from the infusion or make a vinegar (128)

Coenzyme Q-10 (CoQ-10) is an oil-soluble, vitamin-like substance necessary for many bodily processes. It appears the body can synthesize coenzyme Q-10, but with all the demands on the body systems by our toxic world we may need to supplement. For over twenty years many of us have been ingesting the ubiquinone form of CoQ-10 thinking it was beneficial to the heart, kidneys and other organs.

Little did we know that for ubiquinone to be properly utilized, must first be reduced in our bodies to its active metabolite, known as ubiquinol. The uibquinol form of CoQ-10 not only absorbs up to eight times better but also has demonstrated unprecedented anti-aging effects compared to the coenzyme Q-10 (ubiquinone) which most of us have been using. The ubiquinol form is now available in supplements. (129)

Coenzyme Q-10 (Ubiquinol form):
- is a crucial component of the process in mitochondria which converts the energy in carbohydrates and fatty acids into ATP to drive the cellular machinery of the body
- is crucial in promoting heart health, preventing or reversing signs of cardiovascular disease
- acts as an antioxidant, which may cut the risks of cancer and autoimmune syndromes
- is needed for healthy gums
- may be a factor in lowering blood sugar
- may protect against many age-related disorders, including diabetes and various neurological disorders
- plays a critical role in maintaining our supply of vitamin E. When vitamin E gets "used up" in the performance of its duty as an antioxidant protector of our cell membranes, coenzyme Q-10 can "recharge" it, and restore its antioxidant capability. (130)

CoQ-10 levels decline with age, so supplementing might help increase longevity and quality of life. Some drugs given to lower cholesterol have been found to cause a deficiency of coenzyme Q-10. (131)

Food sources: There has been little research to study food sources of coenzyme Q-10; however, we do know it is available in organ meats such as liver, heart and kidney organ meats, wild-caught fish, grass-fed beef, wild game such as bison and venison and pastured poultry. Plant based sources include nuts, seeds and cruciferous veggies providing small amounts. (131)

**Glutathione <u>is not only the master antioxidant but is
also a major factor in detoxification.</u>** Glutathione binds
to toxins such as heavy metals, solvents, and pesticides
and transforms them into a form that can be excreted in
urine or bile. (132)

Glutathione is primarily manufactured in your body
from a combination of amino acids: cysteine, glutamine,
and glycine. Of these, cysteine most determines how
much you can produce. Cysteine is found in several
protein food sources, especially organic whole grains and
beans; pastured eggs, grass-fed meat and whey. (133)

Some believe the secret of glutathione's power is the sulfur
(SH) chemical groups it contains. **Sulfur-rich foods.** (132)

Nutrients needed for glutathione to do its job effectively
are lipoic acid, selenium, zinc, and B vitamins. Foods that
are good glutathione precursors include:

asparagus	spinach
avocados	squash
Brazil nuts	strawberries
grapefruit	tomatoes
okra	turmeric
potatoes	walnuts (134)

The herb milk thistle is an excellent source of the
antioxidant compound silymarin, which may help to
prevent glutathione depletion in the liver. Glutathione is
crucial in the liver for detoxification and can become
depleted from some drugs, alcohol consumption, and
general toxic overload. (135)
Factors which will reduce or deplete glutathione levels in
your body include smoking, alcohol, caffeine, strenuous
exercise, food additives, prescription and over-the-counter
drugs, ultraviolet radiation, and air pollution. (136)

**Note: Glutathione from supplements doesn't seem to be
as effective as from food sources.

Melatonin is a hormone produced in the body by the
pineal gland and in the gastrointestinal tract.

187

- This hormone plays a key role in synchronizing circadian rhythms and helps regulate the sleep-wake cycle in mammals. Darkness stimulates the release of melatonin, and light suppresses its activity.
- Melatonin is a potent antioxidant that protects the body from free-radical damage.
- Melatonin is also one of the hormones that controls the timing and release of female reproductive hormones.

Food sources: oats, rice, dairy products, tomatoes, grape skins, tart cherries, walnuts, olive oil, wine and even beer. (137)

Quercetin is considered one of the most active flavonoids in the plant kingdom. Many medicinal plants owe much of their activity to high quercetin content.
- It is a potent antioxidant which fights free radicals in the body.
- Quercetin inhibits the growth of cancer cells and shows remarkable anti-tumor properties in a wide range of cancers.
- It functions with other bioflavonoids in enhancing the collagen network.
- Quercetin is known for its antiviral activity.
- As an antihistamine it prevents immune cells from releasing histamines, which may help with allergies and other respiratory ailments.
- It may protect against the damage of the "bad" cholesterol.
- It has anti-inflammatory properties and has specifically been found to reduce inflammation of the prostate.
- Quercetin may also help reduce symptoms like fatigue, depression, and anxiety. (138)

Food sources: apples, onions, parsley, sage, citrus fruits, buckwheat, red grapes, red wine, green and black teas, broccoli, leafy greens, cherries, dark berries, beans, and olive oil. (139)

Lutein and **Zeaxanthin** are carotenoids with antioxidant properties which are usually found together in plants. Lutein and zeaxanthin reduce the risk of age-related

188

macular degeneration (AMD) which is caused by steady damage of the retina. These two nutrients are selectively absorbed into the macula in the eyes where they are thought to help prevent retinal detachment and offer protection against "age related macular degeneration disease" (ARMD) in the elderly.

Several years ago I had the beginning of macular degeneration and cataracts. Every day I ate dark berries, included several carotnoid vegetables and fruits as well as taking a lutein/zeathanthin supplement or having calendula petals on my salad. At my next visit the doctor was amazed that there was no longer any sign of degeneration in my eyes. I was delighted!

The pair of nutrients have also been linked with reducing the risk for artery diseases and known to protect against the damaging effects of UV-B radiation. (140) (141)

Food sources for lutein and zeaxanthin include: egg yolks, kale, leafy greens including: romaine lettuce, dandelion, lamb's quarters, arugula, basil, parsley, oregano, thyme,broccoli, Brussels sprouts, zucchini, corn, garden peas, orange peppers, orange squash, oranges, tangerines, red grapes, persimmons, and kiwi fruit. The flower petals of calendula and the Tagetes species of marigold flowers are good sources of lutein and zeaxanthin. (141)

Astaxanthin is a red carotenoid pigment. It is a powerful antioxidant which improves the immune system and protects the eyes from sun radiation. Astaxanthan is found in shellfish, krill oil, red fleshed fish, and red pigmented fruits and vegetables. (142)

Canthaxanthin is a carotenoid with yellow pigments. It is a potent free radical scavenger, and possibly nature's most powerful lipid-soluble antioxidant. It is found abundantly in paprika, green algae, and crustaceans. (143)

Catechins are water-soluble flavonoid phytochemical compounds found principally in green and white tea (Camellia sinensis). Smaller amounts are contained in grapes, black tea, chocolate, and wine. Considered potent antioxidants, catechins are being studied for their potential to prevent heart disease and cancer. (144)

Ellagic acid is a powerful antioxidant which decreases mutations and inhibits damage to the cells' DNA from carcinogens. It also prevents the formation of cancer-causing substances called nitrosamines in the body. It slows tumor growth by blocking the production of enzymes used in cancer cells, inhibits lung and skin tumors, and is considered a vital nutrient in the fight against smoking-related lung cancer. Food sources: blackberries, raspberries, strawberries, pomegranates, cranberries, citrus fruits, apples, grapes, tomatoes, carrots, and nuts, especially walnuts. (145) (146)

Lycopene is a member of the carotenoid family of phytochemicals and is the natural pigment responsible for the deep red color of several fruits, most notably tomatoes.

Scientists have amassed a significant body of research that supports the role of lycopene in human health, specifically in the prevention of cancers of the prostate, pancreas, stomach, breast, cervix and lung, as well as in the prevention of cardiovascular disease, cataracts, and age-related macular degeneration. (147)

Lycopene is a more effective antioxidant than other carotenoids, including beta-carotene. It is especially effective at quenching a free radical called *singlet oxygen*. *Singlet oxygen* is a highly reactive free radical formed during normal metabolic processes that reacts with polyunsaturated fatty acids, which are major constituents of cell membranes. (148)

Due to the fact that lycopene is commonly located in cell membranes, it plays an important role in preventing oxidative damage to the membrane lipids, thereby influencing the thickness, strength, and fluidity of the membranes. Cell membranes are the gatekeepers of the cell, allowing nutrients in while preventing toxins from entering and facilitating the removal of cellular garbage. Maintaining the integrity of cell membranes is therefore a key factor in the prevention of disease. (147)

In addition to its antioxidant activity, lycopene has been shown to suppress the growth of tumors *in vitro* (test tube) and *in vivo* (animal) experiments. One of the ways that lycopene may limit tumor growth is by stimulating cell to cell communication. Researchers now believe that poor communication between cells is one of the causes of the abnormal growth of cells, a condition which ultimately leads to the development of cancerous tumors. (149)

According to a new study conducted by Harvard Medical School researchers in Boston, lycopene has been shown to significantly reduce a woman's risk of heart disease. (150)

Lycopene is believed to play a role in the prevention of heart disease by inhibiting free radical damage to LDL cholesterol. Before cholesterol can be deposited in the plaques that harden and narrow arteries, it must be oxidized by free radicals. With its powerful antioxidant activity, lycopene can prevent LDL cholesterol from being oxidized. (150)

Recent research has suggested that lycopene can boost sperm concentrations in infertile men. In one study, a lycopene-supplemented diet resulted in a statistically significant improvement in sperm concentration and motility amongst the 30 infertile men being studied with six pregnancies following as a result of the trial. (151)

Lycopene is abundant in a variety of foods. 100 grams of fresh tomatoes can contain between .88-4.20 mg of lycopene, while cooked tomatoes, especially when they are concentrated as they are in tomato paste, are an even better source, providing 5.40-150 mg of lycopene per 100 grams of sauce. Adding a bit of olive oil, which contains a good fat, to the tomato paste increases the absorption significantly. Not surprisingly 100 grams of sun-dried tomato in oil provides 46.5 mg of lycopene. (150)

Food sources of lycopene: ripe tomatoes and cooked tomato products, guava, apricots, watermelon, papaya, pink grapefruit, red sweet peppers, red cabbage, mangos, carrots, and cooked asparagus. (152)

Sulforaphane belongs to a group of phytochemicals known as the **isothiocyanates.** Sulforaphane prevents certain enzymes from activating cancer-causing agents in the body and increases the body's production of other enzymes that clean carcinogens out of the system before they can damage cells. Sulforaphane is produced in cruciferous vegetable plants only when two enzymes in separate "sacs" react, myrosinase and glucoraphanin. (153)

di-indolyl-methane (DIM), a lipid soluble metabolite of indole, has immune modulator, anti-bacterial and anti-viral properties. DIM has currently been found useful in the treatment of recurring respiratory papillomatosis caused by the Human Papilloma Virus (HPV) and prevention and treatment of breast and prostate cancer.

Food sources of DIM Sulforaphane and Indole-3-carbinol (I3C): Cruciferous vegetables such as broccoli, cabbage, cauliflower, Brussels sprouts, and kolrabi. (154)

Pterostilbene, a compound found in blueberries, has cancer-preventive properties. It has been shown to inhibit colon and liver cancer. (155)

Plant sterols (phytosterols) are compounds found in plants, have a chemical structure very similar to cholesterol, and when present in the diet in sufficient amounts, are believed to reduce blood levels of cholesterol, enhance the immune response, and decrease risk of certain cancers. They have been found to mitigate allergic reactions, fight cancer, and reduce symptoms of autoimmune disorders. (156)

As part of our immune system, cells called B lymphocytes produce antibodies that deactivate incoming invaders such as bacteria. If the invader is able to get inside our cells, as a virus does, then T-cells take over the fight. Sterols modulate the functions of T-cells by enhancing their cellular division and secretion of lymphokines. (156)

There are at least 250 different plant sterols in natural plants. Plant sterols were highly prevalent in early human diets that were heavily plant-based. Today our diets are often lacking plant sterols.

Beta-sitosterol is one of these remarkable plant nutrients which scientific studies are proving to be a major, safe and non-toxic nutrient for the maintenance of health and for protection against many serious health disorders and diseases. **Beta-sitosterol is among the most effective treatments for prostate enlargement known.** It has a faster onset of action and none of the adverse side effects which are associated with conventional medicines, and it is also less expensive. A 2008 laboratory study published in *Molecular Nutrition and Food Research* found that using beta-sitosterol in combination with the breast cancer drug tamoxifen may enhance the drug's effectiveness. (157)

Isoflavones are a class of phytoestrogens—plant-derived compounds with estrogenic activity. Soybeans and soy products are the richest sources of isoflavones.

Lignans: A lignin is a type of polyphenolic compound, one of four classes of phytoestrogens occurring naturally in some plants. Plant sources particularly rich in lignan phytochemcials (in order of highest to lowest concentration) are flax, sesame, sunflower, and pumpkin seeds. Some lignan compounds are also found in many vegetables, fruits, and botanical-derived beverages such as tea and wine. (158)

One specific lignan compound, secoisolariciresinol diglycoside (SDG), is a precursor to a variety of phytoestrogens with antioxidant properties.

- Some lignan compounds are readily assimilated by the body since they are metabolized by intestinal flora during digestion. These lignans are known as enterolignans and specifically include enterolactone and enterodiol. They are also referred to as the mammalian lignans.
- Pinoresinol is the primary phenol found in extra virgin olive oil. It has been studied for its potential ability to help prevent colon cancer.

- Sesame oil contains several lignans, most notably sesamin, and is being studied for its anti-inflammatory properties. Although much remains to be investigated, evidence indicates that dietary phytoestrogens exert positive, protective effects in humans. (159)

Enzymes are energized protein molecules found in all living cells. They catalyze and regulate all biochemical reactions that occur within the human body. They act as the spark plugs for the vast majority of chemical reactions that make life possible. <u>Over 2,500 different kinds of enzymes are found in living things</u>. (160)

- Enzymes are delicate substances found in <u>all living cells</u> whether animal or vegetable.
- Eating large amounts of processed foods depletes our enzyme bank.
- Enzymes are energized protein molecules which act as catalysts accelerating and precipitating hundreds of thousands of biochemical reactions in the body that control all the life processes.
- Each enzyme has a particular function in the body that no other enzyme can do.
- Enzymes are essential for:
  o digesting food
  o stimulating the brain
  o providing energy to the cells
  o repairing all tissue (161)

There are three groups of enzymes: metabolic. digestive, and food enzymes.

Metabolic enzymes are protein-like substances that act as catalysts in all metabolic actions within your body. In other words, metabolic enzymes are the workers within your body that allow the minerals, vitamins, and proteins to do their job. Metabolic enzymes are your body's labor force, and they are responsible for all the anabolic or catabolic activity in your body. Metabolic enzymes are responsible for repair, formation, and function of each cell within each and every tissue of the body. (162)

194

Over the course of time, these enzymes "wear out" and require replenishing by the body. The storehouse of metabolic enzymes can be exhausted by eating processed, enzyme-deficient foods. The body will use precious metabolic enzymes to digest food rather than for supporting functions in the organs like the liver, spleen and pancreas. Disease is the result. (161)

Digestive enzymes are necessary for the proper breakdown of foods and the proper absorption of the nutrients.

Human digestive enzymes include:
-- Amylase, which breaks down carbohydrates starting with the saliva in the mouth
-- Protease, which helps to digest protein
-- Lactase, which breaks down milk sugar
-- Surcease, which breaks down cane and beet sugar
-- Maltase, which breaks down malt sugar
-- Lipase, which aids in digestion of fats
-- Hydrochloric acid, which is not really an enzyme but is necessary in the interaction of the digestive juices, especially for the digestion of proteins. Elderly people often do not produce enough hydrochloric acid to properly digest food, and taking antacids complicates the problem. (161)

Food enzymes
Each raw food contains the enzymes needed for its digestion. Bananas contain high amounts of amylase because they are a high carbohydrate food which needs amylase to be digested; whereas avocados, which are high in fat content, contain high amounts of lipase, which digests fat. (162)

When we cook (above 118 degrees) or process raw foods they lose most of their enzymes and require the body to provide enzymes for their digestion. So, let's examine an apple. Eaten raw, it has the enzymes needed to digest it. However, when you cook it as in making apple pie or applesauce it now needs to steal enzymes needed for other bodily functions to digest the cooked apple. (161)

To quote the late Dr. Edward Howell, a physician who pioneered enzyme research, "When we eat cooked, enzyme-free food, the body is forced to produce enzymes needed for digestion. This stealing of enzymes from other parts of the body sets up a competition for enzymes among the various organ systems and tissues of the body. The resulting metabolic dislocations may be the direct cause of cancer, coronary heart disease, diabetes and many chronic incurable diseases." (162)

When we eat foods that are deficient in enzymes, the body increases numbers of white blood cells as a defense mechanism. Enzymes are then released from these white blood cells to digest toxins. A diet of enzyme-dead foods causes the white blood cell count to be continually elevated, which causes the immune system to become compromised. The enzymes that are normally held in storage to fight infection are instead drawn out of storage to digest food. This is another example of how interconnected all the body systems are. (160)

Unless you eat a mostly raw foods diet, most health practitioners would recommend taking a combination digestive enzyme supplement.

Caution: Some authorities warn that people taking blood thinners and pregnant women should not take supplements with pancreatin, an animal-derived enzyme found in many supplements, without consulting a physician. (163)

Probiotics and Prebiotics

Probiotics are products containing cultured beneficial bacteria used to replant the digestive tract. There are many brands and combinations, but the most common include lactobacillus, acidophilus, and bifidobacterium. Most people have a compromised immune system, which indicates the digestive system needs serious rebuilding. We have already been introduced to the very fragile ecosystem that exists within the human digestive tract. More than 100 trillion bacteria inhabit the small and large intestines. These organisms play a crucial role in maintaining overall health. In a healthy individual the beneficial bacteria keep the harmful bacteria in balance, aid digestion, and support immune function. <u>This healthy "gut flora" produces valuable nutrients including certain B vitamins, vitamin K, digestive enzymes like lactase, and immune chemicals that fight harmful bacteria and even cancer cells</u>. (164)

The balance of good bacteria is very easily disturbed by factors such as the use of antibiotics, poor nutrition, emotional stress, surgery, hormone supplements, parasitic infestation, infections, and synthetic drugs such as prednisone, cortisone, and chemotherapy drugs. When the level of your good bacteria drops too low, it opens the door for harmful bacteria such as candida albicans to proliferate, creating an environment for diseases to develop. (164)

Prebiotic foods: It may be easy to repopulate the gut using probiotic supplements, but the new flora needs to be fed by prebiotic foods to thrive. These beneficial organisms thrive on fiber and FOS (fructooligosaccharide) sugars found in complex carbohydrates such as legumes, vegetables, fruits, and whole grains. The best sources are bananas, buckwheat, barley, onions, garlic, soy, tomatoes and Jerusalem artichokes. Cultured products like natural unsweetened yogurt and kefir with live cultures; the lignans found in flaxseed, carrots, spinach, cauliflower, broccoli, millet, buckwheat, and green tea; and fermented foods such as sauerkraut all help good bacteria to proliferate. For more on fermented vegetables see Donna Gates' website www.bodyecology.com or read <u>Nourishing Traditions</u> by Sally Fallon.

Our digestive tracts often do not have the right balance of good bacteria due to drugs we take, processed foods, and the chemicals in our lives. Since most of us probably don't eat much fermented food, we may need to supplement with probiotics to maintain a healthy digestive system.

Low stomach acid, called hypochlorhydria, can cause vitamins and minerals, whether from food or supplements, to pass through the system without being properly absorbed. Older people would do well to supplement with Betaine hydrochloride or herbals bitters or a combination digestive enzyme formula. (164)

5. Plants are the Basis of Our Existence

Our bodies are genetically designed to be compatible with the healing substances as found in nature. All foods in their natural form provide nutrients and co-factors that support growth and healing. Nutrients such as proteins, carbohydrates, fats, vitamins, minerals, plant sterols, and phytochemicals provided by food are necessary for growth and the maintenance of life. It is the **synergy** of all the components in a plant that nourishes the body with what it needs. (166)

The **chlorophyll** in green leaves forms the basis of all life on earth. Without this amazing substance, life as we know it, would not exist. Chlorophyll, the green pigment, is the 'green blood' of plants which supplies nutrients to plant cells. It is the chlorophyll molecules of plants that trap the sun's energy, and when we eat green plants this solar energy becomes our energy. (166)

Nutrients in plants are diminished when the food is grown on poor soil or soil that has been chemically treated with synthetic herbicides, pesticides, and fertilizers. Nutrients are lost when food is processed and/or has non-food additives. **Inorganic compounds** are metabolic disrupters of vital nervous, endocrine and immune functions. Even the quality of meat depends on the quality of the food the animal ate and the conditions in which it lived. (167)

Herbs – the Miracle of Nature

Herbs are basic to the human food chain. The use of herbs as medicine goes back to the beginning of man. The historian Diodorus Seculas tells of a belief held by the Jewish faith that when Adam and Eve were driven out of the Garden of Eden, they were instructed by the Creator in the use of herbal remedies and the art of healing. There is evidence that the Egyptians used a high degree of herbal healing. An ancient papyrus describes how herbs were used to heal diseases. (168) When I visited the ancient buildings in Egypt, I have personally seen pictures of herbs carved on the walls from the Early Kingdoms.

199

Greece was the home of Hippocrates, the "Father of Medicine," who used herbs to heal the sick. The story of the use of herbs moves on through the centuries, and the use of herbs is still common practice today in many cultures. Unfortunately, the advent of scientifically created medicines saw the demise of herbal medicine in the early 1900s in the United States. Herbalism was barely kept alive by a few scattered people using it only within their own families or communities.

All naturally living plants are balanced sources of energy. Kitty Campion in Holistic Woman's Herbal says "Herbs are little powerhouses of naturally occurring chemical substances. The advantage of using herbs over man-made chemicals is that nature packages her chemicals in such well balanced and minute amounts that their safe assimilation by the body is assured." She goes on to say, "I believe that plants are not simply the safest way to give medicine but are also the most effective not just because they can be easily assimilated (the green blood of the plant, its chlorophyll, is very similar in its molecular structure to the hemoglobin in our own blood), but because they are capable of working synergistically." (169)

Donnie Yance, a clinical master herbalist who lives and works in Oregon, follows the vitalistic tradition. He explains that both foods and herbs can produce more than one effect in the body including working on the deepest level. He says, "What's very interesting now, with the explosion of science and to the field of herbal medicine, is that we're learning that plants transfer information genetically to our genes that do nothing but add benefit to our health in a genetic level." (170)

It is this synergy that makes herbal combinations so powerful in treating illness, cleansing, and restoring the body. When certain herbs are mixed together the results are much greater than just the sum of the herb's properties. For example, adding cayenne to herbal combinations increases the power of the other herbs and acts as a catalyst carrying the herbs to where they are needed in the body. (171)

It is the use of the whole herb, root, berry, or bark where we get the balance of constituents for use in humans as well as animals. When we fragment herbs, concentrating their chemical constituents, we will surely run amuck. As we are fragmenting herbs, taking only one or two constituents and selling them for a particular purpose, we have lost nature's synergy and don't receive the total benefit of the herb.

Today, there are many herbal products on the market that use only one or two chemical constituents from an herb and advertise it as though it is better than the whole herbal product that nature made. In my opinion, this is treating the herbal factors like drugs. It may work as a drug would to abate symptoms, but will it have all the factors necessary to help the body heal itself?

I think Greg Tilford, in the introduction to his book, <u>Edible and Medicinal Plants of the West,</u> summarizes so well our need to eat green plants. He says, "When we view our universe at the most rudimentary level, we see that all things are composed of energy, and for something to be alive, its collective energy must be continually fed and replenished. Plants provide a critical, life-giving link between what is alive and what is not. Without plants, sunlight could not be transformed into usable energy, and life as we know it could not exist. Through the process of photosynthesis, plants take energy from the sun and convert it into chlorophyll, the basis of assimilable energy that allows the perpetuation and continuance of the food chain. Plants also supply our planet with oxygen, and according to their specific molecular structures, they provide all life with the specialized energetic actions we refer to as medicines. Animals are the oldest herbalists on earth." (172)

I don't think we can improve on Nature.

Why do we need herbs?
1. to prevent disease- herbs are full of nutrients

2. to prevent and fight infectious disease
3. to deal with antibiotic-resistant microbes
4. to prevent and deal with chronic disease
5. to alleviate everyday discomforts

Know your herbs before using! I would never use an unfamiliar herb or wild plant without checking several very reliable sources. If you are interested in using herbs, I recommend that you purchase a good medicinal herbal book or two by reliable herbalists. Some of my favorite herb books are listed at the end of this section.

- Many herbs can be used as foods and remedies.
- Some herbs lend themselves mostly to being used as remedies.
- Some herbs should only be used under the guidance of an experienced herbalist or health practitioner.
- Develop respect for the power of herbs.

Precautions: Always check before using herbs for interactions with any drugs or nutritional supplements you are taking.

- Some herbs are poisonous--avoid them.
- Herbs and drugs don't mix well--always check with your pharmacist or practitioner for interactions.
- Use a reputable guide in dosing yourself.
- Women who are pregnant should not take herbs medicinally unless working with a knowledgeable practitioner.
- Dosage of herbs for infants, children, and the elderly needs to be adjusted.
- Some herbs cause reactions. For example, licorice may raise the blood pressure in some people.

We need to be aware of the side effects of herbs so you may want to become familiar with this website when using herbs. See "List of herbs with known adverse effects" https://en.wikipedia.org/wiki/List_of_herbs_with_known_adverse_effects

Consult your doctor to determine which herbs and nutritional supplements you need to stop before surgery or major dental work.

Herbs and supplements can interact with anesthetics or thin the blood causing excessive bleeding. Most research suggests if you are going to have surgery or major dental work you should stop taking herbs and some supplements a week prior to the treatment.

A few examples are:
1. Echinacea may interfere with some drugs and may impair wound healing.
2. Garlic thins the blood and reduces blood pressure so may cause excessive bleeding.
3. Ginkgo biloba regulates blood flow so may cause excessive bleeding.
4. Ginseng stimulates the system so may cause rapid heartbeat, high blood pressure, excessive bleeding, or low blood sugar.
5. Kava calms the nerves so it may intensify the sedative effects of anesthesia.
6. St. John's Wort may increase or decrease the strength of certain drugs. (173)

The common herb chamomile has anticoagulant compounds called coumarins which thin the blood. If chamomile is used with platelet inhibitors, drugs like Ticlopidine (Ticlid®), Clopidogrel (Plavix®) or Warfarin (Coumadin®), an anticoagulant, or a common aspirin may result in increased risk of bleeding. Chamomile may also increase the blood concentrations of the following drugs causing toxicity: tricyclic antidepressants, Clozapine, Propranolol, Theophylline, and Tacrine. (174)

MORE PRECAUTIONS WHEN USING HERBS

Herbs are not necessarily exotic. They may already be in your cupboard or yard. You'll find herbs are mixed with foods throughout this book.

1. Today it seems fashionable to add herbs to products, BUT WATCH OUT FOR INTERACTIONS.

It is popular for manufacturers to add energizing herbs to the new energy drinks. We have no idea what the long term effects of the combination of ingredients in drinks will be. There is concern about the reaction in the body of the combination of ingredients coupled with caffeine and lots of sugar. There is already a warning not to combine these drinks with alcohol, which has become popular, because people may not feel impaired, but their blood alcohol concentration is still high. This often prompts people to consume larger amounts of alcohol. (175)

2. Understand that no doctor or practitioner knows everything. <u>You need to evaluate the information they give you</u>. Find a second source or opinion.

Become acquainted with herbalists in your area. Finding an herbalist in your area can be tricky, as many are very private about their knowledge. Herbalists are of many types. Some are self-taught, while others may have training in various philosophies. Some concentrate on raising herbs for their own use while others have offices and may recommend and sell commercially prepared herbs. I find they all have much to teach me. They all tend to see the body holistically, knowing that one thing out of balance affects the rest of the body. Herbs are used for their nutritive value and/or as medicine to cleanse and support organs or body systems.

Disclaimer: I am not a medical doctor. The information given is for general educational purposes to provide information on options so you can make good choices.

Learning about herbal remedies DOES NOT REPLACE knowing when to use conventional medicine.

Herbalists know that herbs are food and medicine in a tidy package. Many herbs are sources of important nutrients as well as having medicinal properties. The list below explains some of the medicinal qualities of herbs. Remember, many herbs are foods as well as medicines, depending on how they are used.

Medicinal Properties of Herbs: Below are a few of the common properties of many herbs. To discover the many other properties of herbs see at http://natural-cures-remedies.com/herbs.html

- Alterative - restores proper body function by improving blood composition
- Analgesic - taken or used to relieve pain
- Anthelmintic - helps destroy or expel intestinal worms and parasites
- Antibiotic (anti-bacterial) - kills and/or slows the growth of harmful microorganisms
- Antiemetic – relieves nausea and upset stomach, and helps prevent vomiting.
- Anti-inflammatory – helps reduce inflammation
- Antioxidant – helps increase the uptake of tissue oxygen
- Aphrodisiac – helps impotency problems and strengthens sexual desire and vitality
- Carminative – helps stimulate the digestive system
- Diaphoretic – induces capillary activity and sweating, thus releasing toxins through perspiration
- Demulcent – soothing, coating, mucilaginous herbs
- Diuretic - helps to stimulate kidney and bladder activity, increase flow and elimination of urine
- Emmenagogue - normalizes menstrual flow
- Expectorant – helps remove excess mucous congestion for the chest and respiratory system
- Hemostatic – helps stop bleeding
- Hypotensive – helps lower blood pressure
- Laxative - promotes evacuation of the bowels
- Nervine - tones and strengthens the nervous system
- Sedative - calms the nervous system and reduces stress
- Stimulant – acceleratesand vitalizes body functions
- Tonic – strengthens and tones specific organs
- Vaso-dilator – causes relaxation and expansion of the blood vessels

Sourced from How to Be Your Own Herbal Pharmacist, Linda Rector Page, N.D., Ph.D. (Currently out of print, but some used are available.)

6. Herbs are Foods and Medicine

Herbs are foods that provide concentrated nutrients and medicines in a tidy package.

Many herbs are high in minerals, vitamins and phytonutrients. Most herbs are high in antioxidants. The common herbs with the highest antioxidant activity as of today's research are: oregano, parsley, dill, garden thyme, rosemary, peppermint, cilantro/coriander, and winter savory.
http://www.phytochemicals.info/research/antioxidants-herbs.php

Each herb (as do other plant foods) has its particular combination of nutrients and other factors whose synergy provides the body with the proper fuel. When you raise your own herbs you have an inexpensive and constant supply of fresh, raw herbs which can dramatically change the taste of your meals and your health.

I feel whenever possible we should use the whole herb or whole herb extract, which will provide the synergy of all the factors. When herbs are standardized, we lose that synergy. Our Creator in his infinite wisdom created what we need.

How are we going to use herbs as foods?
Let's Think Raw in salads, juices, drinks, pesto, salsa, and teas; or dry or freeze them.

- Juices made from raw organic vegetables, fruits, and herbs deliver the <u>highest level of concentrated nutrients.</u>
- Salads can be such a delight if you use your imagination. A salad at my house in the summer will contain whatever is available in my garden, including herbs and edible flowers. By adding fresh raw herbs we increase the nutritive value of the salad, increase texture, and add flavors that are amazing.

When using herbs in cooking, add the herbs near the end of cooking time to preserve nutrients.

Don't microwave herbs or water for tea (infusions). I don't microwave anything!! (176)

Dried herbs can be used in foods, teas, oils, capsules, powdered tonics, tinctures, poultices, baths, potpourris, and crafts.

Herbs to consider:
Allium family: onions, garlic, chives, leeks, shallots, and scallions

Garlic, onions, leeks, and chives contain flavonoids that stimulate the production of glutathione (the tripeptide that is the liver's most potent antioxidant). Glutathione enhances elimination of toxins and carcinogens, putting the allium family of vegetables at the top of the list for foods that can help prevent cancer. Here are just a few benefits from members of this family.

Garlic (Allium sativa): a food and drugstore in a clove.
Properties include:

antibacterial	antiparasitic
antifungal	antispasmodic
anti-inflammatory	antiviral
antimicrobial	expectorant
antioxidant	hypotensive (177)

Garlic contains many flavonoid antioxidants like the carotenoids lutein and zeaxanthin, vitamins C and K, and vitamin B-6 (pyridoxine and choline). Garlic is one of the richest sources of minerals such as potassium, iron, calcium, magnesium, manganese, zinc, copper, sulfur, selenium, and germanium.

Selenium is an important cofactor for anti-oxidant enzymes in the body. Manganese is used by the body as a co-factor for the antioxidant enzyme superoxide dismutase.

Garlic has long list of sulfur-containing constituents that help lower our risk of oxidative stress. Thiosulphanates, of which allicin is the most powerful, are activated by mincing or crushing the cloves. Allicin is responsible for most of the medicinal properties of garlic. (178)

Internally:
1. Garlic may prevent heart disease by:
   - Thinning the blood, reducing its tendency to clot.
   - Reducing blood pressure.
   - Opening the blood vessels.
   - Lowering levels of fat and cholesterol in the blood.
   - Lowering serum levels of homocysteine, which is indicated in artery disease.
2. Garlic functions as an antioxidant, thereby counteracting free radicals.
3. Garlic acts as an antibiotic; it will treat infections by killing harmful bacteria and fungi such as:
4. Infections of the mouth, throat, and chest.
5. Infections of the digestive system such as gastroenteritis (stomach flu).
6. Infections of the skin such as athlete's foot and ringworm.
7. Infections of the urogenital area such as thrush or cystitis; specific for Candida infections.
8. Garlic is effective against worms and parasites.
9. Garlic has been known to stimulate insulin production and reduce blood sugar.
10. Garlic is a great antidote for a hangover. Make a garlic/onion broth and drink.
11. Garlic is effective in digestive disorders, diarrhea and liver and gall bladder problems.
12. Garlic is indicated in relieving rheumatoid arthritis.
13. Garlic heats the body and its sulfur encourages the liver to produce bile, which helps the liver detoxify, releasing poisons from the body.

Some studies have shown that people who eat garlic regularly have a decreased risk of colon cancer as it helps to cleanse the colon. (178) (179)

External use: Apply for ringworm of the scalp, carbuncles, swelling, or athlete's foot.

Garlic is most effective when used in its raw form. It must be crushed to release the active component, allicin. When I feel like I'm getting sick I crush a clove of garlic, put it on a spoon, dribble on some olive oil, chew it a few times, and swallow. By following with a cracker or a piece of raw vegetable such as carrot or celery, it's not so bad. Be creative: mix it with a little egg salad or tuna, put it on crackers, and eat it. Mix it in vegetable juices, soups, or green salads such as lettuce and parsley. All these methods will help to eliminate the burning sensation in the mouth or stomach. I find it burns when taken with water. For prevention I try to have a clove of garlic each day, if not raw then lightly cooked in something delicious. If you are concerned about the odor, eating parsley, chewing mint, fennel, or anise seeds seems to tame the smell.

When garlic is boiled, it seems to lose much of the allicin content, so press or mince it and add after the cooking is complete. Cooking crushed garlic lightly (at low temperatures) in oil does not destroy the compounds needed for cardiovascular health but may lessen the antiviral and antibiotic properties. Eat garlic fresh or just warmed in oil for the most health benefits.

Warning: Garlic in medicinal doses may increase the activity of drugs. If you are pregnant or on blood thinning or clot prevention medicines, consult your practitioner before using garlic for other than in culinary endeavors. It should also be noted medicinal amounts of garlic may interfere with insulin metabolism; therefore diabetic therapy may need to be adjusted due to the hypoglycemic effects of garlic. (179)

**Note: Do not store garlic in oil at room temperature. Garlic-in-oil mixtures stored at room temperature provide perfect conditions for producing botulism, regardless of whether the garlic is fresh or has been roasted. Refrigerate!

Onions contain significant amounts of vitamin C, molybdenum, manganese, vitamin B6, folate, potassium, tryptophan, and fiber. Onions contain two powerful antioxidants, sulfur and quercetin. Both help neutralize the free radicals in the body and protect the membranes of the body's cells from damage. (180)

The total polyphenol content of onions is quite high. The flavonoids quercetin and anthocyanins, make up much of the high phenolic content which helps against oxidative stress. Quercetin is the natural flavonoid behind onion's anti-inflammatory and anti-allergic effects. It can also improve cardiovascular health, prevent the oxidation of LDL (bad) cholesterol, and even reduce the risk for cancer. The anti-inflammatory action of quercetin is caused by the inhibition of enzymes, such as lipoxygenase, and the release of histamine, which causes congestion. (180) (181)

A curious thing about cooking onions in liquid at **low to medium temperatures** is the quercetin isn't damaged but survives in the broth. Several servings of onion each week are sufficient to statistically lower your risk of some types of cancer, but eating onions every day would be better yet. Consuming onions may:
- Inhibit the growth of cancerous cells
- Increase in HDL cholesterol (especially when eaten raw)
- Reduce total cholesterol levels
- Increase blood-clot dissolving activity
- Help prevent colds
- Stimulate the immune system
- Reduce the risks of diabetes
- Have antibacterial and antifungal properties
- Reduce the risk of certain cancers
- Help relieve stomach upset and other gastrointestinal disorders (180)

Externally: Raw onion applied directly to the skin will help relieve insect bites, wounds, boils, and bruises. (182)

Leeks, chives, shallots, and scallions have similar healthy properties of the allium family as described above.

Basil (Ocimum basilicum) (183) Properties include:

antibacterial	diaphoretic	febrifuge
antifungal	digestive	nervine
antioxidant	emetic	stimulant
antispasmodic	emmenagogue	
aphrodisiac	expectorant	

Basil is a good source of iron, calcium, magnesium, vitamin A, manganese, potassium, and vitamin C. (184)

Basil is also a good source of antioxidants, especially beta carotene, which helps to prevent free radical damage. It contains a unique array of flavonoids including Orientin and vicenin, two water-soluble flavonoids that protect cell structures as well as chromosomes from radiation and oxygen-based damage. (185)

Basil herb contains exceptionally high levels of beta-carotene, **vitamin A, cryptoxanthin, lutein and zea-xanthin.** These compounds help act as protective scavengers against oxygen-derived free radicals and reactive oxygen species (ROS) that play a role in aging and various disease processes. (184)

The antibacterial properties of basil are in the volatile oils--estragole, linalool, cineole, eugenol, sabinene, myrcene, and limonene. These oils have shown to be very effective in restricting growth of numerous bacteria, including Listeria monocytogenes, Staphylococcus aureus, Escherichia coli, Yersinia enterocolitica, and Pseudomonas aeruginosa. The eugenol in basil qualifies basil as an anti-inflammatory or cox2 enzyme inhibitor. (185)

Basil is a tender annual that loves to be planted near tomatoes. Basils will frost easily, so plant late and harvest early or grow indoors. There are many varities of basil. My favorite to grow is large leaf Genovese basil so I can harvest lots for pesto and drying.

We know basil best in tomato and pesto sauces, but it can be used in so many cuisines. Pesto is a favorite of mine, as it is nutritionally packed with garlic, olive oil, nuts, and various other herbs. If freezing pesto leave out the garlic and add it just before using. Infuse basil in olive oil to preserve to use on salads.

Calendula (Calendula officinalis): Calendula's bright, cheery flowers are a happy addition to any garden. The petals from the flower heads can be used fresh in salads or dried and used for medicinals and skin care preparations. (Some other members of the marigold family have similar properties.)

Nutritionally, calendula petals are high in carotenoids such as beta carotene, lutein, zeaxanthin, and lycopene. **The Linus Pauling Institute reports that lutein and zeaxanthin are the only antioxidants that are found in the retina of the eye, where they protect the eye from the development of cataracts and macular degeneration.** (186) Lycopene is reported to reduce the risk of prostate cancer and heart disease.

Medicinal properties of calendula:

analgesic	antispasmodic
antibacterial	antiviral
anticancer	astringent
antifungal	diaphoretic
anti-inflammatory	emmenagogue
antimicrobial	wound healing
antiseptic	(187)

Externally, calendula is used as an antiseptic to treat wounds. It is used to reduce inflammation and to relieve a variety of skin diseases. Calendula is used as an infused oil, salve, cream or tincture. Salves and creams made from infused oil have a short shelf life. A tincture can be used to make creams, lotions, and salves later.

Healing properties of calendula:
- Due to its antiseptic qualities calendula is one of the best herbs for treating burns, scalds, cuts, abrasions, and infections.
- It can heal wounds very quickly. It can reduce the fluid inside blisters.
- Calendula is used for common sores, bedsores, varicose veins, and hemorrhoids.
- As an antifungal agent, it can be used to treat athlete's foot, ringworm, and candida. (188)

Note: Always cleanse a wound before applying any salve or cream. I keep spray made with calendula oil or tincture, aloe vera gel, vitamin E oil and a few drops of oregano oil on my bathroom counter for whatever skin condition needs attention. I have used this spray for many situations while traveling.

Internally, calendula tea:
- is used for gastro-intestinal disorders, stomach cramps and stomach ulcers, as well as inflammation of the large intestine, dropsy and blood in the urine.
- can help small blood vessels to seal, stopping bleeding and preventing bruising
- works deep inside the body to treat bladder infections, upset stomach, and ulcers
- can bring relief in gall bladder problems (188)

**Warning: Calendula may increase drowsiness if taken with sedative drugs. It should not be taken internally during pregnancy or lactating. (189)

Cayenne pepper (Capsicum frutescens) the ripened dried fruit. **Capsaicin**, the active ingredient in cayenne peppers, is so hot it can make your mouth feel like it's on fire. There are many grades of "heat" from 20,000 to 100,000 Scoville Units. Cayenne is used as a spice with zing, a preventive, and a medicine. Use cayenne in as many foods as you can. Start with a tiny pinch and increase as you can tolerate the heat. A bit of cayenne adds zest to almost any soup, sauce, or casserole.

Cayenne pepper is an excellent source of vitamin A and a good source of vitamin E, vitamin C, vitamin B6, vitamin K, manganese, and dietary fiber.
Some of the properties of capsaicin include:

antioxidant	anodyne–pain killer
thermogenic	anti-cancer stimulant
antibacterial	vasodilator
anti-inflammatory	(190)

Cayenne is used <u>internally</u> to:
- reduce congestion and inflammation
- boost metabolism and aid digestion
- improve circulation
- help to clean out the arteries and reverse atherosclerosis
- thin phlegm and aid its expulsion from the respiratory system
- support the heart, kidneys, lungs, pancreas, spleen, and stomach
- bring relief from arthritis and rheumatism
- ward off colds, sinus infections, and sore throats
- inhibit the growth of H. Pylori, implicated in stomach ulcers
- reduce cholesterol and triglyceride levels
- alleviate nerve pain from trauma of surgery
- increase the effectiveness of other herbs when added to herbal combinations
- protect the heart by reducing cholesterol, triglycerides, and platelet aggregation. It may also help the body dissolve fibrin, which is necessary for blood clots to form.
- relieve inflammation
- raise the metabolic rate, thus burning calories faster (191)

Dr. John Christopher sang the praises of cayenne. He declared: "In 35 years of practice, and working with the people and teaching, I have never on house calls lost one heart attack patient and the reason is, whenever I go in—if they are still breathing—I pour down them a cup of cayenne tea (a teaspoon of cayenne in a cup of hot water, and within minutes they are up and around)." (192)

For the details, read "How To Use Cayenne Pepper To Stop A Heart Attack Fast!"
http://www.naturalnews.com/030566_cayenne_pepper_heart_attack.html

Cayenne can be used as powder in food, in capsules, or as a tincture. I personally know two people who were saved during a heart attack by drinking a glass of water with cayenne in it. I carry a small bottle of cayenne tincture in my purse at all times.

Topically, cayenne can be mixed in a cream or salve and used for pain, diabetic neuropathy, arthritis, shingles, after surgery nerve pain. Do not apply topically on open skin or near the eyes.

**Caution: When handling chili peppers wear gloves and do not rub your eyes. Much of the heat is in the ribs and seeds of the pepper. When working with bulk powder cayenne wear a mask.

Warning: Ingesting cayenne in medicinal amounts may cause an unsafe interaction with many drugs See this website: http://umm.edu/health/medical/altmed/herb-interaction/possible-interactions-with-cayenne

Cilantro (Coriandrum sativum): The green plant is called cilantro and the seeds are coriander.

Properties include:

antibiotic	antioxidant
antibacterial	anti-inflammatory
antimicrobial	chelator (193)

It is rich in several antioxidant phytonutrients such as the polyphenolic flavonoidsquercetin, kaempferol, rhamnetin and epigenin.

- It is a good source of potassium, calcium, manganese, iron, and magnesium.
- It is rich in folic acid, riboflavin, niacin, vitamin A, beta carotene, vitamin C, and it is one of the richest herbal sources for vitamin K.
- It is twice as effective as the commonly used antibiotic drug Gentamicin at killing Salmonella. (193)
- It aids digestion and relieves intestinal discomfort in the stomach.
- It aids in treating the symptoms of arthritis.
- It protects against urinary tract infections.

- It is effective in preventing and treating nausea.
- It helps in lowering blood sugar.
- It helps lowers bad cholesterolwhile raising good cholesterol.
- It is a good source of dietary fiber. (193)

Cilantro is a powerful natural cleansing agent or chelator. It has been effectively used to help **remove heavy metals and other toxic agents from the body.** (194) Find my Cilantro Chelation Pesto recipe in the "Detoxification" section.

Warning: Women who are pregnant, trying to get pregnant, or nursing should consult their health care practitioners before taking cilantro in medicinal quantities.

Dandelion (Taraxacum officinale): <u>Properties include:</u>
antibacterial
anti-cancer   depurative
antioxidant   diuretic
blood purifier   hepatic
cholagogue   stomachic (195)

The whole plant can be used as a medicinal herb internally and externally. The leaves are a nutritious food as well as a medicine. The root is used as a medicine. **The USDA says dandelion leaves rank in the top 4 green vegetables in overall nutritional value.** Dandelions are nature's richest green vegetable source of beta-carotene, from which Vitamin A is created, and the third richest source of Vitamin A of all foods, after cod liver oil and beef liver.

- The most active ingredients found <u>only</u> in dandelions are aeudesmanolide and germacranolide.
- Dandelion leaves are vitamins C, B-complex, and D.
- The leaves are a very good source of potassium, iron, calcium, magnesium, phosphorus and rich in micronutrients micronutrients such as copper, cobalt, zinc, boron, and molybdenum.

- The leaves contain significant pectin, which enhances the detoxifying process.
- The leaves are a good source of inulin, which feeds the good bacteria in the intestines.
- The plant has <u>antibacterial action</u>, inhibiting the growth of Staphococcus aureus, pneumococci, meningococci, Bacillus dysenteriae, B. typhi, C. diphtheriae, and proteus. (195)
- Both the leaves and the root are being used to control of cancer cells.
- Dandelion root is used in many detoxifying combinations for the colon, liver, gall bladder, and urinary system.
- The root detoxifies the liver and stimulates the flow of bile from the liver to the gall bladder. It helps break down liver fats. {References for the above section (195) and (196).

There is encouraging evidence that dandelion suppresses the growth and invasive behavior in several types of cancer. (197)

<u>Traditional uses of dandelion include:</u>
1. As a tonic and blood purifier
2. For constipation
3. For inflammatory skin conditions & joint pain
4. For treating the liver and gall bladder, including hepatitis and jaundice
5. For kidney and urinary disorders
6. To decrease edema associated with high blood pressure and heart weakness. (196)

Caution: Consuming dandelion in medicinal dosages may increase side effects of bipolar medications such as lithium. It may also interfere with the absorption of a class of antibiotics known as quinolones. (195)

Dill Weed (Anethum graveolens): <u>Properties include</u>:
- antioxidant
- antiseptic
- digestive
- carminative
- antimicrobial
- anti-cancer (198)

As a food fresh dill weed is:

- rich in many vital vitamins including folic acid, riboflavin, niacin, vitamin A, beta-carotene, and vitamin C that are essential for optimum metabolism inside the body.
- a good source of minerals like copper, potassium, calcium, manganese, iron, magnesium and the trace mineral vanadium.
- an excellent source of antioxidant activity (199)

Dill oil, extracted from dill seeds, has anti-spasmodic, carminative, digestive, disinfectant, galactagogue (helps breast milk secretion), and sedative properties.
Dill weed (sprigs) and seeds contain many essential volatile oils such as d-carvone, dillapiol, DHC, eugenol, limonene, terpinene and myristicin.The essential oil eugenol in the dill has been in therapeutic usage as local anesthetic and antiseptic. Eugenol has also been found to reduce blood sugar levels in diabetics. (198)

Ginger Root (Zingiber officinale): Ginger has been widely used by Ayurvedic and Chinese traditional healers as well as by western herbalists. It is a warming herb whose active ingredient is gingerol. Forms of ginger: raw grated or powdered ginger can be used as a tea or in fruit or vegetable juices, as a fresh juice, capsules, tablets, tincture; or crystalline ginger may be sucked.

Ginger has qualities that may prevent heart attacks and arthritis pain; aid digestion; prevent colds, flu, and skin cancers; and aid weight loss. Fresh ginger juice is amazing taken at the beginning of a cold or flu.
Properties include:

antioxidant	anti-motion sickness
antibacterial	anti-diabetic
antiviral	anti-inflammatory
adaptogenic	anti-ulcer anti-tumor
digestive	antifungal
anthelmintic	antihistamine
anti-emetic	(200) (201)

218

Below is a smattering of things I have gleaned over the years as to the value of ginger.

- Ginger contains nearly a dozen antiviral compounds, known as sesquiterpenes, which are especially effective at fighting rhinoviruses. As a juice or hot infusion, it stimulates the body to sweat, thus activating the immune system in colds, flu,
- It boosts metabolism and helps reduce toxin build-up in fat cells.
- It is a blood thinner, promotes circulation, and improves vascular health.
- It stimulates secretion of bile from the liver and gall bladder which digests fats.
- It cleanses the colon and reduces spasms and cramps.
- It relieves some types of headaches.
- It is wonderful for relieving bloating and gas.
- It acts as a "bitter," which tonifies the intestinal muscles and stimulates digestion.
- It is effective for flu, vomiting, nausea, and general digestive upset.
- It is helpful in coughs/respiratory tract infections.
- It reduces the vomiting and nausea from chemotherapy or anesthesia in surgery.
- It relieves morning sickness in pregnancy, but it should not be taken for an extended time during pregnancy.
- It reduces the toxicity of other herbs or foods as in food poisoning.
- Ginger offers considerable radiation protection.
- Synergistically, ginger helps other herbs be more effective. Sources for this section (202) 203)

Researchers found that 6-shogaol is active against cancer stem cells at concentrations that are harmless to healthy cells. (202)
Warning: If taking medications of any kind, be aware that ginger may increase the absorption of drugs. Ginger in medicinal levels is not recommended for people taking blood thinning or anti-coagulant drugs, or who have

gallstones. Please consult your practitioner before mixing therapeutic doses of ginger with any drugs. (202)

To learn more about ginger I recommend reading <u>Ginger: Common Spice and Wonder Drug</u> by Paul Schulick.

Horseradish root (Armoracia rusticana): an amazing food and medicine: <u>Properties include</u>:

anti-anemic	antiseptic
antibacterial	diuretic
antibiotic	expectorant
anti-inflammatory	gastric stimulant
anti-parasitic	vasodilator (204) (205)

This root has a moderate level of sodium, potassium, manganese, iron, copper, zinc, and magnesium. It is a good source of vitamin C and has small amounts of B vitamins.

1. The fresh root of horseradish is used as a natural treatment against rheumatic disorders and respiratory disorders.
2. It increases the liver's ability to detoxify and eliminate carcinogens that help in the appearance of malignant tumors in the liver.
3. Horseradish root dissolves the mucus in the nose and thus releases sinus infections.
4. Horseradish also helps in aiding diabetes, mild circulatory problems, water retention, digestion, and toothaches.
5. It stimulates the body's immune system and appetite.
6. It is a very strong diuretic, and has been used by herbalists in calculus (stones). It is useful in the treatment of edema.
7. Horseradish contains powerful antioxidant properties that reduce free radicals.
8. It acts as a natural antibiotic against different types of infections. It reduces urinary tract infections and kills bacteria in the throat which cause bronchitis, coughs, and related problems. Sources for the above section are (204) (205) (206)

Horseradish contains significant amounts of cancer-fighting compounds called glucosinolates (also found in cruciferous vegetables) which increase the liver's ability to detoxify carcinogens and may suppress the growth of tumors. Horseradish has up to 10 times more glucosinolates than broccoli. Two of the most abundant compounds in the horseradish root are sinigrin and gluconasturtiin. (207)

Oregano (Origanum vulgare) is a super antioxidant and multi-medicinal herb. Properties include:

anodyne	carminative
antibacterial	Cox-2 inhibitor
anti-cancer	diaphoretic
antifungal	emmenogogue
antimicrobial	nervine
antioxidant	stimulant
antispasmodic	(208) (209)
antiviral	

Oregano provides vitamins A, B6, C K. It is a very good source of potassium, iron, calcium, manganese, magnesium, dietary fiber, and omega-3 fatty acids. (208)

Antioxidant activity in oregano is due to a high content of phenolic acids and flavonoids. The herb is rich in polyphenolic flavonoid anti-oxidants (carotenes - lutein, zeaxanthin and cryptoxanthin). (211)

When comparing the antioxidant activity of foods and herbs, oregano emerged the clear winner. Dr. Bazilian, author of The SuperFoodsRx Diet: Lose Weight with the Power of SuperNutrients considers oregano a mini salad because "one teaspoon has as much antioxidant power as three cups of chopped broccoli." Oregano had 3 to 20 times higher antioxidant activity than the other herbs studied. Ounce for ounce organo has 42 times the antioxidant activity as apples, 12 times more than oranges, and 4 times more than blueberries. (210) Fresh is even more potent.

Oregano oil is usually used to treat dysfunctions, although a strong decotion of Organum vulgare can also be effective. Be aware that there are several types of oregano in the stores which are fine for flavoring, but Organun vulgare is the most medicinal. (210)

- The herb may increase the motility of the gastro-intestinal tract as well as increase the digestion power by increasing gastro-intestinal secretions.
- A decoction is taken by mouth for the treatment of colds, influenza, mild fevers, indigestion, stomach upsets, and painful menstruation conditions
- Oregano has demonstrated <u>antimicrobial</u> activity against food-borne pathogens such as Listeria monocytogenes.
- Oregano contains many health benefiting essential oils such as carvacrol, thymol, limonene, pinene, ocimene, and caryophyllene. These volatile oils in oregano have been shown to inhibit the growth of bacteria, including Pseudomonas aeruginosa and Staphylococcus aureus. Oregano oil is being studied as an effective alternative to drug antibiotics, which have side effects.
- Oregano essential oil can effectively fight streptococcus, which can cause pneumonia and other infections of the upper respiratory system.
- This amazing super herb can also destroy viruses and fungi, which is why oregano oil is often used during anti Candida (fungi) cleanses.
- Oregano is known to have cancer fighting qualities.
- Oregano is also known to clear giardia. Sources for the above section are (209)(210) (211).

Parsley (Petroselinum crispum): All parts of the parsley plant (leaves, roots, & seeds) can be used for preventive and medicinal remedies. <u>Properties include:</u>

antibacterial	carminative
anti-cancer	diuretic
antioxidant	emmenagogue
antirheumatic	vasodilator (212)

Parsley is among the few plants with the highest antioxidant activity. When parsley is used as a food, it can add significantly to overall well being. Parsley is rich in many antioxidant vitamins, including vitamin-A, beta-carotene, vitamin-C, vitamin-E, zea-xanthin, lutein, and cryptoxanthins. Zeaxanthin and lutein help prevent age-related macular degeneration (ARMD). As an antioxidant,

- Parsley helps to neutralize free radicals in the body.
- Parsley is rich in poly-phenolic flavonoid antioxidants including apiin, apigenin, crisoeriol, and luteolin.
- Parsley is one of the richest herbal sources for vitamin K.
- It is a good source of B vitamins such as folates, pantothenic acid (vitamin B-5), riboflavin (vitamin B-2), niacin (vitamin B-3), pyridoxine (vitamin B-6) and thiamin (vitamin B-1).
- Parsley is a good source of minerals like potassium, calcium, manganese, iron, selenium, zinc, and magnesium.
- Parsley contains many health benefiting essential volatile oils that include myristicin, limonene, eugenol, and alpha-thujene. The essential oil eugenol present in this herb has been in therapeutic use in dentistry as a local anesthetic and antiseptic agent for teeth and gum diseases.
- The volatile oils in parsley can help neutralize particular types of carcinogens that are found in cigarette smoke & charcoal grill smoke.
- Parsley, as a very effective diuretic, is used for flushing out the urinary tract to prevent or treat gravel.
- It is used for flatulent dyspepsia and rheumatic conditions.
- Parsley is known to ease menstrual complaints.
- Parsley leaves are a great breath freshener.

Sources for above section (213) (214).

**Warning: Medicinal amounts of parsley should not be taken when pregnant or when suffering from inflammatory kidney conditions. (214)

Purslane (Portulaca oleracea), a common garden weed, has proven to be one of the world's best plant sources of omega-3 fatty acids being especially high in alpha-linolenic acid. Fresh leaves contain surprisingly more Omega-3 fatty acids than any other leafy vegetable plant. 100 grams (about ½ cup) of fresh purslane leaves provides about 350 mg of alpha-linolenic acid. (215)

Of the 1,300 known food plants, it is one of fewer than 20 plants that have the capacity to meet nearly all of the human body's nutritional requirements. Purslane:
- has all the essential amino acids.
- has 10 to 20 times more melatonin, an antioxidant that may inhibit cancer growth more than any other fruit or vegetable tested.
- is an excellent source of Vitamin A (1320 IU/ per 100 grams of plant material), one of the highest among green leafy vegetables.
- is a rich source of vitamins C and E.
- has some B-complex vitamins like riboflavin, niacin, and pyridoxine.
- is a rich source of carotenoids and glutathione.
- is rich in minerals such as iron, magnesium, calcium, potassium, phosphorous, zinc, silicon, manganese, chromium, selenium, and copper.
- is a source of two types of betalain alkaloid pigments, the reddish beta-cyanins and the yellow beta-xanthins. Both of these pigment types are potent antioxidants and have been found to have anti-mutagenic properties.
- is a source of pectin.

Sources for the above section are from (215) (216) (27).

Ways to use Purslane as a food.
- Fresh, tender leaves can be used as salad.
- Fresh leaves can be juiced with other veggies.
- Steam sautéed stems and leaves served as side dish with fish and poultry.
- It has also been used in soup and curry preparations and eaten with rice.

- It can be stir-fried and mixed with other greens and vegetables.
- It can be pickled and used as a relish.
- Purslane with other ground vegetables can be dried as nutritious leather.

Healing properties of purslane include:

analgesic	blood cleanser
antibacterial	diuretic
antifungal	febrifuge
anti-inflammatory	muscle relaxant
antiseptic	vermifuge
antispasmodic	vulnerary (215)

Purslane is known to:
- Help prevent macular degeneration and cataracts.
- Lower bad cholesterol.
- Protect bones against osteoporosis.
- Stimulate the circulation of blood.
- Reduce inflammation from bee stings and snakebites.
- Aid in treating gastrointestinal disorders.
- Help prevent atherosclerosis, heart attacks and strokes

The root extract is said to be used as an anti-venom for rattlesnakes bites. (216)

To really appreciate purslane one must read The Wonders of Purslane by Elsie Belcheff, Polished Publishing Group, 2012. Elsie is an amazing lady who I have had the privilege to meet on several occasions. She saw potential in purslane and researched to create this great book which entails the research behind this great plant. The book is available on her website, http://www.naturalplantation.com/purslane_facts.html.

Caution: Pregnant women should avoid purslane since it can cause the uterine muscles to contract. (216)

Rosemary (Rosmarinus officinalis) The aerial parts, especially flower tops, contain the phenolic antioxidant rosmarinic acid as well as having numerous other health-benefiting volatile essential oils such as cineol, camphene, borneol, bornyl acetate, α-pinene etc. These compounds are known to have <u>rubefacient, anti-inflammatory, anti-allergic, anti-fungal, and antiseptic properties. (220)</u>

<u>Properties include:</u>

analgesic	antispasmodic
anti-allergic	antiviral
anti-cancer	diaphoretic
antifungal	diuretic
anti-inflammatory	hypertensive
antioxidant	rubefacient
antiseptic	stimulant (218)

1. Rosemary is exceptionally rich in B vitamins, such as folic acid, pantothenic acid, pyridoxine, and riboflavin.
2. It is a good source of vitamin A and Vitamin C.
3. It stimulates the central nervous system, circulatory system, and the pelvic region.
4. It is a proven heart tonic.
5. It aids recovery from stress.
6. It may stimulate the adrenal glands.
7. It scavenges free radicals to neutralize them.
8. It boosts the immune system.

Sources for above (219) (220)

Rosemary is used in foods much as is sage or thyme. Rosemary oil is an ingredient in Thieves Oil, which is a used as a deterrent to viruses. Sniffing rosemary oil is thought to help with memory.

Caution: For the most part, rosemary is considered safe with no side effects. However, pregnant women should avoid consuming large amounts of rosemary because it may lead to uterine contractions and miscarriage. People with high blood pressure should not take rosemary because it may raise blood pressure. (220)

Sage (Salvia officinalis): <u>Properties include:</u>

analgesic	anti-inflammatory	astringent
antibacterial	antioxidant	digestive
anti-cancer	antiseptic	emmenogogue
antifungal	antiviral	nervine (221)

1. Sage is a source of potassium, zinc, calcium, iron, manganese, copper, and magnesium.
2. It is an exceptionally rich source of many B-complex vitamins, such as folic acid, thiamin, pyridoxine, and riboflavin and a good source of vitamins A and C
3. It is a hormonal stimulant.
4. It improves metabolism.
5. It improves cognitive brain function.
6. Sage is often used as a remedy for respiratory infections, congestion, cough, and sore throats.
7. It is an appetite stimulant, aids in soothing indigestion, and may have a beneficial effect on the liver.
8. It is also given for fever, night sweats and urinary problems.

Sources for section above (221) (222)

<u>Culinary uses:</u> Sage combines well with other herbs such as thyme, rosemary, oregano, mint, or parsley to flavor meats. Try the above herbs on wild game. Use sage with thyme in bean soups. Sage blends well with mild cheeses.

**Caution: Sage is a uterine stimulant, so it should be avoided in therapeutic doses during pregnancy. It is also recommended not to use sage in therapeutic doses if you suffer from any type of seizures. (221)

Savory (Satureja speices, winter or summer):
<u>Properties include:</u>

antibacterial	astringent
antifungal	carminative
antimicrobial	expectorant
antioxidant	stomachic
antirheumatic	

Savory, especially the flowering shoots, has many constituents.

- Savory herb is an excellent source of minerals and vitamins that are essential for optimum health. Its leaves and tender shoots are a rich source of potassium, iron, calcium, magnesium, manganese, zinc, and selenium.
- Savory is also rich in many important vitamins such as B-complex group vitamins, vitamin A, vitamin C, niacin, thiamine, and pyridoxine.
- Savory is high in dietary fiber, which helps the digestive system.
- Savory leaves and tender shoots contain incredibly high-quality antioxidants.
- Savory leaves contain many essential volatile-oil phenols such as thymol and carvacrol, as well as linalool, camphene, caryophyllene, terpineol, myrcene, and other terpenoids.
- Thymol in savory has scientifically been found to have <u>antiseptic and anti-fungal</u> characteristics.
- Carvacrol in savory inhibits the growth of several bacteria strains like E. coli, and Bacillus cereus; therefore, it has been used as a healthy food additive for its anti-bacterial properties, pleasant tangy taste, and the marjoram-like smell it gives to food.

Sources for above section are (223) (224).

Tea (Camellia sinensis): White, green, and black tea are good sources of antioxidants.

A study in Hong Kong in 2009 has found the amount of green tea a person drinks is in direct correlation with the length of telomeres on the ends of chromosomes. Telomeres prevent chromosomes from fusing with one another or rearranging, producing undesirable changes that could lead to cancer and other life-threatening diseases. **Research has shown that as cells replicate and age, telomeres get shorter and shorter and that when telomeres finally disappear, the cells can no longer replicate.** The participants with the highest intake, three cups per day of tea, had longer telomeres.

Researchers concluded <u>antioxidative properties of tea and its constituent nutrients may protect telomeres from oxidative damage in the normal aging process</u>. (225)

Researchers at the University of South Florida have found that green tea may protect the brain against the ravages of Alzheimer's disease. EGCG in tea decreases production of the Alzheimer's-related protein beta-amyloid, which can accumulate abnormally in the brain and lead to nerve damage and memory loss. (226)

Studies have suggested that green tea extract induces death in cancer cells, as well as inhibiting the development of an independent blood supply that cancers develop so they can grow and spread. (226)

While green and black tea have great health-giving constituents, **white tea is the least processed tea and has the highest antioxidant levels.** Some of the findings about white tea include:

- It protects the circulatory system by thinning the blood, lowering blood pressure, and reducing cholesterol.
- It increases bone density and strength. White tea may also have beneficial effects for sufferers of arthritis and osteoporosis.
- It is a natural killer of bacteria and viruses.
- It is high in antioxidants that tone the entire immune system, providing protection against a wide range of diseases.
- It may reduce blood sugar and help prevent and/or alleviate the symptoms of diabetes.
- It reduces stress and increases energy.
- It may prevent the activities of the enzymes which break down elastin and collagen, which can lead to wrinkles that accompany aging. These enzymes, along with oxidants, are associated with inflammatory diseases such as rheumatoid arthritis.

- It has shown to reduce the risk of inflammation which is characteristic of rheumatoid arthritis. Source for the above section is (227).

Thyme (Thymus vulgaris): The many varieties of thyme seem to have similar properties, including:

analgesic	antitussive
anticancer	antiviral
antibacterial	expectorant
antifungal	insect repellent
antioxidant	nervine (228)
antispasmodic	

- Thyme leaves are rich sources of potassium, iron, calcium, manganese, magnesium, and selenium.
- The herb is also a rich source of many important vitamins such as B-complex vitamins, vitamin A, C, E, and K.
- Thyme is a great source of vitamin B-6 (pyridoxine), which contributes to the production of GABA (a beneficial neurotransmitter in the brain). GABA is a stress buster.
- Thyme contains a variety of **antioxidants** including carotenes, zeaxanthin, lutein, pigenin, naringenin, luteolin, and thymonin which neutralize free radicals.
- The expectorant and bronchial antispasmodic properties make it effective in respiratory infections.
- Thyme contains an essential oil that is rich in thymol, a powerful antimicrobial, antiseptic, and antibacterial agent. The volatile oil has shown to have antimicrobial activity against a host of different bacteria and fungi including Staphylococcus aureus, Bacillus subtilis, Escherichia coli and Shigella sonnei.
- Rosmarinic and ursolic acids are major terpenoids in thyme that possess anti-cancer properties.
  Sources for the above (229) (230).

Scientists at the University of Manitoba, Canada, wrote that thymol can reduce bacterial resistance to common drugs such as penicillin. (231)

Note: When using thymol oil dilute with a carrier oil such as olive or avocado oil.

How to use thyme:
- As a tea it has been used for headaches, digestive upsets, and coughs.
- Thyme complements beef, fish, poultry and poultry stuffing, lamb, sausages, soups, and stews.
- It is used in herbed butters and herbed mayonnaise. Thyme is also an ingredient in many flavored vinegars.
- It complements many vegetables, including tomatoes, onions, eggplant, mushrooms, and green beans.
- It works well as a flavoring in eggs and cheeses. It combines well with garlic, lemon, basil and oregano in salad dressings, marinades, soups, and casseroles.
- Mix the fresh herb into salads or add to a smoothie. Sources for the above section are (229) (230).

Caution: The herb thyme is entirely safe to use and has no side effects. However, the essential oil of thyme may be irritating to the skin and mucous membranes, and may cause an allergic reaction. Medicinal doses of thyme and especially thyme oil are not recommended during pregnancy as thyme can act as a uterine stimulant. (231)

Turmeric (Curcuma longa): Properties include:

analgesic	antioxidant
anti-amyloidogenic	antiseptic
antibacterial	antiviral
anti-cancer	hepatic
anti-cytotoxic	metal-chelating
anti-inflammatory	neurorestorative
anti-malarial	(232) (233)

The active ingredient most studied in turmeric is curcumin. Turmeric has been used for over 2,500 years in India. The medicinal properties of this spice have been slowly revealing themselves over the centuries. Long known for its anti-inflammatory properties, recent research has revealed that turmeric is a natural wonder, proving beneficial in the treatment of many different health conditions from cancer to Alzheimer's disease. (232)

One of the most comprehensive summaries of turmeric benefits studies to date was published by the respected ethnobotanist James A. Duke, Ph.D., in the October, 2007 issue of *Alternative & Complementary Therapies,* and summarized in the July, 2008, issue of the *American Botanical Council* publication *HerbClip.* Reviewing some 700 studies, Duke concluded, "that turmeric appears to outperform many pharmaceuticals in its effects against several chronic, debilitating diseases, and does so with virtually no adverse side effects." (235) In the research Dr. Duke found turmeric can be used to help prevent or alleviate three major diseases: Arthritis, Alzheimer's disease, and Cancer. To read the details go to http://www.drweil.com/drw/u/ART03001/Three-Reasons-to-Eat-Turmeric.html

Arthritis: Turmeric contains two dozen anti-inflammatory compounds, including six different COX-2-inhibitors (anti-inflammatories) that work as well as many anti-inflammatory drugs, but without the side effects. (235)

Alzheimer's disease: Dr. Duke found more than 50 studies on turmeric's effects in addressing Alzheimer's disease. The reports indicate "that extracts of turmeric contain a number of natural agents that block the formation of beta-amyloid, the substance responsible for the plaques that slowly obstruct cerebral function in Alzheimer's disease." (235)

Cancer: Dr.Duke found more than 200 citations for turmeric benefits related to cancer and more than 700 for curcumin, the component in turmeric most often cited for its healthful effects. (235)
- Turmeric is a major antioxidant. When combined with black pepper, it has been found to control cancer stem cells. (238)

- When combined with cauliflower, it has been shown to prevent prostate cancer and stop the growth of existing prostate cancer.
- Promising studies are underway on the effects of turmeric on pancreatic cancer and multiple myeloma. It may prevent melanoma and cause existing melanoma cells to commit suicide.
- It may reduce the risk of childhood leukemia.
- It may prevent metastases from occurring in many different forms of cancer.
- It has anti-tumoral effects against melanoma cells.
- Turmeric boosts the effects of chemo drug paclitaxel and reduces its side effects.
- It destroys cancer cells both directly, by stimulating apoptosis, and indirectly, by inhibiting telomerase activity, thereby terminating the immortality so typical of cancer cell lines.
- It halts tumor proliferation by inhibiting DNA synthesis in the cancer cells and disrupting their mitotic replication.
- It inhibits the transcription capabilities of at least two major angiogenesis-inducing factors; the curcumin in turmeric halts the formation of the new blood vessels that are essential for tumor growth.
- It exhibits its anti-estrongenic effects by blocking the estrogen-dependent receptors on tumor cells, thereby interrupting the stimulatory effects of estrogen and slowing tumor growth. Most breast cancers are hormone dependent, requiring estrogen as a growth stimulant.

Sources for the above section are (234) (236).

Leading researcher Bharat Aggarwal tells us curcumin, the active component in turmeric, acts against transcription factors, which are like a "master switch," regulating all the genes needed for tumors to form. When we turn them off, we shut down some genes that are involved in the growth and invasion of cancer cells." (237)

233

Other studies have given us many reasons to use turmeric:

- Turmeric is a natural painkiller.
- As an antioxidant, turmeric is a great preventative.
- It is a natural liver detoxifier.
- It may aid in fat metabolism and help in weight management.
- Turmeric can strengthen the blood-brain barrier against attacks that result from auto-immune diseases.
- It has long been used in Chinese medicine as a treatment for depression.
- Turmeric may help in the treatment of psoriasis and other inflammatory skin conditions.
- Externally turmeric is useful in disinfecting cuts and burns, speeds wound healing, and assists in rebuilding damaged skin. (It will discolor the skin.)
- It can be effective in fighting a number of STDs including chlamydia and gonorrhea.

Sources for the above section are (234) (239)

Unfortunately, **curcumin is insoluble in water, thus must be eaen with a fat** such as extra-virgin olive oil, coconut oil, or organic butter. (236)

There are many studies combining turmeric with other factors for better absorption and effectiveness.

Combination examples include:

1. Combining turmeric, black pepper and olive oil.
2. Quercetin, turmeric, and bromelain are often combined especially for inflammatory ills.
3. Combining turmeric with vegetables that contain phenethyl isothiocyanate (PEITC), a naturally-occurring substance, such as watercress, cabbage, winter cress, broccoli, brussels sprouts, kale, cauliflower, kohlrabi and turnips.
4. Formula from Christian Wilde: turmeric, green tea extract, boswellia, black pepper, devil's claw, and bromelain. (238)

I've observed that when supplementing with curcumin it is more effective when taken with turmeric (the parent plant), so that it works in synergy with all the other factors in turmeric.

Cautions: Turmeric should not be used by people with gallstones or bile obstruction. Pregnant women should consult with their physicians before using large amounts of turmeric or curcumin. (234)

7. Mama Linda's Superfoods

Many famous people including Hippocrates have said food is our medicine, so I'm not going to try to separate foods and natural medicines. Many nutritionists and other health writers have their list of superfoods. Hopefully you will create your own after reading this.

All foods need to be raised organically or naturally, from natural seeds, not GMO, in healthy soil without chemicals (pesticides, artificial fertilizers, etc.) for the food to be nutritious. Know the sources of your foods.

I eat a variety of foods every day including meats and eggs from grass-fed animals or wild-caught fish, fermented dairy products, and a variety of vegetables, fruits, seeds, and herbs. We've just begun to understand the nutrients in some herbs, but we need to learn which other plants are nutritional powerhouses.

Nearly every food nature provides is really a superfood because each contains a combination of nutrients that is unique and needed by the body.

I have chosen a few foods that are good sources of the essential amino acids, high in antioxidants and essential fatty acids, and/or have specific nutritional qualities that you may want to add to your eating plan.

- Spirulina
- Quinoa
- Chia seed
- Hemp seed
- Buckwheat
- Purslane
- Wheatgrass

Soy products are good sources of protein, but I don't recommend eating soy products, which I explain in the section on proteins.

Foods below are <u>not listed according to importance, as they are all important</u>.

1. Dark Berries and Other Fruit
All edible berries are good sources of vitamins, minerals, and phytonutrients. I am including berries that we can easily access. <u>Include a variety of berries in your diet</u>

every day. If you can raise them in your landscaping, avoid using any chemicals in your yard. Raspberries and strawberries are probably the easiest to grow in the northern states. Blueberries are a very ornamental bush and are high in antioxidants, but they can be difficult to grow in some areas. We are experimenting with raising wolfberries (gogi berries) in our area because they are very high in antioxidants and other nutrients. So far they are doing well in our Montana climate. If you have no place to raise your own berries, buy them in season from local producers and freeze or dry the extras for later.

Become familiar with the berries that are found growing in your area. Besides the well-known blueberries, consider blackberries, raspberries, bilberries, strawberries, cranberries, seabuckthorn berries, ligonberries, loganberries, honeyberries, dewberries, wineberries, and wolfberries. Explore what may be growing wild in your area, such as chokecherries, buffalo berries, huckleberries, wild cherries, hawthorn berries, serviceberries (June berries), sea berries, currants, or aronia.

Some berries can be eaten raw in hand or frozen, others are better juiced, while others may be made into uncooked freezer jams and preserves. All of these berries are high in antioxidants, vitamins, and other nutrients. Berries lose many of their nutrients when heated. (A word of caution: researchers have found that most supermarket strawberries and blueberries contain large amounts of pesticide, so look for an organic grower.)

Blueberries rank among the fruits with the highest antioxidant capacity (ORAC levels). Blueberries are rich in antioxidants like anthocyanin, vitamin C, B-complex, vitamin E, vitamin A, copper, selenium, zinc, and iron, which boost your immune system and prevent infections. Blueberries may protect against urinary tract infections.

Anthocyanins are the blue-red pigments that neutralize free-radical damage to the collagen matrix of cells and tissues throughout the body which cause cancer and many other diseases. They improve the integrity of support structures in the veins and entire vascular system, thus protecting the heart and the brain from strokes and other age-related brain damage. Anthocyanins enhance the effects of vitamin C to improve capillary integrity.

The constituents in blueberry extract are known to slow visual loss. They can prevent or delay all age-related ocular problems like macular degeneration, cataracts, myopia, and other conditions pertaining to the retina. Blueberries also contain carotenoids such as lutein and zeaxanthin, flavonoids such as rutin, resveratrol, and quercetin, and nutrients such as vitamin C, vitamin E, vitamin A, selenium, zinc, and phosphorus, which are very beneficial and essential for the ocular health. (240) (241) (242)

Raspberries are often not appreciated for their nutritive value. Raspberries possess almost 50% higher antioxidant activity than strawberries. Raspberries contain phytonutrients providing antioxidant, antimicrobial, and anticarcinogenic protection. (243)

The biggest contribution of raspberries' antioxidant capacity is their ellagitannins, a family of compounds almost exclusive to the raspberry, which are reported to have anti-cancer activity. Vitamin C contributes about 20% of the total antioxidant capacity, and anthocyanins, especially cyanidin and pelagonidin glycosides, make up another 25%. (243)

Interestingly, freezing and storing raspberries does not significantly affect their antioxidant activity, but the concentration of vitamin C is cut in half.

Goji berries (Wolfberries) are very high on the ORAC scale (antioxidant level). In China the leaves and young shoots are eaten raw or cooked. They are rich in vitamin A and the leaves also contain about 3.9% protein.
The goji berry is one of the most popular tonics used in Chinese herbal medicine. We are concentrating here on the berries. Nutrients include:

238

- **18 amino acids,** including all of the essential amino acids
- **11 essential minerals and 22 trace minerals**
- **Vitamin A, vitamin C, vitamin B-complex, and vitamin E**
- **5 unsaturated fatty acids,** including the **essential fatty acids** linoleic acid and alpha-linolenic acid
- **Phytonutrients**--5 carotenoids, including beta carotene, zeaxanthin, lutein, lycopene, and cryptoxanthin
- **Polysaccharides and monosaccharides**
- Several **glyconutrients**
- **Betaine**, which is used by the liver to produce choline, a compound that calms nervousness, enhances memory, promotes muscle growth, and protects against fatty liver disease
- **Phenols** with antioxidant properties
- **Physalin**, which is active against all major types of leukemia. It has also been used as a treatment for hepatitis B.
- **Solavetivone**, a powerful anti-fungal and anti-bacterial compound
- **Beta-Sitosterol**, an anti-inflammatory agent. It has been used to treat sexual impotence and prostate enlargement. It also lowers cholesterol.
- **Sesquiterpenoids,** which have anti-inflammatory properties. The sesquiterpenoids contained in goji berries are found to be a powerful **secretagogue,** which stimulates the secretion of the human growth hormone by the pituitary gland.
- **Cyperone**, a sesquiterpene, that benefits the heart and blood pressure. It has also been used in the treatment of cervical cancer.

Sources for section above (244) (245).

Three main components in the goji berry that boost the immune system are:

1. Polysaccharides are well known for their immune-boosting properties.
2. Beta-carotene seems to boost interferon's stimulation on the immune system.

3. <u>Germanium</u> has been found to be critical in boosting interferon levels. (245)

<u>Medicinal properties of Goji berries</u> include:

antibacterial	anti-inflammatory
anti-cancer	antioxidant
antidiabetes	immune stimulating
antifungal	(246) (247)

At present goji berries in the US are quite expensive, since most of them are still imported from China. However, we are discovering <u>goji berries can be grown in gardens</u> in many areas of the US, so hopefully they will soon be available locally. Goji berries are fragile, so they need to be eaten, juiced or dried quickly after picking.
<u>Websites about growing goji berries (wolfberries):</u>

http://forgojiberries.com/HowToGrowGojiBerries.php3
http://www.richters.com/Web_store/web_store.cgi
http://www.saskgojipower.ca/gpage2.html

Tart cherries contain ample amounts of three types of anthocyanin, **a powerful anti-oxidant and anti-inflammatory**. Just 20 cherries provide up to 25 mg (milligrams) of anthocyanins.

One ounce of tart cherry juice has an ORAC value of approximately 4000.
- Tart cherries are rich in the flavonoids queritrin andisoqueritrin, which act as antioxidants and work to eliminate by-products of oxidative stress, thereby slowing down the aging process.
- Queritrin in red cherries has been found by researchers to be one of the most potent anticancer agents.
- They contain ellagic acid, a natural plant phenol known as an anti-carcinogenic/anti-mutagenic compound.
- They contain perillyl alcohol (POH), which is extremely powerful in reducing the occurrence of all types of cancer by binding to protein molecules to stop the signals that stimulate tumor growth and development.

- Cherries are rich in melatonin an antioxidant and it helps with sleep rhythms.
- They have anthocyanins and bioflavonoids which help relieve and prevent arthritis and gout in the body. They also are known to ease migraine headaches.
- The high anti-inflammatory properties of cherries make them an excellent source of pain relief for gout, arthritis, and fibromyalgia.
- Researchers say tart cherries can retard spoilage of ground beef and reduce the formation of potentially carcinogenic compounds in hamburgers.

Sources for above section (248) (249)

Prunes (dried plums)

I never travel without prunes. They provide a quick blood sugar snack and a unique combination of antioxidant phytonutrients, minerals, and soluble fiber. Prunes:

- are a good source of beta-carotene, which is a fat-soluble antioxidant, eliminating free radicals that would otherwise cause a lot of damage to our cells and cell membranes.
- are good sources of vitamin C and vitamin K.
- contain high amounts of neochlorogenic and chlorogenic acids, antioxidants that are particularly effective at combating the "superoxide anion radical." They have also been shown to help prevent oxygen-based damage to fats.
- are high in potassium (1/4 cup has 316 mg) and very little sodium. Potassium-rich foods are known to lower blood pressure and maintain heart function. Potassium may also counteract the increased urinary calcium loss caused by the high-salt diets.
- are known for their soluble and insoluble fiber which prevents constipation, helps normalize blood sugar levels by slowing the rate at which food leaves the stomach and by delaying the absorption of glucose following a meal. Soluble fiber also increases insulin sensitivity which can play a helpful role in the prevention and treatment of type 2 diabetes.

- can be a major player in decreasing the <u>transit time of fecal matter</u> in the intestines. The fiber in prunes decreases the risk of colon cancer and hemorrhoids. Insoluble fiber in prunes also provides food for the "friendly" bacteria in the large intestine. When these helpful bacteria ferment prunes' insoluble fiber, they produce butyric acid, which serves as the primary fuel for the cells of the large intestine and helps maintain a healthy colon.

Sources for section above (250) (251)

Apples have not been given the press they deserve. Whoever said "an apple a day keeps the doctor away" knew something we would do well to heed. Researchers have found that most of an apple's vital nutrients, like pectin and photochemicals, are in the skin of the raw apple. (252)

- Apple pectin is an excellent source of dietary fiber, vitamin C, beta carotene, vitamin B-complex and potassium, as well as small amounts of other minerals. Apples contain a variety of phytochemicals, including quercetin, catechin, phloridzin, and chlorogenic acid, all of which are strong antioxidants. (253)
- In the laboratory, apples have been found to have <u>very strong antioxidant activity, inhibit cancer cell proliferation, decrease lipid oxidation, and lower cholesterol.</u>
- The anti-oxidants in apple pectin help destroy free radicals that are responsible for cellular damage and spread of tumor cells. Through studies, researchers have discovered the apple's cancer-fighting ability may be derived from the procyanidins, a type of polyphenol, found in the skin that protects the fruits against the damaging effects of the sun. Procyanidins trigger signals that lead to cell suicide, thus reducing the growth and spread of cancer. (253)
- Studies have shown that apple pectin is also loaded with <u>acetylcholine</u>, which has a protective action against aging and prevents oxidative and cognitive

damage associated with age. Apple fiber may also play a crucial role of weight control. (255)

- Apples are high in soluble fiber. The fiber content in apple pectin is considered beneficial in improving bowel movement and effective in the management of the bowels. The soluble fiber tones and stimulates a sluggish colon so it can throw out waste matter.
- The phytochemical composition of apples has been found to vary greatly between different varieties of apples. Studies to this point have found the phytochemicals are generally highest in Red Delicious, Fuji, Jonagold, Gala, and Roman Beauty apples. (253)
- **Raw organic apples when eaten alone can help purge old accumulated toxic buildup and rotting matter from the intestines.** (254)

Note: Apples are in the top 12 fruits and vegetables testing for the **most pesticide residue, so buy organic.

2. Incredible Greens
There are many greens in Nature, but the most commonly used as foods are: dandelion, Swiss chard, spinach, romaine lettuce, sorrel, mustard greens, beet greens, collards, kale, arugula (rocket), and cress.

Leafy greens are some of the most nutritious foods. They are high in dietary fiber, chlorophyll, vitamins, minerals and phytonutrients. Everyone needs several servings of mixed raw greens each day.

Dark leafy greens are all good sources of nutrients:

beta-carotene	potassium	omega-3 fats
vitamin C	iron	antioxidants
vitamin K	folate	fiber
calcium	lutein	(256) (257)
magnesium	zeaxanthin	

Each green has specific nutrients needed for health. We've already learned the many nutrients in dandelion greens, so let's look at a few others.

Spinach

- Certain unique anti-cancer carotenoids—called epoxyxanthophylls — are plentiful in spinach and in beets and quinoa.
- Spinach contains significant amounts of vitamin E and B vitamins.
- Spinach is higher in folate than some other greens.

One new category of health-supportive nutrients found in spinach is called "glycoglycerolipids." Recent lab research in laboratory animals has shown that glycoglycerolipids from spinach can help protect the lining of the digestive tract from damage — especially damage related to unwanted inflammation. In recent studies only spinach showed evidence of significant protection against the occurrence of aggressive prostate cancer. (258)

Note: Spinach is best stir/steamed for 1 minute in a bit of coconut or oive oil to help reduce its concentration of oxalic acid. Lightly cooking greens with fat such as olive oil will alsoenhance the availability of carotenoids.

Half a cup of cooked **Swiss chard** provides a huge amount of both lutein and zeaxanthin, supplying 10 mg each. According to Harvard researchers, lutein and zeaxanthin protect the retinas of your eyes from the damage of aging. Both nutrients which are really pigments, appear to accumulate in your retinas, where they absorb the type of shortwave light rays that can damage your eyes. (259)

Beet greens are higher in folate than many other greens. They are also an excellent source of carotenoids, and flavonoid anti-oxidants. Beets are from the same family as Swiss chard so have similar nutrients. The greens have betalain pigments as do red chard and rhubarb. (260)

Arugula, although used as a "green," is actually a member of the Cruciferous Family. Approximately half cup has about 2 1/2 gr. of protein. Arugula:

- Is a rich source of certain phytochemicals such as indoles, thiocyanates, sulforaphane and iso-thiocyanates. Together they have been found to counter carcinogenic effects of estrogen and thus help benefit against prostate, breast, cervical, colon, and

244

ovarian cancers by virtue of their cancer cell growth inhibition, cytotoxic effects on cancer cells.

- Contains **di-indolyl-methane (DIM)**, a lipid soluble metabolite of indole has immune modulator, anti-bacterial and anti-viral properties (by potentiating Interferon-Gamma receptors and production). DIM has currently been used in the treatment of recurring respiratory papillomatosis caused by the Human Papilloma Virus (HPV).
- <u>Is a very good source of folates.</u> 100 g of fresh greens contain 97 mcg or 24% folic acid.
- Is an excellent source of **vitamin A and Beta carotene,** which is converted in the body to vitamin A. Source for section above is (261).

Wheatgrass juice is a complete food with no toxic side effects.
An analysis performed by Harvey Lisle and provided by the Anne Wigmore Foundation found that wheatgrass:
- contains all of the **vitamins and most of the minerals** needed for maintaining the body.
- at harvest is **40-45% protein**. It is a complete protein containing **20 amino acids.**
- has about **30 enzymes.** Enzymes are the necessary regulators of the body. Without enzymes our cells could not function and we would perish.
- is approximately 70% crude **chlorophyll.**
- acts as a natural appetite suppressant, so usually adding wheatgrass juice to your diet will help you to balance your weight at the optimum for you.

For more information read: <u>The Wheatgrass Book</u> or <u>The Hippocrates Diet</u> by Ann Wigmore. (262)

Wheatgrass juice is often used in therapeutic juice fasts. Wheat and barley grass can be grown in flats or bought fresh or powdered.

Barley grass
- has approximately 45 percent protein with 18 amino acids.
- has **18 identified enzymes**

- has one of the highest natural levels of **enzyme SOD (superoxide dismutase),** which is a powerful antioxidant that protects the cells against toxic free radicals.
- is a great source of, **chlorophyll,** a natural detoxifier that rids the intestines of stored toxins.
- is extremely alkaline, so digesting them can help balance the body's alkaline/ acidity ratio.
- is very high in **organic sodium**, which dissolves calcium deposited on the joints and also replenishes organic sodium in the lining of the stomach. (263) (264)

Are wheat grass and barley grass gluten-free?
Yes! The type of gluten that causes reactions in those with celiac disease and gluten intolerance occurs <u>in the seeds of grains</u> of wheat, barley and rye. **Wheat and barley grasses are harvested before the stalk develops when the young leaves are between 12 cm to 16 cm and before the grain stalk has started to develop** is the time it is harvested, dried and powdered. Once the grain stalk has started to develop, the nutrient focus is on growing the stalk and developing the head. This is when the gluten is produced in the stalk and head of the barley.

Caution: Powders - Know your source and how it was processed and at what stage the grass was harvested. For celiacs, it might be best to buy wheat grass grown locally or grow it yourself. (265)

I prefer to grow or buy my green foods locally, but if you can't, supplementing with wheatgrass, barley grass or mixed greens powder can be a great addition to your health. The micro-algea products such as Spirulina, Chloerlla, and Klamath Blue-green Algae might also be a good choice for you.

Klamath Blue-green Algae (Aphanizomenon flos-aquae) and spirulina are blue green algae while chlorella is a green algae. Chlorella has an indigestible cellulose wall which must be cracked to be digestible. All three are superior sources of protein, chlorophyll, vitamins, minerals, and disease-preventive phytonutrients. These are some of the earliest and simplest life forms on the planet, appearing way before animals roamed these lands. They are thought to contain <u>every nutrient required by the human body</u>. (266) (267)

3. Cruciferous Vegetables

Let's settle the confusion over terminology. Cruciferous vegetables, brassicas, cole crops, and the cabbage family all refer to the same group of vegetables: cabbage, broccoli, kale, cauliflower, kohlrabi, Brussels sprouts, bok choy, mustard greens, arugula, collard greens, land cress, horseradish, radishes, rutabagas, turnips, and watercress. (268)

Greens in the Cruciferous family are among the most nutritious vegetables.

They are a very good source of vitamins B1, B2, B6, C, E, and K, as well as fiber, calcium, iron, copper, and manganese. Their biggest claim in nutrition is having high levels of phytonutrients. (268)

The greens in the cabbage family have almost three times as much calcium as phosphorus. This ratio is very beneficial, since high phosphorus consumption has been linked to osteoporosis.

Cruciferous vegetables contain **enzymes** that help the liver manufacture and transfer glutathione to our bodies' cells. Glutathione is considered the master antioxidant because it replenishes and recycles spent antioxidants for more activity to protect cells from oxidative damage. (269)

Cruciferous greens are at the top of the list in **sulforaphane** content in foods. Sulforaphane is a chemical that increases your body's production of enzymes that disarm cell-damaging free radicals and reduce your risk of cancer. Sulforaphane is produced in cruciferous vegetable plants only when two enzymes in separate "sacs" react, myrosinase and glucoraphanin. Stanford University scientists determined that sulforaphane boosts your levels of these cancer-fighting enzymes higher than any other plant. (270) (271)

Broccoli sprouts are the richest food source of **glucoraphanin**, the precursor to sulforaphane, or SFN, also known as glucoraphanin sulforaphane. Three-day old broccoli sprouts are concentrated sources of this phytochemical, offering 10 to 100 times more of it, by weight, than mature broccoli plants or cauliflower. (271)

Savoy and red cabbage and raw Brussels sprouts are also high in glucosinolates, a sulforaphane precursor. A 1/2-cup serving or 44 g of raw Brussels sproutsprovides approximately 104 mg of total glucosinolates. (271)

Another food-based chemical that has shown promise against cancer stem cells is **phenethyl isothiocyanate (PEITC). This chemical is produced from the reaction of a compound and an enzyme that occur in cruciferous vegetables**, such as broccoli and cabbage. This reaction actually takes place simply when the vegetables are chewed, which means that eating cruciferous vegetables causes the human body to be exposed to PEITC. (272)

Indole-3-carbinol (I3C) Broccoli has long been lauded as an anti-cancer food, largely for its high levels of cancer-fighting plant chemicals called glucosinolates, which the body metabolizes into powerful anticarcinogens. The Carcinogenesis Study recently presented at the National Cancer Research Institute Conference proposed that a naturally occurring phytochemical in cruciferous vegetables called indole-3-carbinol (I3C) may be preventative against cancers of the breast, prostate and ovaries. Scientists from the University of Leicester, believe that I3C may induce apoptosis (programmed cell death) in breast cancer cells. After conducting an in vitro study, the researchers proposed that I3C could also make cancer cells more susceptible to traditional pharmaceutical treatments. (269) (273)

As great as these vegetables are, <u>regular consumption of **raw** cruciferous vegetables is **not** a good idea.</u> There are two reasons to temper your consumption of raw cruciferous vegetables.

1. They contain irritants to the large intestine that, when eaten raw, can cause bloating, gas, and abdominal cramping. These irritants are neutralized by cooking or fermentation (as in the case of sauerkraut or kim-chee). Having raw broccoli or cauliflower with dip at a party once in a while is not a problem, although it might make you feel uncomfortable.

2. The isothiocyanates found in cruciferous vegetables are goitrogenic compounds that have been associated with decreased thyroid function by interfering with the body's ability to use iodine thus depressing the thyroid gland. These compounds can be neutralized by lightly cooking or fermenting.

https://www.womentowomen.com/thyroid-health/goitrogens-and-thyroid-health-the-good-news/

Kale is a top food source for at least **four glucosinolates**, and once kale is eaten and digested, these glucosinolates can be converted by the body into cancer-preventive compounds. Kale's glucosinolates and the isothiocyanates (ITCs) made from them have well-documented cancer-preventive properties, and in some cases, cancer treatment properties as well. New research has shown the ITCs made from kale's glucosinolates can help regulate detoxifying at a genetic level. The ITCs may also help protect the stomach lining from bacterial overgrowth of Helicobacter pylori. (274) Kale contains health-promoting phytochemicals, **sulforaphane** and **indole-3-carbinol,** that appear to protect against prostate and colon cancers.

- **Di-indolyl-methane** (DIM), a metabolite of indole-3-carbinol has been found to be an effective immune modulator, and anti-bacterial and anti-viral agent through its action of potentiating "Interferon-Gamma" receptors.
- Kale is very rich source of **beta carotene**, **lutein** and **zeaxanthin**. These carotenoids have strong anti-oxidant and anti-cancer activities.

249

- This leafy vegetable is a good source of many B-vitamins such as niacin, B-6 (pyridoxine), thiamin, and pantothenic acid that are essential in activating the enzymes necessary for metabolic process to provide energy for the body.
- Kale can provide you with some special cholesterol-lowering benefits if you will cook it by steaming. The <u>fiber-related components in kale do a better job of binding together with bile acids in your digestive tract when they've been slightly cooked</u>.
- Researchers can now identify over 45 different flavonoids in kale. Two flavonoids, kaempferol and quercetin, combine both antioxidant and anti-inflammatory benefits in way that gives kale a leading dietary role with respect to avoidance of chronic inflammation and oxidative stress. (274) (275)

4. **Sprouting Seeds**
Sprouts provide a different form of nutrition than that found in grown vegetables. Broccoli sprouts concentrate phytochemicals found in mature broccoli. Researchers estimate that broccoli sprouts contain 10-100 times the power of mature broccoli to boost enzymes that detoxify potential carcinogens. The reason for these amazing results may be the rich concentration of sulforaphane, which protects against oxidative (free radical) damage in cells. Try various sprouts: broccoli, kale, radish, alfalfa, bean, or sunflower. (276)

5. **Beet root**
Beetsroot provdes a unique source of betalains. Betanin and vulgaxanthin are the two best-studied betalains and have been found to have outstanding anti-inflammatory, antioxidant, and detoxifying effects. Lab studies show <u>betanin pigments can impede tumor cell growth in tissues</u>. Betacyanin, the pigment that gives beets their rich, purple-crimson color, is also a powerful cancer-fighting agent.

- Beet fiber seems to increase the activity of two antioxidant enzymes in the liver, glutathione peroxidase and glutathione-S-transferase.

- Beets are a source of B-vitamins, especially folate, potassium, manganese, iron, copper, phosphorus, and magnesium. (277) Beet root is known:

- to boost the body's natural defenses in the liver, regenerating immune cells
- to accelerate bile secretion
- to accelerate cell growth and restore a cell's nucleus
- to help to regulate blood pressure
- to strengthen skin and vein walls
- to speed the formation of red corpuscles, thus improving cellular oxygenation
- to purify and detoxify the liver, kidneys, and bladder
- to help to relieve constipation
- to have anti-inflammatory activity
- to be one of the best sources of both <u>folate and betaine</u>, which work together to lower your blood levels of homocysteine, an inflammatory compound that can damage your arteries and increase risk of heart disease
- to contain silica, which is vital for healthy skin, fingernails, ligaments, tendons, and bones
- to remove heavy metals and toxins from the brain
- to purify the blood and to have anti-carcinogenic properties (277) (278)

Beet juice was found to be a potent inhibitor of the cell mutations caused by nitrosamines, cancer-causing compounds produced in the stomach from chemicals called nitrates. Nitrates are commonly used as a chemical preservative in processed meats. (278)

Yellow beet root is a source of carotenoids, especially lutein, needed by the eyes.

Eat beets raw by grating into salads or juicing them. Cooking decreases their antioxidant power. Raw beet juice is part of many detoxifying protocols. (278)

6. Avocados
Avocados are nutrient dense, containing essential vitamins, minerals, and phytonutrients. Avocados provide significant amounts of vitamin K, folate, potassium, lutein, magnesium, and vitamin B6.

251

Avocados contain the <u>highest amount of the carotenoid lutein</u> of all commonly eaten fruits, as well as measurable amounts of related carotenoids, zeaxanthin, alpha-carotene and beta-carotene, plus significant quantities of tocopherols (vitamin E). Avocado is a rich source of Beta-Sitosterol. (279)

Carotenoids are fat loving, so combining avocado (a fat) with vegetables increases absorption of carotenoids such as lycopene, lutein, alpha-carotene and beta-carotene from vegetables. A study conducted by researchers at The Ohio State University found:

- Subjects who ate avocado with salsa absorbed nearly 4.5 times more lycopene from the salsa than those who didn't eat avocado.
- Subjects who ate avocado with salad absorbed 8.3 times more alpha-carotene and 13.6 times more beta-carotene from the vegetables than those who didn't eat avocado.
- Subjects who ate avocado with salad absorbed four times more lutein than those who ate only salad.

Avocados are an excellent source of essential fatty acids. 1 cup of avocado contains: 253 milligrams of alpha-linolenic acid, an omega-3 fatty acid, 3886 milligrams of linoleic acid, an omega-6 fatty acid, and oleic acid, a monounsaturated omega-9 fatty acid. (279 (280)

7. <u>Quinoa</u>
Quinoa belongs to the chenopod family, which includes beets, chard, and spinach, and provides an interesting mix of phytonutrients.

It is gluten free and often cooked as a substitute for potatoes or pasta with a meal. Other good news:

- It is high in protein, including <u>all nine essential amino acids, and especially high in the amino acid lysine, which is essential for tissue growth and repair</u>. It is a good protein source for vegetarians.
- Quinoa is low on the glycemic scale, thus helps control blood sugar spikes.

- Quinoa is a good source of magnesium, manganese, folate, and riboflavin and also contains iron, copper, and phosphorus.
- Lignans are in abundance in quinoa. Lignans are converted by friendly flora in our intestines into mammalian lignans, including one called enterolactone that is thought to protect against breast and other hormone-dependent cancers as well as heart disease.
- New research lists several anti-inflammatory phytonutrients in quinoa including: polysaccharides, hydroxycinnamic and hydroxybenzoic acids, flavonoids like quercetin and kaempferol; and saponins including molecules derived from oleanic acid, hederagenin, and serjanic acid.
- Quinoa is higher in fat content than most cereal grasses and provides valuable amounts of heart-healthy fats like monounsaturated fat (in the form of oleic acid). Quinoa provides small amounts of omega-3 fatty acid. (281) (282)

8. <u>Seeds and Nuts</u>

Several types of nuts and seeds are natural sources of **beta-sitosterol**. Pistachio nuts, almonds, hazelnuts, filberts, and macadamia nuts provide 100 to 199 mg per 3.5 oz. serving, while pecans have 96 mg and English walnuts 64 mg. Roasted pumpkin seeds and squash seeds have 13 mg per 3.5 oz. serving. (283)

Nuts and seeds are great sources of protein, essential fatty acids, and minerals. Keep a balance of omegas and eat what fits your type and conditions. (Individuals with herpes may need to avoid nuts high in arginine.)

Flaxseed – There are known to be **27 anti-cancer compounds** including fiber, pectin, vitamin E, magnesium and sitosterol in flaxseeds. (285) Elaine Magee on Webmd asks, "Is flaxseed the new wonder food? Preliminary studies show that it may help fight heart disease, diabetes and breast cancer". (284) Flax hull lignans contain some of the most promising anti-cancer phytochemical lignans known to man. (285)

Recent research has found flaxseed lignans have anti-tumor, antioxidant, and weak estrogenic activity. They are potentially the richest source of phytoestrogens in the human diet. In addition to having anti-cancer properties, lignans also have anti-viral, anti-bacterial, and anti-fungus properties. (285)

Flaxseed is an excellent source of lignans, which, when converted in the gut to phytosterols, deactivate potent estrogens and testosterones that contribute to cancer growth. Flaxseed seems to encourage the creation of good estrogen, while at the same time discouraging bad estrogen from developing. Eating about an ounce of ground flaxseed each day will affect the way estrogen is handled in postmenopausal women in such a way that offers protection against breast cancer, but will not interfere with estrogen's role in normal bone maintenance. Two tablespoons of ground flaxseed contain 3.5 grams of omega-3s, a healthy serving of magnesium, fiber, and high lignan content. (285)

Flaxseed hulls contain potent nutrients that have the potential to enhance immune system functioning and are effective against many different cancers as well as diabetes, lupus, and other chronic disease. (286)

Lignans in the hulls of flaxseed are also a good source of alpha-linolenic acid, which is converted by the body into omega-3 fatty acids. Omega-3 fatty acids improve cell function in the lining of the heart and blood vessels, lower triglyceride levels, and inhibit platelet clumping. Omega-3 fats are used by the body to produce Series 1 and 3 prostaglandins, which are anti-inflammatory hormone-like molecules which can reduce the inflammation that is a significant factor in conditions such as asthma, osteoarthritis, rheumatoid arthritis, and migraine headaches. (286)

Flaxseed may also protect against radiation. A study from the Perelman School of Medicine at the University of Pennsylvania found that flaxseed might also have a role in protecting healthy tissues and organs from exposure to radiation and significantly reduces damage even after exposure. (287)

Since the valuable lignans in flaxseed are found in the outer shell of the seeds, when the seeds are refined into oil **only a trace of the lignans ends up in the finished oil.** Although pressing the oil increases the concentration of alpha-linolenic acid (ALA), the **valuable lignans are NOT in the oil**. **Unrefined organic flaxseed oil contains around 55% Omega-3.** The American Dietetic Association lists flaxseed oil as the richest source of ALA (alpha linolenic acid), the parent compound of Omega-3 fats. ALA is converted in the body to EPA (eicosapentaenoic acid) and DHA (docosahexaenoic acid). (286). Flaxseed oil is very perishable and goes rancid easily, so keep it refrigerated.

I personally use flaxseed oil in detoxifying but choose to use ground flaxseed each day for the whole complex of nutrients. I grind enough flaxseed for a few days and keep it in a glass jar in the refrigerator so it stays fresh and is ready for whatever I decide to concoct. My favorite uses are: on cereal or plain yogurt with fresh fruit; in a smoothie, sprinkled on salads, or tossed on a casserole as it comes out of the oven. In baking I add it muffins, cookies, crackers, or breads.

Chia seed - Many people have not been introduced to this powerhouse food the Aztec warriors used as they went into battle. The word "chia" comes from the Mayan language meaning strength. Chia seeds are a balanced blend of protein, carbohydrates, fats, nutrients, and fiber. It is said that 1 tablespoon of chia can sustain a person for 24 hours. Athletes have reported that chia seeds help them perform at optimal levels for much longer periods of time. (288)

Chia seed is a very important food for a storage plan.

- Chia seeds have one of highest levels of Omega-3 of plants tested, naturally containing more than 60% Omega-3 fatty acid. The body converts Omega-3 from chia into EPA and DHA. The high concentration of Omega-3 helps to lubricate joints and keep them supple. Additionally, Omega-3s are converted into prostaglandins, which are known to have both pain relieving and anti-inflammatory effects.

- Chia seeds are a complete protein source providing <u>all the essential amino acids.</u> Compared to other seeds and grains, chia seed provides the highest source of protein, between 19 to 23 percent protein by weight.
- One of the exceptional qualities of the chia seed is its hydrophilic properties, having the ability to absorb more than 12 times its weight in water. Its ability to hold onto water offers the ability to prolong hydration. Fluids and electrolytes provide the environment that supports the life of all the body's cells.
- The soluble fiber in chia seed cleans the intestines by transporting debris from the intestinal walls so that it can be eliminated efficiently and regularly.
- Chia contains Vitamin C and Vitamin E, but the real secret is the cinnamic acids that guard the Omega-3 oils from oxidation.
- Chia seeds supply significant amounts of iron, calcium, niacin, magnesium, zinc and phosphorus.
- Chia seeds are an excellent source of antioxidants, containing even more antioxidants than fresh blueberries.
- Chia seeds contain strontium which is needed for healthy bones, helps to assimilate protein, and produces high energy. (288) (289)

<u>How to use chia seed:</u> Whole chia seeds can be sprinkled on your cereal, salads, or yogurt. Seeds can also be ground and mixed into smoothies or added to baked goods. I like to add 3 tablespoons of seed to a pint of purified water and stir often with a fork so it doesn't clump. Keep this chia gel in the refrigerator to add to cereals, smoothies, baking, puddings, etc.

Chia is not just for people, but dogs, cats and even horses will benefit by the elements found in the seed and oil.

Sesame seeds have the highest total phytosterol content of all nuts and seeds, while English walnuts and Brazil nuts have the lowest. The seeds are:

- especially rich in <u>mono-unsaturated fatty acid oleic acid</u> which comprise up to 50% fatty acids.
- a very good source of dietary proteins with fine quality amino acids that are essential for growth. Just 100 g of seeds provide about 18 g of protein.
- a very good source of manganese, calcium, and copper, they are also a good source of magnesium, iron, phosphorous, zinc, selenium, and dietary fiber.
- a very good source of B-complex vitamins such as niacin, folic acid, thiamin (vitamin B1), pyridoxine (vitamin B6) and riboflavin. (290) (291)
- a rich source of the lignan, sesamin. <u>New research indicates that a "novel synergistic effect" of newly discovered lignans interacting with vitamin E accounts for "the anti-aging effect of sesame."</u> The lignans evidently help prevent the decomposition of sesame tocopherols (vitamin E compounds), preserving the antioxidant potency of vitamin E. According to a Japanese review of sesame research, "Sesame lignans also showed other useful functions, such as acceleration of alcohol decomposition in the liver, antihypertensive activity, immunoregulatory activities, anticarcinogenic activity, and others." (292)

Hemp seed - <u>Shelled hemp</u> seed is basically 34.6% protein, 46.5% fat, and 11.6% carbohydrate. Few other plant sources provide balanced protein with <u>all the essential amino acids in a favorable ratio for digestibility</u>. <u>Shelled seed</u> is 40% more nutritious than whole hempseed. When the hull is removed, the percentage of essential nutrients rises. The protein content increases by 8% (to more than 30%), and the total fat content goes up 17% (to more than 47%). The ratio of EFAs remains the same, though. (293)

Shelled hemp seeds are unique because they have the **correct ratio ofessential amino acids**. 65% of the protein occurs as the easily digestible storage protein, edestin, and 35% of the protein content is albumin. Edestin is so compatible with the human digestive system that in 1955 a Czechoslovakian Tuberculosis Nutrition

Study found hemp seed to be the <u>only food that</u> <u>successfully treated tuberculosis,</u> a disease in which nutritive processes become impaired and the body wastes away. (294)

Shelled hemp seeds contain <u>essential amino acids</u> with a high content of <u>sulfur-containing methionine and cysteine,</u> <u>which are usually low in vegetable proteins.</u> The absence of trypsin inhibitory activity is a major advantage over the type of protein found in soybeans. (293)

The globulins contained in hemp seeds are one of the seven classes of 100% pure amino acids. Globulins make up the portion of seed between the embryo and the seed coat, and they are a fraction of all animal and human blood. Edestin globulin comes from seed; globulin is in blood plasma. Globulin and albumin are classified as globular proteins. All the enzymes, antibodies, many hormones, hemoglobin, and fibrogin are made from globular proteins. (293)

<u>Shelled hemp seed provides</u>:
- The perfect ratio of omega fatty acids (3 omega-3`s to 1 omega-6)
- Major minerals: potassium, calcium, sulfur, iron, and zinc. It is especially high in magnesium.
- Important trace elements found including strontium, thorium, arsenic, and chromium
- High levels of B-vitamins
- A good source of the antioxidant vitamin E in the form of alpha-, beta-, gamma-, delta-tocopherol and alpha-tocotrienol
- A source of lecithin, a type of liquid found in the protective sheaths surrounding the brain and nervous system. Lecithin helps in the breakdown of fats and enhances liver activity and enzyme production.
- Choline, which is produced from lecithin. It is needed for nerve impulses from the brain throughout the nervous system and for liver and gall bladder function.
- Inositol, which promotes hair growth, reduces cholesterol levels, prevents artery hardening, and is calming to the nervous system.

- Phytosterols or phytoestrogens that affect cholesterol absorption, hormone regulation, and cell metabolism
- A good source of dietary fiber. (293)

Hemp seed is low on the glycemic index.

Hemp seed is NOT PSYCHOACTIVE and cannot be used as a drug. (293)

Raw Pumpkin seeds (papitas) provide a wide variety of nutrients for overall health. They are:
- the most alkaline-forming seed.
- approximately one-third good quality protein. (100 g seeds provide 30 g of protein).
- a source of monounsaturated fat They are high in omega-6, <u>so balance with a food high in omega-3.</u>
- a good source of vitamin K
- a good source of vitamin E containing about 35.10 mg of tocopherol per 100 g.
- an excellent source of B vitamins: thiamin, riboflavin, niacin, pantothenic acid, vitamin B-6 and folates.
- a good source of minerals including zinc, phosphorus, magnesium, manganese, iron and copper. (296) (297)
- high in zinc content, which reduces the risk of osteoporosis. (298) Zinc stimulates immune function and is important for good prostate health. (299)
- a good source of magnesium, which is needed by the body for over 300 actions including the creation of ATP (adenosine triphosphate, the energy molecules of your body), the synthesis of RNA and DNA, the pumping of your heart, proper bone and tooth formation, relaxation of your blood vessels, and proper bowel function.
- a source of **L-tryptophan,** which helps with good sleep and with lowering depression. Tryptophan is converted into serotonin and niacin. Serotonin helps us sleep.
- a source of cucurbitacins, a chemical substance in pumpkin seeds, known to prevent the body from converting testosterone into a much more potent form of this hormone called dihydrotestosterone. Without dihydrotestosterone, it is more difficult for the body to

produce more prostate cells, and therefore more difficult for the prostate to keep enlarging. (296) They are:

- very effective as a vermicide. They are known to paralyze intestinal parasites like tapeworms, helping to expel them from the body. An old German cure for intestinal worms was ground pumpkin seeds mixed with milk and honey. (298)
- very low on the glycemic index.
- a good source of fiber
- a good source of monounsaturated fat, but low in omega-3's and high in omega-6.

Except where noted the sources for above section are (296) (297) (299)

The phytosterols inpumpkin seeds are known to lower cholesterol. Pumpkin seeds also reduce inflammation in arthritis without the side effects. (299)

Amaranth seed has nine amino acids, but is missing histidine and is low in leucine and threonin, but contains high levels of **lysine** and **methionine**, two essential amino acids that are not commonly found in grains or other plant sources.

Amaranth is a good source of:

- important **minerals**. The seeds provide five times the iron and calcium of whole wheat and they have twice as much magnesium. Amaranth seeds contain twice as much magnesium as calcium, which is significant because most grains are higher in calcium.
- vitamins B2, B3, and B5 and a very good source of vitamin B6 and folic acid.
- **tocotrienols, a vitamin E fraction** with numerous cardiovascular benefits, including cholesterol-lowering activity in humans.
- **fiber content** that is 25 percent higher than whole wheat.
- has significant amounts of **phytosterols, especially beta sitosterol,** which may reduce high cholesterol and decrease symptoms of an enlarged prostate.

Research is showing beta sitosterol may play a big role in preventing chronic degenerative disease. (300) (301)

Cumin (Cuminum cyminum) – seeds are used as food and medicine.Cumin seeds have the ability to increase glutathione tissue levels. **Glutathione** is not only the master antioxidant, but is a major factor in detoxification. Glutathione binds to toxins such as heavy metals, solvents, and pesticides, and transforms them into a form that can be excreted in urine or bile. Scientists have recently proved cumin to have anti-cancer properties, as it has the ability to kill free radicals. (302)Nutritional factors include:

- Cumin seeds are a rich source of many flavonoid phenolic anti-oxidants such as carotenes, zea-xanthin, and lutein.
- They contain very good amounts of B-complex vitamins such as thiamin, vitamin B-6, niacin, riboflavin, and other vital anti-oxidant vitamins like vitamin E, vitamin A, and vitamin C.
- Cumin seeds are excellent sources of minerals like iron, copper, calcium, potassium, manganese, selenium, zinc and magnesium. (303)

Medicinal Properties of Cumin seed:

Alterative	Disinfectant
Anticongestive	Diuretic
Antifungal	Emmenogogue
Antimicrobial	Expectorant
Antioxidant	Hepatic
Carminative	Stimulant
Decongestive	Relaxant

(302) (304)

As a medicinal: Cumin seeds such contain health-benefiting essential oils as cuminaldehyde (4-isopropylbenzaldehyde), pyrazines, 2-methoxy-3-sec-butylpyrazine, 2-ethoxy-3-isopropylpyrazine, and 2-methoxy-3-methylpyrazine.

Cumin seeds:

- Act as a bronchodilator, anti-congestive, & expectorant, for respiratory disorders

261

- Are used as a gargle to treat laryngitis
- May help the body reduce blood glucose levels and increase insulin sensitivity
- May decrease cognitive disorders
- May reduce total cholesterol, triglycerides, and pancreatic inflammation
- Increase your metabolism and improve the absorption of nutrients
- May improve immune response
- May, in extract form, increase bone density and improved bone structure
- Are used as poultices to treat swellings of the breasts or testicles (302) (305)

Cumin is high in fiber and contains a compound that stimulates your digestive system to secrete bile acids and pancreatic enzymes that aid the digestive process. The benefits of cumin **enhance the liver's detoxification** enzyme, and **act like a natural laxative** that can help in treating constipation. (305)

**Cumin can be grown in many areas, but in climates with short growing seasons it must be started inside to ensure a seed harvest.

9. Legumes
This category includes the most common beans (kidney, red, black, white, pinto), chickpeas (garbanzo beans), soybeans, dried peas, lentils, lima beans, and black-eyed peas.

Beans and lentils are great foods, but I discovered we don't all digest all legumes well. It seems to depend on your blood type. For information on which legumes to eat for your blood type visit http://www.mercola.com/forms/beans_legumes.htm. (306)

Beans are unique because they are high protein foods but also have significant phytonutrients.
- Except for soybeans, legumes do NOT provide all the essential amino acids so must be served with a food that provides those missing amino acids, such as corn

or grains, if you're not eating meat at the same meal. (307)

- Legumes have varying phytonutrient content. In general, beans and lentils have the same potent anti-inflammatory antioxidants—flavonoids and flavonals—found in tea, fruits, grapes, red wine and cocoa beans. In particular, the reddish and darker flavonal pigments in bean and lentil seed coats exert more antioxidant activity, 50 times greater than vitamin E. Black beans have more antioxidant activity than other beans. (307) (308)
- One study found anthocyanins were the most active antioxidants in the beans. The level of anthocyanins in black beans was about 10 times the amount of overall antioxidants in an equivalent serving of oranges and similar to the amount found in an equivalent serving of grapes, apples, and cranberries. (308)
- Legumes are good sources of selenium, zinc, phosphorus, calcium, potassium, folate, and molybdenum. (307)
- Beans are among the richest food sources of saponins, chemicals that help prevent undesirable genetic mutations. (307)
- Legumes are low in fat (except for soybeans) but high in complex carbohydrates and dietary fiber. (307)

There are individual differences among the nutrients in various legumes, so plan to use a variety in your meal planning. There is more information on soybeans in the "Proteins/Amino Acid" section.

10. Buckwheat
Though buckwheat is usually thought of as a grain, it is actually the seed of a broadleaf plant related to rhubarb. Buckwheat has many health providing qualities.

- Buckwheat is only about 11% protein, but is considered a "complete protein" because it has the 8 essential amino acids in the proper proportion. It is especially high in lysine and arginine.

- It is high in minerals: especially zinc, copper, and manganese.
- It has a low fat content which is mostly monounsaturated fatty acids—the type that makes olive oil so heart-healthful.
- It is largely insoluble similar to the fiber in oats which is considered heart-healthy.
- It contains <u>no</u> gluten.
- It is high in magnesium providing 86 milligrams per one-cup serving.
- It is also high in "resistant starch," which enhances colon health, and serves to reduce blood sugar levels.
- It contains <u>rare carbohydrate compounds called fagopyritols (especially D-chiro-inositol), of which buckwheat is by far the richest food source yet discovered</u>. They are known to reduce blood glucose levels in diabetic rats, a promising finding that should lead to similar research in human diabetics.
- Buckwheat has significant flavonoids, particularly rutin, which extends the action of vitamin C, and provides lipid-lowering activity. <u>Rutin also acts as an ACE inhibitor</u> contributing to buckwheat's ability to reduce high blood pressure.
- It contains lignans which are converted to beneficial flora in the intestines.

Sources for above material (309) (310).

Soba noodles popular in Asia and used in the US as a wheat substitute in gluten-free diets are made from buckwheat. (Check ingredient labels, as I found some soba noodles also had wheat.)

11. Raw Chocolate (Cacao)
Until recent years we had no idea of the valuable nutrients in chocolate, including antioxidants, protein, essential minerals, and beta-sitosterol. (311)

Raw chocolate (or cacao) contains the highest concentration of antioxidants in the world.

These antioxidants include flavonoids such as polyphenols, catechins, and epicatechins, the same antioxidants that are present in red wine and green tea. (311)

- Dark chocolate with at least 45 to 69 percent cacao solids contains significant amounts of beta-sitosterol. Scientific studies suggest that beta-sitosterol may offer certain health benefits. (312) Studies show the flavonols in cacao stimulate your body's <u>production of nitric oxide, boosting blood flow to your heart, brain, and other organs</u>. One study found **cacao thins your blood just as well as low-dose aspirin!** Wow!
- **Cacao is one of the best food sources of magnesium** and is a good source of potassium, iron, zinc, manganese, copper, the trace mineral, chromium, phenethylamine, tryptophan, and serotonin.
- Cacao is the only plant found so far that is a source of Anandamide, an endorphin that the human body naturally produces after exercise. Anandamide is known as the "bliss chemical" because it's released in your brain when you're feeling great.
- Cacao usually contains about 1% theobromine a chemical relative of caffeine, but is not a stimulant. Theobromine dilates the cardiovascular system and is one of the major reasons why cacao is a valuable part of a heart-healthy diet. Theobromine is also an effective anti-bacterial substance that kills the primary bacteria that cause cavities.

Today we have a variety of choices in the cacao content of dark chocolate and powdered cocoa. Unsweetened baking chocolate is even healthier, with 66 to 86 mg of beta-sitosterol per 3.5 oz serving. (311) (312) The secret is to find chocolate with the highest cacao and least sugar for your purposes.

12. <u>Fermented and Cultured Foods</u>

Most of us are familiar with yogurt, kefir, and sauerkraut, which are all great cultured foods if properly made. We want to avoid products with added sugars or anything processed. Even adding salt, which is antimicrobial, can

265

interfere with the culturing process in which we want the good bacteria to grow.

Weston A. Price, the nutritional pioneer who studied and observed isolated cultures around the world, discovered that cultured foods were an integral part of most, if not all native diets. His findings revealed that traditional peoples cultured everything from grains, seafood, and flesh meats, to dairy products, fruits and vegetables. (313)

There's growing evidence that there's a special connection between the gut and the brain. They found that giving probiotics can cause changes in mood and mental health, suggesting these "good" bacteria might have potential as a treatment for depression and other psychiatric maladies. (314)

In Gut and Psychology Syndrome, Dr. Natasha Campbell-McBride, MD draws great correlations between the health of the gut and many of the learning disabilities that children develop such as autism. (315)

Today, we know that the regular consumption of cultured foods introduces beneficial microbes into the intestinal track to aid in digestion and detoxification, provide enzymes, vitamins and minerals, balance our internal bio-systems, and boost immunity. The sour flavor of cultured foods will help curb cravings for sweets and other processed, devitalized foods. (316)

What are Raw Cultured Vegetables? Raw cultured vegetables are unheated, cultured (which refers to the fermentation process) vegetables that have been either cut, ground, or shredded and left in a sanitary container for a about a 7 day period at a temperature maintained in the range of 59° to 71°. This process allows for the proliferation of lactobacilli (healthful micro-flora that are naturally present in vegetables and also in our digestive tract), which break down the sugars and starches found in the vegetables, aiding the pancreas and intestines in proper digestion. The difference between raw cultured vegetables and commercially available heated sauerkraut is that the heat destroys much of the lactobacilli and healthful enzymes. As long as they are refrigerated and eaten within six months of being created, raw cultured vegetables are a flavorful self-sustaining culture of these essential enzymes and lactobacillus cultures that do not dissipate with reasonable shelf life. (317)

Caution: If you want to culture your own vegetables I recommend you use one of these two books as your guide. If the process is not done correctly in very sanitary conditions unwanted pathogens may develop.
Body Ecology Diet by Donna Gates
Nourishing Traditions by Sally Fallon

13. Other Foods to Include in your Diet
Apple Cider Vinegar
Before we begin with the accolades for Apple Cider Vinegar (ACV) I must caution you that for some people especially O Blood Types, ACV may not work as well for you as for others. I kept trying to make it work for me, but I finally realized that NO vinegar is good for me. (318)

It is important to use only raw, organic apple cider vinegar, the kind with the "mother" (looks like cobwebs in the vinegar) in the bottom of the bottle. The two step fermentation process that apples go through to form vinegar retains all the nutritional benefits of the apples plus gaining the extra acids and enzymes from fermentation. (319)

Real raw, organic apple cider vinegar:
- is rich in potassium, phosphorus, organic sodium, magnesium, sulphur, iron, copper, natural fluorine, silicon and other trace minerals
- is rich in malic acid, which plays an essential role in the production of energy and helps remove high levels of phosphorous and aluminum from the body.
- has been used for centuries as an energizing tonic and elixir. It is thought that apple cider vinegar has such curative abilities because it causes one's pH levels to become more alkaline.

267

- has anti-fungal, anti-bacterial, and anti-viral properties, primarily coming from the malic acid and acetic acid portion of the vinegar. It is a natural antibiotic germ fighter which fights E Coli and other bacteria. (319) (320) (321)

Many people feel their ACV/ honey tonic every morning really helps them. To save tooth enamel drink ACV mixtures through a straw.

Don't be confused by the <u>distilled</u> apple cider vinegar, which is clear and pretty but little more than a flavoring. In the distilling process it lost whatever positive characteristics it had. Some imitations of apple cider vinegar include colored distilled white vinegar. Read the labels.

Below are several <u>external</u> applications in common use:
1. When diluted with water 50/50, it is often used as a toner for the face. Caution should be used when applying as cider vinegar is very dangerous to the eyes.
2. A bath of apple cider vinegar is said to reduce the effects of sunburn. If the sunburn is localized, a vinegar-soaked cloth applied to sunburn may also help.
3. Many women have tried a douche of apple cider vinegar as a remedy for yeast infections.
4. It is known to prevent dandruff and itching scalp.
5. Apple cider vinegar can be used as a cleanser. (319)

For more about the uses of apple cider vinegar you might want to read the book <u>The Miracles of Apple Cider Vinegar Health System</u> by Paul and Patricia Bragg or search online.

Molasses
Molasses is the syrup that remains after the sugar has been extracted from sugar cane or beet juice. Regular molasses is the first or second boiling of cane sugar syrup, while blackstrap is the third boiling of the syrup.

Unsuphured blackstrap molasses is the thickest form of molasses, the darkest, and the most dense including calcium, copper, iron, magnesium, manganese, potassium, and selenium. It contains all the minerals, vitamins and trace elements lost in the refining process that makes refined sugar such an empty food. (322)

A tablespoon of blackstrap molasses contains:
- as much calcium as a glass of milk
- as much iron as ten small eggs
- more potassium than virtually any other food
- minerals such as magnesium, manganese, and copper
- B vitamins and vitamin E (323)

Blackstrap molasses can offer a temporary energy boost by providing carbohydrates that are quickly converted into energy in the body. Being high in iron, it can also increase your energy by helping to replenish your iron stores. Often menstruating women are more at risk for iron deficiency, so boosting iron stores with blackstrap molasses is a good idea. Iron is an integral component of hemoglobin, which transports oxygen from the lungs to all body cells and is also part of key enzyme systems for energy production and metabolism. Pregnant or lactating women find their need for iron has increased. Growing children and adolescents also have increased needs for iron, especially adolescent girls. (322) (324)

Being a good source of variety of minerals, blackstrap molasses is important for bone health. The great late Dr. John Christopher believed that just three tablespoons of blackstrap molasses would greatly improve the following conditions. (325)
- Arthritis
- Ulcers
- Dermatitis and eczema
- High blood pressure
- Constipation and colitis
- Varicose veins
- Anemia
- Bladder troubles
- Nerve damage

Dr. John Christopher recommended 1 teaspoon to 1 tablespoon of blackstrap molasses in water per day. (325)

Raw Honey and Bee Products

- Raw honey provides quick energy
- Raw honey has phenolics, which have antioxidant properties. The darker the honey the more antioxidants.
- Honey is a source of minerals like magnesium, potassium, calcium, sodium chlorine, sulfur, iron and phosphoorus..
- Honey contains vitamins B1, B2, C, B6, B5 and B3, as well as C, D, E, K and beta-carotene, and enzymes, all of which change according to the qualities of the nectar and pollen.
- Raw honey contains antibiotic and antiviral capabilities, which prevent infections by killing the bacteria in and around your wounds and on burns. Honey's ability to heal wounds and treat infections has been used by many cultures through the years. Material above (328)

Caution- Honey contains a **bacterium that might be harmful in infants**. Honey should never be fed to children younger than one year old, as it could lead to food poisoning.

Royal jelly is a creamy white secretion produced by worker honey bees for the queen bee. It typically contains about 60% to 70% water, 12% to 15% proteins, 10% to 16% sugar, 3% to 6% fats, and 2% to 3% vitamins, salts, and amino acids. Its composition varies depending on geography and climate. This product gets its name from the fact that bees use it for the development and nurturing of queen bees. (331)

Royal jelly is considered to be a superfood for humans because it is rich in nutrients, especially acetylcholine, and is believed to invigorate mental clarity and to improve memory. Royal jelly is the only compound in nature that contains pure acetylcholine. (331)

Bee Propolis is created by honey bees from resins collected from various plants and trees. They mix the resins with beeswax and amino acids and use the mixture to form structures within the hive, similar to the way that we use cement. (333)

In its rawest form bee propolis has up to 500 times more bioflavonoids than oranges. **Propolis has antibiotic, antifungal, antibacterial, antiseptic, antifungal and antiviral properties**. It is a valued wound healer, immune stimulant, and it is even being used on certain types of cancers. (333)

8. Proteins, Amino Acids, Fats, and Carbohydrates

The importance of amino acids is often overlooked.
I was astounded to learn there are approximately 40,000 distinct proteins which must be made from only 20 amino acids to provide for all the needs of the body. Amino acids can best be described as the construction blocks from which protein is made.

There are nine amino acids generally regarded as essential for humans, which means they must be supplied by their diet. They are tryptophan, lysine, methionine, phenylalanine, threonine, valine, leucine, histidine, and isoleucine. Nonessential amino acids that can be synthesized in the body are alanine, aspartic acid, arginine, asparagine, GABA, cysteine, glutamic acid, glutamine, proline, serine, and tyrosine.

When we eat foods with dietary protein it is broken down into its amino acid forms which are then used by the body to **build specific proteins** as needed. Amino acids from proteins are used to make **neurotransmitters** that allow your brain to network and communicate.

Neurotransmitters are the brain chemicals that motivate or sedate, focus or frustrate. **Amino acids can excite or calm your brain as well as nourish your brain throughout its lifetime**

Proteins are substances, which make up muscles, tendons, ligaments, organs, glands, nails, hair, vital body fluids, and bones. Enzymes and hormones which regulate bodily process are actually proteins. Proteins form the structural basis of chromosomes, through which our genetic information is passed from parent to offspring. As you can see, proteins are really an essential component of all aspects of the body.

The more than 20 amino acids each have unique characteristics and yet are capable of being fitted together into an almost limitless variety of proteins. Amino acids have a direct interaction with vitamins and minerals. **Amino acids enable vitamins and minerals to perform**

272

their specific jobs in the body properly. (335) Source for
the section on amino acids above.)

Amino acids work on virtually every infection including even MRSA and CRKP.

Therefore, by eating a variety of foods like nuts, grass-fed
meats and dairy products, beans, and seafood you will
provide the body with the needed amino acids to fight
infection. (336)

**Amino acids are needed for cell growth, maintenance
and repair.** Eating too little protein can be very serious,
as <u>all the body systems need protein</u> to keep structurally
sound and to function. <u>After just three days without
protein your body will begin to break down muscle and
vital organ to meet its daily protein needs.</u>, You can only
survive so many days without protein before you'll literally
eat your body from the inside out! (335)

<u>A complete protein includes all of the essential amino
acids.</u> Good quality, organic meats have the essential
amino acids and need to be a part of the diet. Most
vegetable proteins are incomplete providing only some of
the amino acids. However, as we learned in "Superfoods,"
spirulina, quinoa, chia seed, hemp seed, buckwheat,
purslane, and wheatgrass have all the essential amino
acids in the proper proportion. (337)

Can people get too much protein? Usually not, if eating
quality protein foods with a variety of vegetables. The
extreme use of body builder proteins, liquid protein
drinks, or foods containing mostly textured soy protein
can put an extra burden on the body. Concentrated
protein products should not replace eating proper meals,
because they may give you an imbalance of amino acids.

<u>Magnesium</u> is necessary for the synthesis of protein, so
the protein you are eating may not be fully utilized by the
body if there is a magnesium deficiency. Magnesium
deficiency is estimated to be as high as 68% in the US.
(338)

We often take for granted that our bodies will do what needs to be done to keep us healthy without realizing the importance of giving it the needed nutrients. Below are a few examples to help you understand what individual amino acids contribute to your health.

Lysine
- Lysine is a basic building block for all protein in the body.
- Lysine is necessary for helping the immune system produce antibodies necessary for warding off viral infections.
- Lysine is beneficial for regulating glands.
- It assists in controlling acid/alkaline balance and with the assimilation of all amino acids.
- Lysine enhances the assimilation and absorption of calcium and ensures the formation of cartilage, bone, connective tissues, and collagen.
- Lysine helps to build muscle and repair tissues.
- Lysine specifically inhibits the replication of the herpes virus.
- Lysine is necessary for niacin metabolism. A lysine deficiency can result in the niacin deficiency disease pellagra. (339) (340)

Caution: If you are pregnant or breastfeeding, or have heart disease consult your health care professional before using L-lysine supplement.

Tryptophan is an essential amino acid that is transformed into important stress-protective neurotransmitters such as serotonin and melatonin. "Serotonin deficiency syndrome" is one of the most common and widespread disorders in human psychobiology in the today's world. Studies of humans and animals conducted over the past 30 years show that serotonin nerve circuits that promote feelings of well-being, calm, personal security, relaxation, confidence and concentration may be not reaching the brain due to a lack of tryptophan. (341)

274

Tryptophan is found in protein foods and is particularly plentiful in chocolate, oats, bananas, dried date, milk, cottage cheese, meat, fish, turkey and peanuts. However, tryptophan is heat sensitive and therefore is absent in conventionally-processed foods. For a better understanding of the role of tryptophan please see "L – Tryptophan - Nature's answer to Prozac," by James South MA at http://smart-drugs.net/ias-tryptophan-article.htm

Work with a practitioner to find if you need to supplement with tryptophan.

Carnosine is an important dipeptide, or small protein, made up of two amino acids, alanine and histidine, which are responsible for its <u>antioxidant action</u>. Carnosine is found in all protein-rich **animal products** such as dairy products, eggs, beef, poultry, and pork.

- Carnosine has been found to have incredible healing properties.
- Carnosine has been shown to be useful in children with autism for improving speech, socialization and behavior.
- Carnosine can oppose glycation which is a process where sugar and protein molecules combine to form a tangled mess of tissue. Glycated tissue is tough and inflexible, leading to wrinkling not only of the skin, but also of important internal organs.
- Carnosine has been shown to retard cancer growth.
- Carnosine is neuroprotective against permanent cerebral damage.
- It protects against alcohol-induced oxidative stressand chronic liver damage.
- It has been found to inhibit diabetic nephropathy.
- It has been found to be helpful in chelating heavy metals out of the body.
- It's been found to be beneficial in preventing and treating cataracts of the eyes and cloudiness in the eyes. (343)

Glutamine (NOT to be confused with glutamate)
(344) (345)

- Glutamine has marked anti-inflammatory and moderate analgesic activity.
- Glutamine is used at a high metabolic rate by both lymphocytes and macrophages.
- Immune suppression can result when levels of glutamine are decreased in both muscle and plasma during sepsis, injury, burns, surgery, and even endurance exercise.
- Probably glutamine's greatest benefit is in assisting intestinal integrity. It prevents deterioration of gut permeability, which is so important for absorption of nutrients as well as immune health.
- Glutamine provides life-saving action in hepatic damage from drugs such as acetaminophen.
- Glutamine is important in the production of muscle tissue.

Food sources of glutamine include: cabbage, spinach, beets, beef, chicken, fish, beans, and dairy products.

Taurine (346) (347) is the most abundant of all the amino acids present in humans, but it is also deficient in more people than any other amino acid. Taurine must be synthesized from methionine, which is found in greatest concentration **only** in animal products. The conversion of methionine to cysteine and then to taurine requires vitamin B-6; therefore, if vitamin B-6 is deficient, not enough taurine will be produced.

- Taurine plays a major metabolic role in regulation of the electrical charge on cell membranes, a role synergistic with magnesium.
- Taurine drastically counteracts or down-regulates the body's stress reaction, helping stabilize carbohydrate metabolism, insulin levels and epinephrine levels, and muscle tension.
- As a mild sedative to the nervous system, taurine assists in reducing pain, as well as assisting in regulation of serotonin, prolactin, growth hormone, immune function, and cholesterol metabolism.

- Taurine is also necessary for the management of potassium levels in tissues such as the heart.
- Recent research indicates that taurine may be a very important amino acid for thinning bile.
- Heart muscle and the retina of the eye contain the highest concentration of taurine, but high levels are also found within white blood cells.
- Deficiency of taurine may alter immune functions and increase the cells' susceptibilities to damage from free radicals.
- Taurine has recently been used therapeutically for such problems as epilepsy, cardiac arrhythmias, and cholesterol-saturated bile. (348)

Vegetables and grains do not contain taurine. It is found only in animal products. (347)

Meat, poultry, seafood, and eggs provide all the essential amino acids. Many sources recommend soy products for people who don't eat meat. From my studies, it seems only fermented soy products are a good choice.

The foods below are not only **good plant protein sources of the essential amino acids**, but are also high in antioxidants and essential fatty acids. So far my study has found the following plant foods are complete proteins, thus having **all the essential amino acids in the proper proportions.** (349)

Spirulina	Hemp seed	Wheatgrass
Quinoa	Buckwheat	Wolfberries
Chia seed	Purslane	(Goji berry)

Eating a variety of incomplete sources, such as beans, peas, lentils, whole grains, nuts, seeds, and vegetables, throughout the day should provide the essentials. However, I have found the type and amount of protein needed by your body is somewhat determined by your blood type. We are all different and have different nutritional needs.

Spirulina and chorella (blue-green algae) are over 60 percent protein.

Sprouted seeds - each type of sprout has differing proportions of nutrients, so it's best to eat a variety of sprouts.

Common Plant Sources of Essential Amino Acids
Histidine: Apple, pomegranates, alfalfa, beets, carrots, celery, cucumber, dandelion, endive, garlic, radish, spinach, turnip greens

Arginine: Alfalfa, beets, carrots, celery, cucumbers, green vegetables, leeks, lettuce, potatoes, radishes, parsnips, nutritional yeast

Valine: Apples, almonds, pomegranates, beets, carrots, celery, dandelion greens, lettuce, okra, parsley, parsnips, squash, tomatoes, turnips, nutritional yeast

Tryptophan: Alfalfa, Brussels sprouts, carrots, celery, chives, dandelion greens, endive, fennel, snap beans, spinach, turnips, nutritional yeast

Threnoine: Papayas, alfalfa sprouts, carrots, green leafy vegetables such as celery, collards, kale, and lettuce (especially iceberg), lima beans, Nori, a sea vegetable

Phenylalanine: Apples, pineapples, beets, carrots, parsley, spinach, tomatoes, nutritional yeast

Methionine: Apples, pineapples, Brazil nuts, filberts, brussels sprouts, cabbage, cauliflower, chives, dock (sorrel), garlic, horseradish, kale, watercress

Lysine: Lima beans, kidney beans, potatoes, corn, apples, apricots, grapes, papayas, pears, alfalfa, beets, carrots, celery, cucumber, dandelion greens, parsley, spinach, turnip greens

Leucine: Avocados, papayas, olives, coconut, sunflower seeds

Isoleucine: Avocados, papayas, olives, coconut, sunflower seeds (349)

Amino acid deficiencies affect every tissue in the body, most importantly in the brain. The best reading I've found on understanding proteins is Heal with Amino Acids and Nutrients by Billie J. Sahley, Ph.D., C.N.C. and Katehrine M. Birkner, C.R.N.A.,Ph.D.

Red meat is not the enemy!

From years of study and evaluating the research, I feel red meat has gotten a bad rap. Contrary to what some would have us believe, humans have been eating meat in varying amounts for as long as we have recorded history. (350)

How much protein you need depends upon your individual type. The first things to consider in eating meat are your blood type and metabolic type. Next consider how that meat was raised. Personally, I have found I do well on wild or grass-fed beef but quickly have digestion problems when I eat feedlot-raised beef.

A feedlot diet is not the normal food for cattle. They are grass eaters. The feedlot diet is often centered around crushed, steamed corn kernels and a protein supplement made of molasses and urea to which are added liquid vitamins, synthetic estrogen, antibiotics, and a little alfalfa hay and corn silage for roughage, and everything mixed in a giant mixer. Often cattle are fed things that are not on their food chain which disturbs their digestive process causing weakness and disease. Crowded, filthy feedlots create weak, diseased animals. Antibiotics given with the feed is the only way to keep them alive. Feedlot beef is often very contaminated with pesticides, herbicides, nitrates, antibiotics, GMO foods and hormones. (351)

Grass-fed meat - A study done at Iowa State University in August 2001 found that grass-fed organic beef has a much higher Omega-3 to Omega-6 ratio than fish. It has higher levels of B vitamins and almost all other nutrients and it doesn't have the antibiotics, hormones, and other additives that are put in the mix for feedlot cattle. How poultry and pork are raised is equally important. Yes, I do eat pork. It's the conditions under which any animals are raised and their diets that affect how the meat affects me. (351)

The Magnificent Egg

Again we have followed the wrong drummer. The poor egg, along with butter and other natural fats, has been blamed for high cholesterol. Little was understood about the real role of cholesterol in the body at the time, so it was easy for those who wanted to make money on the newly designed (created foods) to persuade people to discard their old ways and eat the new supposedly safer foods.

Eggs have been given a bad rap. In restaurants I hear people ordering egg white omelets and I want to start lecturing right there. Yes, the whites contain protein, but the other nutrients are in the yolk. Eating only the egg whites can cause a biotin deficiency. Nature provides balance in eating the whole egg cooked as lightly as possible. Fresh eggs have not been found to be a cholesterol problem, however, dehydrated eggs have been highly processed and may contain oxidized or rancid cholesterol which is harmful to the body. Baking mixes and bakery goods often have powdered eggs, powdered milk, powdered butter, or powdered cheese. This is another reason to make your foods from whole ingredients. (352)

Wm Campbell Douglass II cited three studies which affirm that eating eggs does not raise cholesterol. (353)

1. A University of Washington study found that adding two eggs per day to the National Cholesterol Program's recommended daily diet had NO EFFECT on plasma LDL - even among those with elevated LDL!

2. Finnish research involving over 21,000 male subjects found that dietary cholesterol was NOT associated with coronary heart disease risk.

3. A pair of large epidemiological studies (involving over 117,000 participants) showed that the adjusted risk of cardiovascular disease was identical whether subjects ate less than one egg per week or seven.

I feel we have a whole generation that has been robbed of their last good years. They were told not to eat eggs or butter because they raised cholesterol which led to cardiovascular disease. Now we know differently, but the lack of vital nutrients may have contributed to Alzheimer's disease, macular degeneration, and other deficiency triggered diseases.

- Organic or free-range eggs are a nearly perfect food, providing a rich source of many crucial nutrients, some of which are found in only a few foods. (354) They provide:
- Protein, a good source of essential amino acids
- B-vitamins, specifically:
  -Folate (folic acid)—needed for heart, vascular, bone and brain health
  -Choline—Choline deficiency can cause deficiency of folic acid, another B vitamin critically important for health. The flexibility and integrity of fat-containing structures of the cell membranes depends on choline. Choline is a source of two fat-like molecules in the brain, phosphatidylcholine and sphingomyelin, which account for an unusually high percentage of the brain's total mass. Choline also has an impact on cardiovascular health since it is one of the B vitamins that helps convert homocysteine, a molecule that can damage blood vessels, into other benign substances.
  -Eggs are also a good source of vitamin B12, another B vitamin that is needed to control homeocysteine levels.
  -Biotin - Egg yolks have one of the highest concentrations of biotin found in nature. (355)
- Betaine found mostly in eggs and liver has been shown to substantially decrease homocysteine levels indicated in cardiovascular disease.
- Vitamin D - As early as 1929, researchers tested a variety of foods for vitamin D content and found the second most potent source of vitamin D was egg yolk.
- Vitamin A which is essential for growth and repair of body tissue

281

- <u>Carotenoids</u>—Lutein and zeaxanthan are carotenoids known to help prevent macular degeneration and other aging eye syndromes.
- <u>Vitamin K</u> is necessary for blood coagulation
- <u>Selenium</u> is a trace mineral and a powerful antioxidant against cancer and age related conditions
- <u>Sulfur</u> - Egg yolks are one of best food sources of natural sulfur.
- <u>Calcium, potassium, and iron</u> and other minerals are in the magnificent egg.
- <u>Omega 3 fatty acids</u> - If the eggs are from free-range chickens that eat a natural diet, they will have high omega-3 content. (355)

The white of the egg appears to be an especially good source of proline, an amino acid which is important for tissue repair, collagen formation, arteriosclerosis prevention and blood pressure maintenance.

A study found that women who ate at least 6 eggs a week had a lower risk of breast cancer by 44% compared to women who ate only 2 eggs a week. (355)

Eggs provide phospholipids, which are fats combined with phosphorous. They are critical building blocks that, along with glycolipids, cholesterol, and proteins, form the basis of the membranes surrounding each and every cell in the body. Phospholipids are especially abundant in your brain and in the myelin sheaths of nerves. They are normally synthesized in the body, but the aging process slows down the synthesis, so by middle-age, you may no longer process a sufficient amount. Eating eggs can provide badly needed phospholipids as we age. They are also important for the growing child. (355)

Research is finding there is a significant difference in the nutritional value of eggs from hens that are pastured (allowed to roam and eat a normal diet of green plants, bugs, seeds, and worms and live in the sunshine) as compared to eggs from caged hens who never see sunshine and are fed a diet corn, soy, and/or cottonseed meals to which additives are added. Caged chickens are often unhealthy because of their cramped, unsanitary conditions and unnatural diet. Antibiotics may be added to their food to keep them alive. To help chickens grow faster and increase profits, they may be given hormones. The eggs from these chickens may have traces of toxic substances which can cause sensitivities in people and/or add to the toxic load in our bodies. Also these eggs are not as rich in Omega-3s. (356)

"Free range" is a term used today which may only mean that chickens are not caged but are kept in a confined area so they are not allowed to roam and eat a natural diet. Organic hens may be caged but are given organic foods. Read the carton to see if the chickens have been fed antibiotics and hormones. (356)

Not only have studies shown that eggs do not significantly affect cholesterol levels in most individuals, but the latest research suggests eating whole eggs may actually result in significant improvement in one's blood lipids (cholesterol) profile.

Eating eggs may help lower risk of a heart attack or stroke by helping to prevent blood clots. A study published in the October 2003 issue of <u>Biological and Pharmaceutical Bulletin</u> demonstrated that proteins in egg yolk are not only potent inhibitors of human platelet aggregation, but also prolong the time it takes for fibrinogen, a protein present in blood, to be converted into fibrin. (355)

<u>Cooking eggs:</u> Raw eggs may pose a salmonella hazard, so lightly cook the eggs.

Soy Products

The soy controversy over the value versus the dangers of soy products in the human diet continues to rage. Soybeans do contain essential amino acids, and during the last few decades there has been much hype about substituting soy for meats supposedly to avoid saturated fats and to eat lower on the food chain. Much of the hype led us to believe that cholesterol from saturated fat caused heart disease which we now know was just hype to sell products created from soy.

Supposedly by avoiding meat we were eating lower on the food chain to help the planet. I'm not so sure we have helped the environment, and I think we have damaged our bodies by turning to soy instead of eating meat, eggs, and dairy. Also, the increased demand for soy products has been a factor in creating genetically modified strains and in the use of more and more pesticides which have polluted our earth. (357)

There are many concerns connected with using processed soy products. Below is information from an article, "Confused About Soy?—Soy Dangers Summarized" from the researchers at the Weston Price Foundation that explains the dangers of soy thoroughly.

High levels of phytic acid in soy reduce assimilation of calcium, magnesium, copper, iron and zinc. Phytic acid in soy is not neutralized by ordinary preparation methods such as soaking, sprouting and long, slow cooking. High phytate diets have caused growth problems in children.

- Trypsin inhibitors in soy interfere with protein digestion and may cause pancreatic disorders. In test animals, soy containing trypsin inhibitors caused stunted growth.
- Soy phytoestrogens disrupt endocrine function and have the potential to cause infertility and promote breast cancer in adult women.
- Soy phytoestrogens are potent antithyroid agents that cause hypothyroidism and may cause thyroid cancer. In infants, consumption of soy formula has been linked to autoimmune thyroid disease.
- Vitamin B_{12} analogs in soy are not absorbed and actually increase the body's requirement for B_{12}.
- Soy foods increase the body's requirement for vitamin D.
- Fragile proteins are denatured during high temperature processing to make soy protein isolate and textured vegetable protein.

- Processing of soy protein results in the formation of toxic lysinoalanine and highly carcinogenic nitrosamines.
- Free glutamic acid or MSG, a potent neurotoxin, is formed during soy food processing and additional amounts are added to many soy foods.
- Soy foods may contain high levels of aluminum which is toxic to the nervous system and the kidneys.

References for above data found in (358)

There were times when I consumed soy products regularly, but I rarely use them today after understanding the dangers of soy. Fermented soy, which is the form most used by Asians, seems to be an acceptable alternative.

Nuts and seeds are a good source of protein, minerals, and good fats. However, it is best for most people to use them in moderation. People who are prone to herpes infections may need to avoid most nuts because nuts have high levels of arginine that can trigger an outbreak. If they do eat nuts, supplementing with lysine may balance the arginine. (359)

Legumes (dried beans, peas, chickpeas, and lentils)
Legumes can be a good source of protein for some people, but each legume has individual characteristics which affect its acceptance by the body. O blood types, for example, don't digest many legumes well. (360)

ScienceDaily.com summarizes the results of a study on the antioxidant activity of various types of beans and compared the antioxidant activity of 12 different types of dry beans. It found that black beans had more activity per gram than any of the other beans in the study. The second highest antioxidant activity went to red beans, followed by brown, yellow and white. (361)

There is much controversy among health practitioners as to which foods are best for certain conditions. Some health practitioners feel that beans are an ideal food for diabetics. I don't find that to be true for me. I need meat.

No one is an expert, although some will strongly indicate that they have the answers. Mostly, we are all constantly experimenting to find better ways to be well. Find what works for you.

Fats - Separating the Good from the Bad Resources for this section (362) (363) (364)

Twisted thinking! Before 1920, when people were eating butter, cream, eggs and red meat coronary heart disease and clogged arteries were rare in America. It was in the 1950s when medical science decided high cholesterol was a risk of heart disease. It was about that time they also decided saturated fats were causing the high cholesterol. We were told to use vegetable oils instead of butter and not to eat red meats due to their saturated fat content.

For decades we were told that saturated fat would cause cardiovascular disease, so we avoided anything with animal fat, thinking that margarine and vegetable oil were safer alternatives. Then we started to hear about unhealthy "trans-fats" and the confusion mounted. Trans- fats are fats that have been altered through the chemical process of hydrogenation of oils. Trans-fats are found in processed foods such as ready-made cakes, chips, pastries, pies, chocolates, sweets and ice cream.

Interestingly, the consumption of foods containing saturated fats dropped drastically. However, during the same time period, the **incidence of coronary heart disease rose dramatically.** It rose so much that by the mid fifties, heart disease was the leading cause of death among Americans. (365)

Are you confused about what fats to eat? There certainly is a plethora of confusing information in the media concerning fats and cholesterol, so I hope this section will clarify the situation.

The basic facts are:
1. Many experts agree that fats don't make you fat.
2. Fats provide a source of energy for body processes.

3. Fats are crucial to the transport and absorptions of fat-soluble vitamins such as A, D, E, and K throughout the body.
4. Fats help to balance the body's chemistry and provide padding as protection for vital organs.
5. Essential fatty acids, sometimes referred to as vitamin F, are necessary for body processes and can only be obtained through diet.
6. The body needs saturated fat. It is essential that infants and children receive <u>saturated fat</u> for proper development.
7. Fats are needed for proper brain and nerve function.
8. <u>Trans-fats</u> are damaged fats created through the processing vegetable oils.

"Low-fat" as a philosophy has led us down a twisted path. It is true the American diet has too much "bad" fat, but through the years experts have not agreed on what is "bad fat". We need fats, especially essential fatty acids. About 20 years ago some researchers decided saturated fat was causing cardiovascular problems. In actuality, it is altered fats called <u>trans-fats and oxidized fats that cause most of the problems.</u> (366)

Feeling good is actually a symptom of high cholesterol. (364)

Cholesterol is a good guy. Cholesterol is a substance vital to the cells of all mammals. The production of cholesterol increases when you eat lower cholesterol foods and decreases when you eat high cholesterol foods. (367)

- Some say there is **no scientific evidence** that cholesterol over 200 will cause heart disease, and that **there is no evidence that too much animal fat and cholesterol in the diet promotes atherosclerosis or heart attacks.** (366)
- Cholesterol is not the cause of heart disease but rather a **potent antioxidant**, a weapon against free radicals in the blood and a repair substance that helps heal arterial damage (although the arterial plaques themselves contain very little cholesterol).

287

- Cholesterol is so important in keeping good health that **all the cells in the body contain it**. The brain, all the nerves, and the spinal cord are richly supplied with cholesterol. Cholesterol is the foundation of most hormones.
- **Cholesterol is converted into Vitamin D by sunlight** and is the precursor for steroid hormones like the testosterone we all need to grow and the estrogen women need to be feminine.
- The liver manufactures about 1,000 mg of cholesterol per day, even if you consume no cholesterol at all. Of that amount, about 800 mg becomes bile salts to help with digestion.
- **Cholesterol protects your arteries.** Excess homocysteine is a killer because it literally eats away at your artery walls. Your body responds by slapping on cholesterol to patch the holes. If it didn't, blood vessels in your brain might burst, and you'd die of a massive stroke! It would be even better to avoid the holes and the patches by consuming adequate B vitamins which regulate homocysteine.
- It was found in postmortems to measure what statins really do to arteries, that the arteries of people who had used statin drugs were far more plugged than those who had not.
- **Low cholesterol has been linked to depression and foggy memory.**
- **Low cholesterol may increase your chances of dying from infectious disease.**
- Researchers at Texas A&M University have discovered that **lower cholesterol levels can actually reduce muscle gain with exercising.**
- People who are under great stress **will have higher cholesterol because the nervous system needs the cholesterol for their well-being.**
- **Lowering cholesterol below 200 can actually be dangerous**. There is evidence that cholesterol below 200 can be linked to strokes, aggressive behavior, and depression. (364)

The vast majority of the cholesterol circulating in our blood is manufactured in the liver. Only a small amount comes from the diet. Cholesterol manufactured by the liver is obviously not rancid and, therefore, not oxidized. The cholesterol in fresh, natural foods, likewise, is not oxidized, but foods that have been overly processed may contain oxidized (altered) cholesterol.

When the body is deficient in certain B vitamins (especially B 12, pyridoxine, and folic acid), homocysteine builds up in the bloodstream and converts cholesterol to oxidized cholesterol (oxycholesterol), which can lead to direct damage of the walls of your arteries.

Processing can cause the cholesterol in natural foods to oxidize. The foods with the highest oxidized cholesterol content are dried cheese, powdered whole milk, powdered eggs, powdered butter, hard meats, and products made with these ingredients. We also get oxidized cholesterol when we fry foods using vegetable oils. The diet many of us eat consisting of white flour products, margarine, processed vegetable oils leaves the body very deficient in B vitamins, causing even good <u>foods to be oxidized and become a health risk</u>. (367)

Oxycholesterol (oxidized cholesterol) is a toxin to the body which damages arteries and causes strokes and heart attacks. (367)

Saturated Fats - In general, the main sources of saturated fat are animal products: red meat and whole-milk dairy products, including cheese, sour cream, ice cream and butter. However, there are also plant-based sources of saturated fat, principally coconut oil and coconut milk, palm kernel oil, cocoa butter, and palm oil. Saturated fats are:
- essential for of all body tissues
- a major part of the phospholipid component of cell membranes
- the preferred fuel for the heart
- used as a source of fuel during energy expenditure

- used by the body to increase HDL concentrations
- modulators for genetic regulation and prevent butyric acid which is indicated in cancer
- useful antiviral agents (caprylic acid)
- effective against cavities, anti-plaque and anti-fungal agents (lauric acid)
- useful to actually lower cholesterol levels (palmitic and stearic acids)
- beneficial effects on thrombogenic and atherogenic risk factors (stearic acid) (362)

Essential fatty Acids: (368)
There are basic two essential fatty acids: Omega 6 - linoleic acid (LA) and Omega 3 – alpha linolenic acid (ALA).

Omega 3 can be converted in the body to eicosapentaenoic acid (EPA) and docosahexaenoic acid (DHA). The best direct sources of EPA and DHA are fish oils, especially cod liver oil and salmon oil.
- Omega-3 oils are crucial to preventing not only cancer, but also heart disease and many other diseases.
- The human brain is also highly dependent on DHA.
- People with depression, memory loss, and schizophrenia have shown low levels of DHA.
- It's been found that women whose diets provided the high amounts of omega-3 fatty acids had a lower risk of dry eye syndrome compared with those who consumed few omega-3 rich foods.
- Omega-3 fats can help reduce the inflammation that is a significant factor in conditions such as asthma, osteoarthritis, rheumatoid arthritis, and migraine headaches.
- Omega-3 fats are used by the body to produce Series 1 and 3 prostaglandins, which are anti-inflammatory hormone-like molecules. (369)

Experts feel the ratio of Omega-3 to Omega 6 should be close to 1:1, which is what they have found in studying the diet of our ancestors, who ate wild meat and naturally grass-fed meat, which are high in Omega 3s.

Omega-6 fatty acids are needed by the body, but our modern diet has upset the ratio of Omega-3 to Omega-6 so badly that most of us are getting too much Omega-6. Most Americans' diet ratio is between 1:20 to 1:50 because we eat many foods made with soy, corn, and safflower oils. (371)

When consumed in excess Omega-6 fats produce Series 2 prostaglandins, which are pro-inflammatory molecules produced from other fats, notably the omega-6 fats, which are found in high amounts in animal fats, margarine, and many vegetable oils including corn, safflower, sunflower, palm, and peanut oils. (372)

Good food sources of omega-3 fatty acids: Sardines, wild salmon, flaxseeds, chia seeds, walnuts, hemp seed, goji berries, avocados and purslane. (370)

Some of the functions of essential fatty acids in the body include: (373)
- Construction and repair of cell membranes and capillaries
- Lowering triglyceride levels
- Helping eradicate plaque from the walls of arteries
- Lowering blood pressure
- Increasing the rate at which the body burns fat
- Assisting in the function of glands and balancing hormones
- Helping the body manufacture hemoglobin
- Assisting in the manufacture of cholesterol while at the same time helping to remove excess cholesterol from the blood
- Altering the production of leukotrienes, which aggravate inflammation in the body
- Nourishing skin, hair, and nails
- Assisting in the body's production of electrical currents vital for regular heart beat
- Inhibiting the growth of yeast organisms in the body by helping the oxygen flow to cells

Today, many fish are not considered good sources of Omega-3 due to contamination, so it may be necessary to take fish oil supplements. Critically research your source of fish oils and also supplement with at least 400 IU of Vitamin E when supplementing essential fatty acids. (373)

Below is a list which may help you sort through the fats. (368)

Super-unsaturated – Omega-3s
LNL - Alpha-linolenic Acid - found in flax, hemp seed, canola, soy, walnuts, chia, pumpkin seeds, kukui (candlenut), purslane, and dark green leaves
SDA - Stearidonic Acid - found in black currant seeds and other wild seeds
EPA - Eicosapentaenoic Acid – found in oils of cold water fish such as salmon, trout, mackerel, sardines
DHA - Docosahexaenoic Acid - found in oils of cold water fish such a salmon, trout, mackerel, sardines
Comparing Seeds: % Omega-3
Chia - Salvia hispanica 62.3
Flax - Linum usitatissimum 54.6
Hemp - Cannabis sativa 19.9

Polyunstaurated – Omega-6s
LA - Linoleic acid found in safflower, sunflower, hemp, soybean, walnut, pumpkin, sesame, and flax
GLA - Gamma-linolenic Acid - absent in mother's milk; borage richest source, followed by black currant seed oil and evening primrose oil
DGLA - found in mother's milk
AA - Arachidonic Acid - found in meats and other animal products.

Monounsaturated – Omega-9s
OA - Oleic Acid - found in olive, almond, avocado, peanut, pecan, cashew, filbert, and macadamia oils, also in land animal fats and butter. This can also be produced in the body.

Monounsaturate
- POA - Palmitoleic Acid - found in tropical oils, especially coconut and palm kernel. Our body converts POA into several other forms of fats.

- SA - Stearic Acid - found in beef, mutton, pork, butter, cocoa butter, and shea nut butter
- PA - Palmitic Acid - found in large quantities in tropical fats: coconut, palm, palm kernel
- BA - Butyric Acid - found in butter
- Arachidic Acid - found in peanuts

Olives and olive oil - While extra virgin olive oil is widely recognized as a heart-healthy oil, it also contains lignans, which further contribute to the beneficial nutritional profile of this functional food. The lignin pinoresinol is the primary phenol found in extra virgin olive oil. The anti-cancer value of this compound has been observed in studies when introduced to cancer cells in vitro. In addition to apoptosis (cellular death) of the cancer cells occurring, it was noted that the best results were achieved with low concentrations of pinoresinol, as they are found naturally in extra virgin olive oil. (374)

Krill oil - Krill are shrimp-like crustaceans eaten by the blue whale. Krill oil extracted from krill contains the important omega-3 fatty acids, EPA and DHA. Krill oil also has a high amount of a potent antioxidant called astaxanthin, along with small amounts of vitamin A and vitamin E. Avoid krill oil if you are allergic to shellfish. (375)

Black Currant Seed Oil contains 14% alpha-linolenic, 12% gamma-linolenic 47% linoleic, and 2.7% stearidonic acids. (376)

Black currant seed oil contains a more complete range of EFA containing linoleic acid and alpha linolenic acid, plus GLA the unique stearidonic acid. GLA is important because it is the source of prostaglandins, the biological regulators of:
- the menstrual cycle
- the skin
- the body's immune system
- the minute-by-minute control every cell and organ in the body

293

Since black currant seed oil is 44 – 51 % Omega-6 which is pro-inflammatory, it should be taken with a high source of Omega-3. (377)

Hemp oil has perfectly balanced 1:3 ratio of naturally-occurring Omega-3 and Omega-6 essential fatty acids and quite a good taste so is welcome on salads or wherever you would use oil as a condiment. Don't use the oil in cooking, as unhealthy by-products are formed when it is heated to high temperatures. (378)

Lecithin a lipid, as a type of fat needed by every living cell in the human body. Cell membranes, which regulate the passage of nutrients into and out of the cells, are largely composed of lecithin. The protective sheaths surrounding the brain are composed of lecithin, and the muscles and nerve cells contain this essential fatty substance. Lecithin is <u>a natural component of butter and eggs</u> that assists in the metabolism of cholesterol and other fats. I use sunfolower or egg lecithin as <u>soy lecithin may have significant levels of glutamate</u>.

Lecithin:
- improves brain function
- protects against cardiovascular disease
- aids absorption of several vitamins by the liver
- enables excess fats to be dispersed in water and removed from the body
- promotes energy
- helps repair damage done to the liver by alcoholism and other toxic overload

Lecithin is a source of phosphatidyl choline which is needed to make a vital neurotransmitter for memory, control of sensory input memory, and muscular control. (379)

Bile contains lecithin, which helps to emulsify large fat particles and turn them into tiny particles with a greater surface area for the fat-splitting lipase enzyme to work on. Supplementing with lecithin as granules or capsules improves emulsification and can help people with poor tolerance of fat, especially people who have had their gall bladders removed. (380)

Egg yolks, sunflower seeds, and soy are good sources of lecithin, while minor sources include brewer's yeast, grains, legumes, fish, and wheat germ. Lecithin can be bought in supplement form.

Trans-fats – We don't need them!
Trans-fatty acids are deformed fat molecules which can damage the cells and cause a fatty acid deficiency by inhibiting enzymes that cause fatty acids to be changed into essential molecules.

The body cannot use trans-fatty acids so they simply collect around fatty tissues and the body's organs. They take up space where essential fatty acids normally would be, but do not perform any useful function. (381)

When I stir-fry, I dribble a little olive oil or coconut oil in the pan, toss in the vegetables to coat, then add a tablespoon of water, cover and turn down the heat. Cook only a few minutes.

Saturated fats are better for regular frying as they are more stable than most liquid vegetable oils. Butter and coconut oil are the best for light frying. Never fry on high heat, which changes the fats to carcinogens.

Avoid using hydrogenated or partially hydrogenated fats including margarine, shortening, and many vegetable oils. They are heavy on omega-6 fats, which worsen the ratio with omega-3. Hydrogenated sunflower, corn, soy, safflower, and canola oil are almost always used in anything processed. If you choose to use vegetable oils, use cold-pressed or expeller pressed oils which fewer trans-fats.

Summarizing thoughts about fats for good health:
- Eat a good balance of Omega-3s and Omega-6s. Aim for a 1:1 ratio.
- Use only cold pressed non-refined oils (keep refrigerated).

- Avoid margarine which is made from hydrogenated fats and refined oils.
- Avoid hydrogenated fat: peanut butter, white shortening, partially hydrogenated vegetable oils or the products made from them (almost everything that is a packaged, processed product). You can buy nut butters that are not hydrogenated at a health food store.
- Avoid processed oils from the supermarket, as they are usually heated and refined.
- Avoid anything that is "French fried".
- Be aware that labels may be deceiving, as some say "No trans-fats.", but Read the small print.
- Avoid processed food
- Use the most recommended fats, which are cold pressed extra virgin olive oil, avocados, coconut oil, hemp oil, and organic butter. (368)

FAT DOES NOT MAKE YOU FAT, BUT SIMPLE CARBOHYDRATES DO! (382)

Carbohydrates The diet pendulum keeps swinging. The truth is, we need complex carbohydrates as found in most vegetables with the fiber and nutrients for complete metabolism. It's the simple carbohydrate foods made with refined sugar and white flour that are a nail in the coffin of the nation.

Simple carbohydrates are sugars. All simple carbohydrates are made of just one or two sugar molecules. They are the quickest source of energy, as they are very rapidly digested. Some food sources of simple carbohydrates include any product using these ingredients: table sugar, brown sugar, corn syrup, high fructose corn syrup, honey, maple syrup, molasses, jams, jellies (including fruit drinks, sodas, and candy). (383)

Complex carbohydrates are made of sugar molecules strung together like a necklace or branched like a coil. They are often rich in fiber, thus satisfying and health promoting. Complex carbohydrates are commonly found in whole plant foods and, therefore, are also often high in vitamins and minerals. These whole plant foods are great sources of complex carbohydrates: green vegetables, whole grains, starchy vegetables, and legumes. (383)

As a diabetic I have found it most important to avoid all simple carbohydrates and make sure I get good fats, protein, and a variety of fruits and vegetables that provide the phytonutrients, vitamins and minerals my body needs. Processed food is a burden on the body.

Grains Are Not the Staff of Life.

Grains were not part of early man's food chain, so many people have difficulty digesting them.
For several decades whole grains were thought to be very healthful foods and in comparison to white flour products, they are much more nutritious. However, we have already discussed the reasons modern wheat is not a healthful food.

Grain sensitivities are much more common than people realize. Children with middle ear infection may have dairy and/or gluten sensitivity. Dr. Braly and Mr. Hoggan in Dangerous Grains say, "a variety of highly prevalent gastro-intestinal diseases such as canker sores, cancers, irritable bowel, Crohn's disease, ulcerative colitis, esophageal reflux often benefit from a gluten-free diet." (384)

Neurologist Dr. David Permutter, author of Grain Brain, says, "The problem with gluten is far more serious than anyone ever imagined. Modern...structurally modified, hybridized grains contain gluten that's less tolerable than the gluten that was found in grains cultivated just a few decades ago". (385) Gluten is a two-part "sticky" protein made up of the peptides gliadin and glutenin. It is found in grains such as wheat, rye, barley, and others. It's considered sticky because it holds together the nutrient stores of the plant. This stickiness is why it's so commonly used in processed foods as a binder and filler.

Gluten is causing your body to attack itself. (386)

Gliadin is the primary immunotoxic protein found in wheat gluten and is among the most damaging to your health. Gliadin gives wheat bread its doughy texture and is capable of increasing the production of the intestinal protein **zonulin,** which in turn opens up gaps in the normally tight junctures between intestinal cells, causing Leaky Gut Syndrome.

From Paleo Mama we learn in "Grains — Especially Whole Grains — Increase Intestinal Permeability," that Leaky gut is a condition that occurs due to the development of gaps between the cells (enterocytes) that make up the membrane lining your intestinal wall.

- These tiny gaps allow substances such as undigested food, bacteria and metabolic wastes, that should be confined to your digestive tract, to escape into your bloodstream —hence the term Leaky Gut Syndrome.
- Once the integrity of your intestinal lining is compromised and there is a flow of toxic substances "leaking out" into your bloodstream, your body experiences significant increases in inflammation.
- Also, your immune system may become confused and begin to attack your own body as if it were an enemy (autoimmune disorder).
- Most often leaky gut syndrome is associated with inflammatory bowel diseases like Crohn's and ulcerative colitis, or celiac disease, but even healthy people can have varying degrees of intestinal permeability leading to a wide variety of health symptoms. This is influenced by the foods you choose to eat. (387)

From the article "What is Wrong with Grains" at http://paleoleap.com/what-is-wrong-with-grains/, we also learn some other problems with wheat:

- **Calories:** Wheat is one of the biggest sources of calories in the average person's diet.
- **Amylopectin A:** Modern wheat contains a super starch, amylopectin A, that is a super gluten, very fattening and super inflammatory.

- **Phytates:** Wheat contains phytates which bind to dietary minerals and prevent their absorption.
- **Chemicals:** The chemical pesticides and fertilizers that are approved and considered safe for human consumption such as disulfoton (Di-syston), methyl parathion, chlorpyrifos, dimethoate, diamba, and glyphosate are **designed to create neurological fragmentation in insects.** How do you think they affect the human body?
- **Irradiation:** Wheat was one of the first foods approved by the FDA for irradiation as a way to control insects. Irradiated food can lower immune resistance, decrease fertility, damage the kidneys, depress growth rates, and reduces vitamins A, B-complex, C, D, and K.
- **Loss of Nutrients:** According to the Weston A. Price foundation, many of the nutrients in wheat are lost by modern industrial processing. (388)

Another difference in the grains of the past and those of today is that in early times the grains were soaked, sprouted, or fermented. These processes broke down the anti-nutrients in grains (such as gluten, lectin, and phytic acid) so they were more digestible. These methods also made the nutrients in grains much more bioavailable. To learn more about this please read http://wellnessmama.com/3807/sprouted-soaked-fermented-grains-healthy/

Another difference was bread of early times was prepared using slow rise methods such as from sourdough starter rather than the quicker methods of today. (389)

In early times when wheat was raised on fertile soil with no chemicals it had significant fiber and was a source of protein. However, when wheat was refined to create a nice white flour, the bran and germ containing many of the nutrients were milled out. In addition, to make flour whiter it is bleached with bromate and chlorine dioxide (which are toxic chemicals), which can change the quality of the protein, making it even more difficult to digest. To compensate for the nutrients lost in the milling process, the flour is enriched with a few synthetic vitamins and minerals which are not necessarily in the form or ratio that is good for health. (390)

White flour is now used in most bakery goods and many other packaged foods. It is high on the glycemic index (GI), which means it causes a quick rise in blood sugar levels. A steady intake of high GI foods causes a gradual insensitivity to insulin, which can lead to Type 2 diabetes, weight gain, and other health issues. (390)

If you want to avoid gluten and buy gluten-free foods, be sure to read the label. There are now breads that are gluten free; however, many of the non-gluten flours are higher in sugars. When baking gluten-free bread and goodies I include flour from rice, corn, amaranth, quinoa, sorghum, tapioca, potato, millet, beans, and buckwheat, and I add xanthan gum. Other ingredients that add texture and nutrients to gluten-free breads are ground flaxseeds, chia seed gel, and other ground seeds and nuts.

One of my favorite recipe books is <u>Wheat-Free Recipes & Menus</u> by Carol Fenster, Ph.D.

Foods Summary

The Recommended Daily Allowances (RDA) of nutrients set by our government many years ago really had very little scientific basis. The RDAs are so minimal as to barely keep one alive, certainly not healthy today when our bodies need to constantly use nutrients to detoxify the pollutants in our foods and environment. To complicate matters, although we all need all the nutrients, the amount of each nutrient needed can vary greatly from person to person.

The charts in this book will help you plan the foods you need to eat to have a variety and a balance. Remember, the vitamins in packaged foods are often synthetic in origin and may not be easily absorbed by the body. ; there are usually few, if any, phytonutrients in processed food.

While science has identified many nutrients such as vitamins, minerals, antioxidants, and other phytochemicals, there are many more that have not been identified. We would do well to respect the synergy of how nutrients work together. Everyone needs to eat a variety of foods, including raw fruits and vegetables, to get all the nutrients that the body needs.

We already discovered the building materials for a healthy cell in the section "Priorities for Survival". Most of these nutrients cannot be made in the body, so we must get them from foods, drinks, or supplements.

Foods are the primary source of the nutrients our bodies need.

Supplements can never replace food because supplements are only isolated components of food without the factors which have yet to be identified which together create synergy. We supplement only to assure we are getting enough nutrients for our bodies to be able to constantly detoxify our polluted environment. Amost always supplements should be taken with food which will provided the enzymes for their absorption.

Prepare and eat real food made from fresh ingredients as much as possible. Eat organic whenever possible. Plan to eat according to your particular type, though this can be challenging when planning family meals for several different types. Consider which foods give you the biggest bang for your shopping bucks, and start making a few changes at a time by choosing from the list below:

1. Organic vegetables - raw, steamed, stir-fry, or baked.
2. Wild, free-range, or organic meat and poultry.
3. Fresh, organic fruits, especially dark berries, apples, and bananas.
4. Natural fish only from northern, less polluted waters.
5. Nuts and seeds - according to your type (fresh, raw and organic, if possible)
6. Fresh green and/or vegetable juices or combined fruit and vegetable juices.
7. Good fats: butter, cocnut oil, olive oil, avocado oil, flaxseed oil. (Yes, you do need fats!)
8. Eggs from free range chickens which are not fed antibiotics, hormones, and eat their natural diet.

301

9. Garlic - eat it raw and use it in cooking.
10. Liberally use herbs which will add nutrients to salads, juices, and other foods.
11. If you are using dairy and have access to raw milk products, they are the most digestible. If not, use organic products and/or fermented such as plain yogurt and kefir.

When we prepare and eat fresh organic vegetables and fruits either from our gardens, the local farmers' market, or other local growers, we are:

- Eating fresher, more nutritious food. Much of the produce in the supermarket is picked and packaged when it is firm and unripe so it will stand the long shipping and is often sprayed with chemicals to improve shelf life. Since most fruits and vegetables don't develop their full array of vitamins, antioxidants, and phytonutrients until they are fully ripe, what we find in supermarkets is often lacking
- Eliminating the throw-away packaging of processed food.
- Keeping the dollars in our local economy.
- Saving precious non-renewable petroleum by avoiding long distance transportation
- Encouraging local sustainable agriculture

I realize advocating that we not eat manufactured food is suggesting a change to the dynamics of industry. <u>For the health of our bodies and the earth, I feel we need to change how our society is doing things</u>. We need to encourage local organic, sustainable agriculture.

Looking at the quantity of digestive aids sold each year, the number of cases of intestinal disease such as colitis, IBS, diverticulitis, and colon cancer we can quickly see that we are not properly digesting and absorbing what we eat.

PART C: DETOXIFYING

1. MAJOR HEALTH INDICATORS

I am NOT a medical doctor, so I cannot and will not attempt to cure anyone or anything. If you have read previous sections of this book you know that **it is my goal to guide you to find what you need to build your body to prevent disease and to deal with whatever diseases come along.** You may want and/or need to use various types of practitioners as your resources.

Our conventional medical system is overworked, so it is very important for each of us to become more aware of our bodies and our symptoms. **Learn when a symptom may be telling you that something is serious and needs immediate medical attention, as well as when a change in diet or lifestyle is indicated.** (Go back and review "We Were Created to be Well" in Part A)

You've heard throughout the book that I feel almost all disease can be prevented by nutrients, detoxifying the body, and some lifestyle changes. Specific diseases may need individualized protocols, but basically disease comes from cellular toxicity and breakdown. It is easier to prevent disease than to treat it. Typical medical treatment may merely palliate symptoms or may suppress the disease, causing it to manifest differently.

Constipation and inflammation are markers for disease.

CONSTIPATION AND COLON HEALTH: Constipation is not a topic that is likely to be the center of everyday conversation. Dr. Norman W. Walker in his book, Colon Health: Your Key to a Vibrant Life, says, "Constipation is your body's greatest enemy." Since he lived to be 115 years of age, I have a tendency to listen to what he says.

The word constipation comes from the Latin word "constipatus" which, translated, means "to press or crowd together, to pack, to cram." When the feces are not regularly eliminated they may become packed in the bowel. Walker goes on to say, **"Constipation is the**

number one affliction underlying nearly every ailment." (1) Even when we think we are not constipated, we may be. I recently read we in the US spend $400 million a year on over three hundred different brands of laxatives. That says we are in trouble.

The terms bowel, intestine, and gut are used interchangeably in this section. The small intestines include the duodenum, jejunum, and ileum. The large bowel or large intestine is also called the colon. The colon may become damaged resulting in diseases such as colitis, diverticulitis, irritable bowel syndrome, inflammatory bowel disease, Crohn's Disease, and cancer.

Have you ever wondered why there has been such a rise in cases of colon cancer in the last decade?

How does the colon become damaged?

1. Not drinking enough water to keep the digesting food lubricated and moving
2. Eating devitalized, processed food and failing to nourish the digestive organs
3. Eating a diet low in organic vegetables and fruits and not providing the digestive tract with friendly bacteria
4. Not providing the soluble and insoluble fiber necessary to feed good bacteria and sweep the colon
5. Using antibiotics which kills friendly flora and leaves candida albicans to grow rampantly, thus hindering digestion, absorption, and immune response (2)
6. Failing to evacuate when the urge comes, which allows toxic material to sit in the colon where it putrefies; then the small intestine can't empty. It is natural for the body to eliminate after every meal, so three bowel movements a day would be normal if you eat three times a day.
7. Interaction of genetic and/or environmental factors or infections with the body's intestinal immune system causing many white blood cells to accumulate in the inner lining (mucosa) of the gut. These white cells release chemicals that lead to tissue injury such as inflammation. (3)

When the intestinal tract is not healthy, the immune system is compromised, which compromises the health of the entire body.

Dr. Bernard Jensen, in <u>Tissue Cleansing Through Bowel Management</u>, says, "In the fifty years I've spent helping people to overcome illness, disability and disease, it has become crystal clear that poor bowel management lies at the root of most people's health problems." (4)

A diet for your blood type containing the nutrients and fiber your body needs, along with a simple herbal colon cleanse at least once a year, will usually keep the colon healthy. When you have a physical you may want to ask for a simple stool sample to check butyrate levels instead of the more invasive colonoscopy to check colon health.

Your appendix is necessary! Modern medicine makes the assumption that you don't need your appendix, and doctors have routinely removed the little rascal when they were doing other abdominal surgeries. Turns out they were wrong! Surgeons and immunologists from Duke University Medical School now believe your <u>appendix produces and protects the good bacteria in your gut</u>. (5)

The removal of the appendix helps explain the problem in modern society with yeast overgrowth. Normally, the appendix acts like a "good bacteria factory." Since good bacteria are constantly being assaulted by infectious disease, antibiotics, chlorinated water, birth control pills, stress, sugar, and many environmental factors, the person without an appendix has no way to repopulate good bacteria except by supplement. Without good bacteria being replaced regularly, the unfriendly bacteria such as candida can take over in the digestive tract and often other organ systems. (6) (7)

Of course there are times when the appendix becomes infected and must be removed for the safety of the patient. These people will need to supplement probiotics (good bacteria) to repopulate the gut and eat prebiotic foods to keep it healthy.

INFLAMMATION

Inflammation is the body's normal response to stress and leads tohealing. If you cut your finger, inflammation is part of the healing process in which damaged tissues are cleaned up and the area protected from infection. If your body is attacked by a virus, often there is a fever, which is the outward sign the immune system has gone to work. However, chronic inflammation is <u>not</u> a good thing.

Dr. Blaylock says, "Newer and rapidly accumulating evidence now indicates that when inflammation continues for too long or is too intense, it can be very destructive, and even result in other diseases. It turns out that two physiological processes play a major role in inflammation: the immune system and the prostaglandin system. They interact with each other and either enhance inflammation--or reduce it. Now there is growing evidence that one or both of these systems stops functioning correctly in many people and gets stuck in the inflammation mode. A process meant to speed recovery in fact goes into overdrive, causing potentially far greater problems." (8)

High levels of free radicals, mostly generated by the immune system and then released into the tissues and blood, are found in inflammation. Several factors influence this process, such as your diet, toxins, infections, injury, stress and heredity. (8)

Inflammation is a symptom in many chronic diseases. Your body's response to stress, whether from your diet, lifestyle, or the environment, may express itself in several ways. For example, Jack Challem, health and medical writer says in his book, <u>The Inflammation Syndrome</u>, "Elevations in blood sugar spontaneously generate free radicals which stimulate inflammation." (9)

Inflammation is the common factor in such debilitating conditions as Alzheimer's, heart disease, cancer, arthritis, and autoimmune syndromes. Many times people with arthritis and asthma have low levels of anti-inflammatory antioxidants (such as vitamins E & C), Omega-3 fatty acids, and other important nutrients." (9)

We've already learned that a lack of B vitamins is indicated in a rise of homocysteine and inflammation of the vascular system. (10)

2. The Destruction Team

We have determined that the cells need to be well fed for the body systems to be healthy. Many times our bodies are not getting all the nutrients needed, and to compound the problem, the body is trying to neutralize many substances which were never meant to enter our bodies. The immune and lymph systems, as well as the liver, all become stressed.

We've learned how food additives, refined sugar, high fructose corn syrup, trans-fats, and many other ingredients found in food can alter the body's chemistry. Now, let's take a look at how chemicals, heavy metals, and other non-natural things in our environment affect our bodies.

The following is a list of some of the major stressors (toxins) with which our bodies must deal:

- Our toxic food supply, made of:
  - o Chemicals - pesticides, herbicides, artificial fertilizer, and preservatives
  - o Genetically Modified Organisms (GMOs)
  - o Irradiation
- Toxins in our home and work environments
- Toxins in personal care products
- Fluoride
- Chlorine
- Heavy metal toxicity from mercury, arsenic, lead, etc.
- Other stresses on the body
  - o Infection
  - o Parasites
  - o Fungus and yeast overgrowth
  - o Nicotine, alcohol, and drugs
  - o Radiation, EMFs, and cell phones
  - o Dangers of microwaving
  - o Vaccinations (11)

People living in the last three decades have been exposed to an unprecedented number of chemicals and other toxins which are foreign to the body.

Understanding how to cleanse the body of these invaders is paramount to good health.

3. CLEANSING AND DETOXIFYING

Disclaimer: This information is for educational purposes to help you understand options for health. Please work with your doctor or a holistic practitioner.

Fasting and cleansing are not new concepts. Most early cultures had seasonal rituals and various methods for cleansing. Fasting, hot rocks, sweat lodges, steam baths, and mineral baths were among their ways to keep healthy. There are references to fasting in the Bible and other historical texts indicating it was common for early people to fast at certain times of the year. Somehow they knew the body needed to be cleansed inside.

We periodically have our cars serviced: the radiator flushed, the oil changed and a new filter installed, and the transmission fluid changed. Do we periodically cleanse our systems: the colon, the liver, the blood and circulatory system, the digestive system, or the kidneys? After a couple of weeks of herbal cleansing, I always feel so much better.

The human body handles toxins by storing, neutralizing, transforming, or eliminating the invaders from the body. Detoxification involves some dietary and lifestyle changes.

While working with an herbalist I started to understand that a toxic body can't be healthy. In this section you will find many of the things I did to cleanse my body.

Detoxification therapy can include:
1. Eating nutrient-dense foods to increase natural detoxification
2. Dietary flushes based on your blood or metabolic type
3. Fasting and juice fasting

4. Herbal cleanses
5. Chelation, the process of removing a toxin such as a heavy metal from the bloodstream by means of a substance, such a EDTA that will bind with it so it can be eliminated from the body.
6. Hydrotherapy (steam, soaks)
7. Heat/light therapy (infrared hothouse or sauna)
8. Body work (massage, acupuncture, chiropractic, etc.)
9. Meditation, counseling, spiritual awakening (11)

Dr. Sherry Rogers in Detoxify or Die writes, **"The secret to health is getting your body so chemically unloaded and nutrient primed that it heals itself."** (11)

The work of detoxifying this intensive chemical exposure can cause serious nutrient deficiencies. Inability to adequately detoxify the body has often resulted in chronic disease. Dr. Rogers reminds us that **"disease is not a drug deficiency."** Therefore, drugs cannot solve the toxic situation. (11)

The most elemental cleansing happens when you eat nutrient-dense foods on a daily basis. As we've discussed earlier, raw organic foods or foods closest to their natural state are best-digested and most nutritious. Most of the foods and herbs listed as "superfoods" are not only super nutritious but also help detoxify the body. Let's take another look at some that are especially helpful in cleansing.

Reference for foods that detoxify below. (16)

Foods that are superstar detoxifiers

Beet root has many detoxifying forces and nutrients to rebuild the body. It contains the powerful antioxidant betacyanin, which gives beetroot its deep red hue. Research shows it boosts the body's natural defenses in the liver, regenerating immune cells, and has liver, spleen, gall bladder, and kidney cleansing properties. It also helps purify and build the blood. In addition, beet juice has anti-carcinogenic properties. (12)

Beet root (especially beet root juice) will help stop the creation of endless free radicals, which are made in **malformed red blood cells**. The body makes blood cells even if it does not have enough of the needed raw materials; thus, malformed red blood cells are produced. It's thought malformed red blood cells put out about 100+ free radicals per minute of their existence; they are free-radical factories that need to be destroyed. They pollute the blood unimaginably quickly. Beet root will not only detoxify but will also force the correct making of new blood cells. (13) You may want to explore the "Mini Beet Protocol" developed by Robert von Sarbacher, to be found on http://robertvon.com/mbp.html.

Garlic is <u>one of the best detoxing foods on the planet</u>. Garlic contains flavonoids that stimulate the production of glutathione, the liver's <u>most potent antioxidant</u>. Glutathione enhances elimination of toxins and carcinogens. Glutathione helps stimulate the liver to produce detoxification enzymes that help filter toxic residues from the digestive system. (14)

Berries and other fruits are high in <u>antioxidants</u>, vitamins, and other nutrients, as well as fiber. Their high fiber and liquid contents help eliminate toxins.

Green foods are very high in antioxidants, vitamins, minerals, chlorophyll, and fiber. There are a great variety of green foods: barley grass, wheatgrass, kale, spinach, chard, arugula and other leafy greens, blue-green algae, spirulina, chlorella, and alfalfa.

Chlorophyll rids the body of harmful environmental toxins from smog, heavy metals, herbicides, cleaning products and pesticides. (15)

Citrus fruits are good sources of bioflavonoids, vitamin C, potassium, and folate. Citrus is a good source of pectin, a water-soluble fiber which aids the body in flushing out toxins and stimulating enzymatic processes in the digestive tract. Lemon juice aids the liver in its cleansing processes. Many people start each morning with a warm glass of lemon water drunk through a straw to protect the enamel on their teeth.

Sprouting grains, seeds and legumes makes them more digestible by removing the anti-nutrients which inhibit the absorption of nutrients.

Sprouts are an excellent source of dietary fiber, vitamins, minerals, and protein. They are easily digestible and stimulate the detoxification enzymes in the digestive tract. If the sprouts are exposed to sunlight, chlorophyll develops, which aids in purifying the blood.

Research shows that broccoli sprouts are fifty times more nutritious than the full-grown broccoli. Researchers found broccoli sprouts contain high levels of glucoraphanin, also known as sulforaphane glucosinolate (SGS). SGS is considered a cancer preventative and boosts the immune system. "Three-day-old broccoli sprouts consistently contain 20 to 50 times the amount of chemoprotective compounds found in mature broccoli heads' production of Phase 2 enzymes, which are part of the body's antioxidant system." (15) Below is a great site to learn about sprouting. http://www.sproutpeople.com/

Cruciferous vegetables: Eating broccoli and cauliflower will increase the amount of glucosinolate in your system, adding to enzyme production in the liver. These natural enzymes help flush carcinogens and other toxins out of our bodies, which significantly lowers our risk of cancer. Eating cabbage helps stimulate the activation of two crucial liver detoxifying enzymes that help flush out toxins. Try eating kimchi, coleslaw, cabbage soup, and sauerkraut for variety.

Green tea is a great detoxifier due to the antioxidants, especially catechins, which are known to increase liver function.

Mung beans have been used by Ayurvedic doctors for thousands of years but are not commonly seen in western diets. They are incredibly easy to digest and absorb toxic residue on the sides of the intestinal walls. They are easy to sprout and make a delightful soup.

311

Seeds and nuts are excellent protein options. Many of the seeds and nuts are more digestible when soaked, sprouted, or freshly ground. Flaxseed, pumpkin seeds, almonds, walnuts, hemp seeds, sesame seeds, chia seeds, and sunflower seeds are all excellent options.

Omega-3 oils provide alpha-linolenic acid while lubricating the intestinal walls, allowing the toxins to be absorbed by the oil and eliminated by the body. Use hemp, avocado, olive, or flaxseed oil while detoxifying.

Turmeric is the liver's favorite spice. Try sprinkling turmeric and dill weed on eggs, or add turmeric to soups, stews, or veggie dishes for an instant liver pick-me-up. Turmeric helps boost liver detoxification by assisting enzymes that actively flush out known dietary carcinogens. Since turmeric is not water soluble it needs to be combined with a fat such as olive oil or coconut oil and black pepper. Turmeric has high levels of curcumin, which is useful for increasing glutathione levels. (17)

Vitamin C is one of the best detox vitamins, as it transforms toxins into digestible material.

Glutathione is not only the master antioxidant. It is also a major factor in detoxification. Glutathione binds to toxins such as heavy metals, solvents, and pesticides and transforms them into a form that can be excreted in urine or bile. (18)

Glutathione is primarily manufactured in your body from a combination of amino acids: cysteine, glutamic acid, and glycine. Of these, cysteine most determines how much glutathione you can produce. Cysteine is found in several food sources, especially whole grains, beans, eggs, and meat. Nutrients needed for glutathione to do its job effectively are lipoic acid, selenium, zinc, and vitamin B2.

Glutathione is crucial in the liver for detoxification and can become depleted from acetaminophen, alcohol consumption, and general toxic overload. Smoking, caffeine, strenuous exercise, food additives, prescription and over-the-counter drugs, ultraviolet radiation, and air pollution are factors that can also reduce or deplete glutathione levels in your body. (18)

The herb **milk thistle** is an excellent source of the antioxidant compound silymarin, which may help to prevent glutathione depletion in the liver. (19)

Selenium is necessary for the formation of glutathione in the body. Selenium is a good chelator of heavy metals. Studies have shown selenium effectively scours the body of toxic mercury buildup and mitigates its neurotoxic effects. (20) These heavy metals have two unpaired electrons that are looking for any molecules that are short two electrons. Since selenium is short two electrons, it can be used to chelate some of the worst of the heavy metals: mercury, lead, nickel and cadmium. Once chelated these metals are excreted from the body. Foods rich in selenium include Brazil nuts, whole grain cereals, oats, walnuts, legumes, tuna, beef, poultry, cheese, and eggs. (20)

**Quoted from Natural News, "Most glutathione supplements are shown to possess poor bioavailability and, in the most extreme cases, can even affect our bodies' production of natural glutathione." (21)

Cilantro, also known as coriander or Chinese parsley, has been proven to chelate toxic metals from our bodies in a relatively short period of time. (22)

My variation of Cilantro Chelation Pesto to detoxify heavy metals.
- 4 cloves garlic (glutathione, selenium, & sulfur)
- 1/3 cup Brazil nuts (selenium)
- 1/3 cup sunflower seeds (cysteine)
- 1/3 cup pumpkin seeds (zinc and magnesium)
- 2 c packed fresh cilantro (antioxidants, vitamin A)
- 2/3 cup flaxseed oil (good essential fats)
- 4 tablespoons lemon juice (vitamin C)
- 2 tsp. dulse powder (B6, B12, iodine, and other minerals)

(Adding chopped turmeric root or a tablespoon of dried turmeric will increase the overall health benefits.)

In food processor, chop garlic, nuts and seeds; add oil and lemon juice alternately with cilantro; add dulse and process until pesto consistency. Store in glass jar in the refrigerator or fill small containers and freeze.

Two teaspoons of this cilantro pesto daily for three weeks is purportedly enough to increase the urinary excretion of mercury, lead, and aluminum, thus effectively removing these toxic metals from our bodies. I usually use a tablespoon daily for 1 week. It's delicious on salads, toast, baked potatoes, sandwiches, and pasta. Consider doing this cleanse often as it is easy and tastes good.

Taking chlorella (or other greens providing chlorophyll) at the same time will help the body eliminate the metals.

Even when we are eating good organic foods, we still may need to occasionally do some herbal cleansing and hit the infrared sauna, do some soaks, or have body work to remove the toxins from the environment and the products we use.

NOTE - Before we begin to discuss detoxifying and cleansing protocols, I want to make you aware of some things I have noticed about doing cleanses.

1. Diabetics should always check with their physican before contemplating a cleanse. (23) A great website is http://www.diabetesselfmanagement.com/blog/juicing -is-it-for-you/
2. If you are on medications, you need to check with your primary care provider before you begin any major cleanse or detoxification protocol. It's possible the effectiveness of the drugs may change during the detoxification process.
3. Understand that fasting and other methods of cleansing will often cause reactions as the body is ridding itself of the unwanted toxins. These may include skin eruptions, headaches, cramping of bowels, nausea, diarrhea, or dizziness. These symptoms should be temporary, but be sure to communicate with your health practitioner during the process if you have concerns. If symptoms become

severe, call your doctor or 911 immediately. It is rare that cleansing procedures would cause any severe side effects.
4. People with certain conditions should not use infrared devices. Check with your practitioner.
5. When detoxifying children, work with an experienced practitioner.

There are many philosophies, programs, and products for cleansing available. Some are more expensive than the process needs to be, so shop around. It is always best to work with a holistic practitioner who will guide you in finding what you personally need.

Some routines are quite simple and will not interrupt your routine, while others are more intense and may require you to lessen your activity, stay at home, or even check into a center for a week or more. You will speed the process if you start to change your diet before you begin any cleanse. Making the following changes will help you detoxify faster.

Drink:
- Purified water- drinking plenty of water is very important during any cleansing procedure. Water softens material and aids in transporting toxins out of the body.
- Vegetable juices or vegetable/fruit juice combinations.
- Herbal teas

Eat:
- Lots of vegetables (sprouted, raw, baked, steamed,) and a variety of fruits. Juicing vegetables gives concentrated nutrients, but if you don't have time to juice vegetables and grasses, buy some powdered green drink to help the process.
- Lean organic or grass-fed meat, lightly cooked eggs, and plain yogurt or cultured vegetables.

Avoid:
- Refined foods—anything made with white flour, white sugar, or highly processed foods, including canned foods, frozen entrees, packaged meals, & fast foods.

- Refined grain products. This might be a time to try going wheat or gluten-free, which may often make considerable difference in your digestive health.
- All products made with hydrogenated oils or shortening, including most bakery goods.
- All processed meats, such as bologna, bacon, ham, etc. Decrease other meat consumption during the cleansing process. Meat takes more energy to digest, and you want your energy to go into cleansing.
- Dairy products, as they form mucous, which interferes with clearing the intestinal tract. Cultured dairy such as plain yogurt and kefir are acceptable.
- Alcohol, coffee, soda, and fruit drinks before and during cleanses. Decide to use less after your cleanse.

Cleansing the Colon

Start with your diet
Everyone can benefit from a colon cleanse, but if you aren't having two or three good, easy bowel movements most days, you probably have a congested colon.

It is usually best to start with a colon cleanse with liver-supporting herbs. We already know the importance of a clean colon. Much of our disease starts in the colon when the toxic waste is not regularly and completely eliminated, allowing the toxins to be reabsorbed by the body. Once we know the colon is working properly, then cleansing the other systems is more effective. A good practitioner will recommend herbal combinations that he or she feels are best for you to cleanse, detoxify, and heal the colon.

Most colon cleansing protocols will have a Formula A which makes sure the colon is emptying several times a day and a "B" formula, which will draw material from the walls of the colon and heal the walls of the colon.

Usually you can start Formula A at any time, as it won't have any major impact on your daily routine. **It is very IMPORTANT that you have taken Formula A long enough to make sure the bowels are moving well and**

**often, several times a day, BEFORE you add Formula
B. Some cleanses only use one formula. Follow the
directions for the formula you buy.**

As soon as you start a colon cleanse, start taking milk
thistle tincture (two droppersful three times a day is the
usual recommendation) to support the liver during the
cleansing process.

Usually after a week on Formula A you will add Formula B
which will draw toxins out of your body, so you may feel
sensations such as nausea, strange taste in your mouth,
and slight headache and some minor cramping normal. If
you have major cramping, vomit, or have severe diarrhea
call your health professional to readjust the protocol.

In some protocols, after your two to three week regimen of
"A" and "B," there is a maintenance program, usually
called formula "C," along with a parasite formula to take
for two weeks. If you are including fruits, vegetables, and
other foods with fiber, after a couple of weeks you will
want to wean yourself off the "C" formula. If you start to
feel sluggish and don't have several bowel movements a
day, some dietary changes may need to be made.

I don't recommend trying to mix powdered herbs for these
formulas, as it is NOT cost effective and very messy. I'm
listing the herbs usually used in colon cleansing. My
favorite colon cleansing protocol includes the following
herbs, which I learned about from studying Dr. Richard
Schultz's writings. (24)

Formula A
Aloe vera leaf -Aloe barbadensis
Senna leaves and pods - Cassia angustifolia
Cascara sagradabark - aged
Rhamnus purshiana – turkey rhubarb
Berberis vulgaris - Barberry root bark
Ginger rhizome - Zingiber officinalis
Garlic bulb - Allium sativum
Cayenne pepper - Capsicum (90,000 Scoville units)

Formula B
Ground flax seed - Linum usitatissimum

317

Apple fruit pectin- Malus communis
Pharmaceutical grade bentonite clay
Psyllium seed and husk - Plantago psyllium
Slippery elm inner bark - Ulmus fulva
Marshmallow root - Althaea officinalis
Peppermint leaf - Mentha piperita
Activated charcoal - Salix alba (25)

** It is very important to start taking a probiotic such as acidophilus or mixed cultures to repopulate the entire intestinal track during and after the cleanse and continuing for a couple of months. Remember to add prebiotic foods to your daily diet.

Parasite cleanse: Whether we want to believe it or not, most of us have parasites living in our bodies. A parasite combination can be taken during the first two or three weeks of the colon cleanse. Black walnut hull tincture, wormwood capsules or tincture, and clove bud powder in capsules are recommended by many herbalists. Continue the clove capsules for an additional two weeks to kill any eggs that may be left.

Enemas and Colonics: Colonics and enemas are therapies used to cleanse the colon by introducing water into the colon through to rectum. Enemas have been used for many years before certain surgeries or just as a cleansing procedure. Enemas use a single infusion of water into the colon, which cleanses the lower part of the colon. Kits are available in the local drug store for you to use on yourself. Some holistic health practitioners use enemas along with other detoxifying procedures.

Colonics involves multiple infusions of water that are gently forced along the entire length of the colon. Colonics need to be done by a professional who has the proper equipment. (26)

Liver/Gall Bladder Cleansing
Your liver is one of the most vital organs you possess. If it is damaged, your body cannot function properly. Without it, you cannot survive. Your liver performs tasks such as:

318

- Manufacturing a full quart of bile daily to break down fat. Bile is the yellowish green fluid that's stored in your gallbladder.
- Filtering harmful toxins and substances out of nearly 100 gallons of recycling blood every day and allowing nutrients to get to your cells
- Producing more than 13,000 crucial chemicals and hormones including cholesterol, testosterone, and estrogen
- Managing over 50,000 enzymes to maintain a healthy body
- Regulating blood sugar levels and preventing dangerous spikes and lows
- Storing essential vitamins and minerals—including vitamins A, D, K and B12—to help keep your bones from crumbling
- Detoxifying all internal and external environmental pollutants

When your liver can't cleanse your blood, all the toxins you ingest and absorb are passed unchecked into your bloodstream, where they can poison your kidneys, lungs, skin, reproductive organs, bones, and every cell in your body.

Dr. Michael Cutler says, "If your liver didn't continually remove metabolic trash and toxins from your blood, you would be dead in a matter of hours!" The reference for the above section is (27).

Gallstones are a serious warning of liver problems. I have found dissolving the stones is a more healthful option than having surgery. When your liver can't make enough bile to remove the toxins, it encapsulates and stores the toxic materials, which can affect and harm your body for years to come. Some of these toxins become hard mineralized stones stored in your gall bladder and commonly known as gallstones.

When the liver is congested from processed food, additives, drugs, other chemicals, and negative thinking it cannot provide the other natural services for the body. We must detoxify and rebuild the liver. There are many herbal combinations to help detoxify the liver/gallbladder. Below some I use in an herbal tincture combination to support and help the liver detoxify: **milk thistle, dandelion root, and barberry root**. Other combinations of herbs may be more effective for your personal needs. I do an herbal liver cleanse several times a year and often take milk thistle alone when I'm stressed or if I'm feeling toxic. (28)

There are many liver/gall bladder fasts and cleanses. Diabetics should always check with their physician before doing any cleansing.

My apple juice fast to flush the liver and gallbladder:

The malic acid in the apple juice starts to dissolve solidified bile (slush and stones). The pectin and other wonderful nutrients in the apples help to detoxify and support the liver.

Shop for a dozen organic apples, 1 gallon of organic apple juice, purified water, 2 or 3 lemons, and extra virgin olive oil.

For three days ingest only organic apples and organic apple juice, though you may have a cup herbal tea or purified water if very thirsty. If you are on necessary medications take them as usual, but don't take nutritional supplements during the fast. (Some people have success doing this protocol for only two days. I have always done it for three days.)

Near bedtime of the last day, squeeze ¼ cup fresh lemon juice and mix it with ¼ cup olive oil. While standing, drink the mixture completely within five minutes. Think positive thoughts about how this concoction is going to help your health.

Lie down immediately on your right side and try to sleep in this position for at least 5 hours. This position gets the concoction into the gallbladder to do the flushing. I have found after a few hours I needed to eliminate. Each person will react differently. You should flush out greenish slush and maybe some stones. Typical bile is greenish, so that is normal. (29)

Start your new day with apple juice, and eat lightly for the rest of the day. Choose vegetable salads with light oil dressing. By evening you can add a little protein (chicken or fish) or complex carbohydrate such as a baked sweet potato or lightly stir-fried vegetables.

Some people enjoy the benefits of a simple 2- or 3-day apple detox:
- It helps the body eliminate built up toxins and sludge.
- It is a natural way to remove the toxins causing acne or other skin problems.
- It may lessen or eliminate bad breath.
- It often results in shedding a few pounds.
- It may help adjust your eating habits.
- It improves your body's nutrient absorption.
- It should increase your energy throughout the day.
- It may help curb your desire for cigarettes. (30)

Procedure: You simply eat only raw, unpeeled organic apples and drink only water or herbal tea for 2 or 3 days. Plan it for over a week-end or when you can relax and lessen your activities. During the detox, fatigue, muscle aches, headaches, abdominal bloating, gas, constipation, and loose bowel movements may occur.

To be most effective, you will want to prepare a few days before the detox. Cut down on simple carbohydrates, tea, coffee, alcohol, and soda, reduce the size of meals, and increase your consumption of raw vegetables and fruits.

After you start, your only food can be raw, unpeeled organic apples. You are permitted unlimited quantities and all varieties. You may also have 1 cup of organic apple juice per day if you like. The only other beverages allowed are water and herbal tea but absolutely no sugar or honey or anything else in your tea. If you eat or drink anything other than apples, water, and herbal tea, you will interfere with the detoxifying process. No, I cannot tell you the science behind this, but it works for me.

321

After your detox fast ends, ease back into a normal diet with a bowl of mixed fruit, a smoothie, vegetable soup, or steamed vegetables. Hopefully your normal diet will include only foods that are nutrient dense. Avoid all processed foods.

**Note: Since apples are in the "Dirty Dozen" list of produce testing for the most pesticide, you <u>must use organic apples </u>for this to be effective. (31)

Caution: As with any detoxifying procedure, pregnant women and people with blood sugar problems such as diabetes or with conditions such kidney, heart or liver disease <u>should not undertake this fast without discussing it with your health care provider.</u>

Blood Cleansing. Blood cleansing herbs can be taken alone or at the same time as other cleanses. Some herbs that are used are garlic, red clover blossoms, cayenne pepper, chaparral dandelion root, echinacea root, hawthorn leaf, licorice root, pau d'arco, sarsaparilla, and yellow dock root. If you use Chaparral in a combination, limit its use to a week, as it is very powerful. (28)

Kidney/bladder cleansing uses these supporting herbs: uva ursi, juniper berries, corn silk, marshmallow root, and parsley leaf or root.(28)

Below is a site with information on cleansing by Hulda Clark. (32)
http://curezone.com/cleanse/liver/huldas_recipe.asp

Candida yeast: remedies and notes
In the gastro-intestinal tract there is a constant battle between good and bad bacteria. Candida yeast/fungal overgrowth has been found to be a common occurrence in many disorders and is often lurking in people who cannot figure out what is wrong with them.

<u>Symptoms vary but might include:</u>
- an incapacitating fatigue
- problems with concentration, brain fog, and short-term memory

- flu-like symptoms such as pain in the joints and muscles
- extreme tightness in the shoulders and neck
- hyper-acidity/acid reflux
- blisters in the mouth/tongue/throat
- poor sleep, never feel rested
- "crawling" skin
- white coated tongue
- dark circles under the eyes
- chronic sinus problems and headaches (33)

Remedies to relieve yeast infections can be divided into <u>three groups</u>:

1. <u>Herbs that kill candida</u>: goldenseal root or Oregon grape root, garlic*, oregano oil, caprylic acid, grapefruit seed exact, black walnut hull, mugwort, pau d'arco, and olive leaf extract. Coconut oil is also effective against candida. (34)
2. <u>Herbs that support the immune system</u>: echinacea, astragalus, and garlic*.
3. Probiotics to restore normal intestinal flora: Lactobacillus acidophilus, L. bifidus, etc. Take probiotics at bedtime and/or the first thing in the morning. Probiotics need to be taken in large quantities as well as with soluble fiber to rebuild the intestinal terrain. Also add prebiotic foods to your meals whenever you can.

*Garlic serves the dual purpose of immune support and killing yeast.

Caprylic acid is very effective in an anti-yeast protocol. Buy caprylic acid in a timed-release capsule because the intestine quickly absorbs caprylic acid. We want gradual dispersion, allowing the entire gastrointestinal tract to be coated.

Do a liver cleanse and a colon cleanse either before or with candida treatment.

** *Often candidasis exists with parasites, so a parasite cleanse may also be necessary.*

Foods to avoid until candida is under control:
- <u>All forms of sugar,</u> alcohol, fruits, white flour products
- Yeast and gluten
- Vinegars and other fermented products
- Dried, processed or pickled meat
- Aged or processed cheeses (mold)
- Peanuts, peanut butter and pistachios (mold)
- Coffee, black tea, sodas
- Processed food

Eat a high protein diet—<u>Candida cannot live on protein</u>—and non-starchy vegetables.

Antifungal herbs for sitz baths or douching are soothing and healing. Use a strong infusion of chamomile, lavender, and calendula flowers. (28)

Juicing: Almost any combination of raw vegetables, fruits and herbs can be juiced. I use what is in season or what I have. Try carrots, beets, asparagus, apples, celery, and one of the Brassicas -broccoli, cabbage, kale, Brussels sprouts, or cauliflower—with wheatgrass, spinach, chard, or dandelion leaves and purslane if available. Adding some parsley, turmeric, and/or oregano enriches the juice with mega nutrients plus added flavor. The synergy of the combination of these foods will help your liver purge toxins during the cleansing process.

Many of these foods and herbs are high in naturally-occurring sulfur and glutathione, which help the liver detoxify harmful chemicals. Try a variety of combinations.

For information on the health benefits of juice fasting I recommend http://www.hippocratesinst.org/or <u>The Hippocrates Diet and Health Program</u> by Ann Wigmore.

<u>**I repeat, discuss any fasts or protocols with your holistic practitioner.**</u>

1. You may not be able to tolerate the changes that detoxifying will cause.

2. Those with anemia may not be able to do this protocol because they are too weak and need a nutritional program to build the blood before detoxifying.
3. If you are taking drugs, be sure to check with your doctor before doing this cleanse, as it may change the action of the drugs.
4. If you are diabetic, pregnant or nursing, don't do detoxifying procedures unless you are working closely with a knowledgeable practitioner. (35)

Hydrotherapy refers to using water to revitalize, maintain, and restore health. Baths or soaks, saunas, steam baths, foot baths, sitz baths, and the application of cold and hot water compresses are all used to help elimination. Often your practitioner will ask you to alternate hot and cold water.

I first learned about the cold/heat treatment when studying John Christopher's materials. Cold water is stimulating and causes superficial blood vessels to constrict, shunting the blood to internal organs. Hot water is relaxing, causes blood vessels to dilate, removing wastes from body tissues. Alternating hot can cold water also improves elimination, decreases inflammation, and stimulates circulation. (36)

I have found soaks to be an important part of my maintenance program. Start a soak by steeping a pot of ginger or yarrow tea (at least 2 cups). These herbs will raise your internal temperature and induce perspiration. You can add a bit of honey if it is too bitter. Drink a cup of tea while the tub is filling, then a cup while soaking. Soak for 30 minutes, adding hot water to keep it as warm as you can stand. Your body may lose several cups of liquid during the soak as you sweat out the impurities.

- Relaxing: Try a warm bath with 6-8 drops of lavender essential oil
- Heavy petrochemical detox: add 1 pint 3% hydrogen peroxide (regular drugstore variety) to the water.
- Radiation detox: One pound each of sea salt and soda to a tub of very warm water. Soak for 30 minutes. Shower with warm water to remove the salt &soda

When finished, wrap in a large towel and a blanket to continue to sweat. Continue to drink herbal tea or water, as your body has lost considerable fluids.

Far Infrared therapy - Infrared light is part of the sun's invisible spectrum. One of Far-Infrared light's characteristics is the ability to penetrate human tissue easily.

In her book, "The Science of Far Infrared Therapies," Dr. Toshiko Yamazaki explains that one of the reasons FIR (Far Infrared) has beneficial results in a variety of illnesses is the ability of FIR waves to remove toxins, which are often at the core of many health problems. Conventional saunas heat the air in the chamber to a very high temperature, which in turn heats our body. The Infra red sauna works differently: activated by heat, the Far Infared sauna emits FIR energy that is absorbed by human cells, causing a physical phenomenon called "Resonance." Neither oxygen molecules nor nitrogen molecules in the air block the FIR wave; therefore, the FIR infrared rays penetrate directly into our bodies. (37)

"Infrared heat is the only heat that penetrates deep enough and hot enough to melt subcutaneous fat, (at 40C or 104F), which is where the body stores dangerous toxins and acids, and literally shakes them lose so they can be directly expelled safely out of the body through our sweat," says David Floyd, CEO of LuxSauna Inc.

In studying the safety of using Far Infrared devices I can find no dangers related to the rays. However, there are dangers if the person does not understand the process or has health situations such as indicated below.

Who can use far-infrared devices such as a sauna?

Healthy adults who follow the procedures usually have no problems. The elderly should use it only under a practitioner's supervision. Children can use it briefly if they are hydrated, have good nutrition, and are supervised. Do not bring pets into a FIR sauna.

Completely avoid using a sauna in the case of existing
medical conditions such as:
- Stroke
- Severe aortic stenosis
- Recent myocardial infarction (heart attack)
- Unstable angina pectoris
- Lupus erythematosus, if you are on steroids (interferes
with blood circulation)
- Brain tumors
- Multiple sclerosis
- Silicone implants (38)

Check with your doctor about sauna use if you have:
- Pacemakers (check with doctor and/or manufacturer)
- Pins, rods and other implants, such as cochlear
  implants
- Diabetes (and definitely start slowly and monitor your
  blood sugar)
- Any heart condition.

**While the above are some of the conditions which may
pose dangers through sauna use, definitely check with
your doctor about your specific medical condition(s) and
any drugs you are taking.

Things to consider when using a sauna:

- **Dehydration** and inadequate fluid replacement: Make
  sure you are hydrated and have a large glass of water
  in the sauna with you; drink several glasses of water
  after a session. As you sweat your body will lose
  electrolytes (minerals), so replace with a liquid mineral
  supplement of a mineral rich juice.

- **Do not drink alcohol or take recreational or OTC
  drugs** before or while in the sauna.

- **Overheating effects**: Limit those first sessions until
  you know how your body is going to react. If you
  suspect you're overheating, get out of the sauna and
  into a cool shower.

- **Effects of past use of any drugs especially
  psychedelic and other mind-altering drugs**: Any

327

drugs you have used in the past, including prescription drugs, may have left residues which may be released during the sauna process. If you know you have used psychedelic and other mind-altering drugs in the past, you may experience a full-blown "trip" as residues of the drug are released from where they were stored in the tissues into your bloodstream again. If you know you might have this experience you should NOT be alone. Have a knowledgeable adult with you as you do the sauna detoxifying and for several hours after to help you through the experience.

- **Risks for chemically sensitive people**: During any detoxification program the body will be bringing chemicals out of tissues and organs and moving them into the bloodstream, which may cause very nasty effects for some chemically-sensitive people.

Eating organic raw apples with the skins (before or after) is very helpful in avoiding the side effects of detoxification. Juiced or blenderized greens will also help and will provide needed vitamins and minerals.

More than 800 fire-fighters and police officers that were poisoned at the World Trade Center 911 disaster site were successfully detoxified through a sauna detox program in New York City. (39)

PART D—A GLIMPSE AT ILLNESSES OF TODAY

We've already discussed cancer and infectious disease, so now let's look at a few of the other major issues facing people today.

1. Protecting the Cardiovascular system
2. Blood Sugar Issues
3. Autoimmune Disease
4. What Has Society Done to Our Children?
5. Alzheimer's Disease

1 PROTECTING THE CARDIOVASCULAR SYSTEM

A heart attack can happen to anyone from teens through elders, even to those with low cholesterol and those who are very physically fit. This tells us there are many different factors involved in cardiovascular disease. Men used to be considered more vulnerable to heart attacks, but that isn't true anymore. Now more women than men die of heart disease each year in the U.S. (1)

The staff at the Mayo clinic has published the following good information to help us deal with heart attacks.

WARNING SIGNS: *Know the warning signs of a heart attack so you can act fast to get treatment for yourself or someone else. The sooner you get emergency help, the less damage your heart will sustain.*

CALL FOR IMMEDIATE HELP IF YOU EXPERIENCE:
- **Persistent chest pain that is not relieved by nitroglycerin**
- **Severe and persistent shortness of breath**
- **Fainting**

INFORM YOUR DOCTOR OR NURSE AS SOON AS POSSIBLE IF YOU EXPERIENCE:
- **Increasing shortness of breath and tolerating less and less activity**
- **Consistently awakening short of breath**
- **Needing more pillows to sleep comfortably**
- **Rapid heart rate or worsening palpitations**

The most common heart attack symptom in <u>women</u> is some type of pain, pressure or discomfort in the chest. But it's not always severe or even the most prominent symptom, particularly in women. **Women are more likely than men to have heart attack symptoms unrelated to chest pain**, such as:
- Neck, shoulder, upper back or abdominal discomfort
- Shortness of breath
- Nausea or vomiting
- Sweating
- Lightheadedness or dizziness
- Unusual fatigue

These symptoms are more subtle than the obvious crushing chest pain often associated with heart attacks. This may be because women tend to have blockages not only in their main arteries, but also in the smaller arteries that supply blood to the heart—a condition called small vessel heart disease or microvascular disease. <u>It is well known that taking aspirin may not be an effective preventive for women</u>. (1)

The National Heart Lung and blood Institute tells us:
"Not everyone having a heart attack has typical symptoms. If you've already had a heart attack, your symptoms may not be the same for another one. However, some people may have a pattern of symptoms that recur. The more signs and symptoms you have, the more likely it is that you're having a heart attack.

Act Fast. - The signs and symptoms of a heart attack can develop suddenly. However, they also can develop slowly—sometimes within hours, days, or weeks of a heart attack.

Call 911 for help right away if you think you or someone else may be having a heart attack. You also should call for help if your chest pain doesn't go away as it usually does when you take medicine prescribed for angina.

Do not drive yourself to the hospital. Call an ambulance so that medical personnel can begin life-saving treatment on the way to the emergency room." (2)

RECOGNIZING A STROKE—ask these 4 questions to identify a stroke:
S- Ask the individual to **S**MILE.
T- Ask the person to **T**ALK, to SPEAK A SIMPLE SENTENCE.
R- Ask him or her to **R**AISE BOTH ARMS.
O- Ask the person to "STICK **O**UT THEIR TONGUE. If the tongue is "crooked" or if it goes to one side or the other, <u>that is also an indication of a stroke.</u>

If he or she has trouble with any one of the above tasks, call 911 immediately and describe the symptoms to the dispatcher.

The goal is to Keep the entire vascular system healthy.

Most conditions are preventable and/or treatable naturally. Our goals include:

- Strengthening the heart muscle
- Lowering inflammation throughout the body
- Strengthening and cleaning the blood vessels (veins, arteries, and smaller vessels)
- Improving circulation of the lymph and the blood
- Controlling the viscosity of the blood
- Managing your blood pressure
- Understanding and lowering triglycerides

The heart is a muscle, so as with all muscles, it needs to be exercised. Walking briskly every day can be the easiest way to work that heart and improve circulation. (1)

Risk Factors in Cardiovascular Disease

Atherosclerosis is often a big factor in cardiovascular disease. Inflammation is the fundamental cause of

331

atherosclerosis. Arterial damage is caused by several factors including high levels of homocysteine, trans-fatty acids, chemical toxicity, lack of essential fatty acids, and lack of vitamin C.

A high level of <u>homocysteine</u> in the blood has been positively correlated with pathological buildup of plaque in the arteries and the tendency to form clots - a deadly combination. High levels of homocysteine are usually an indication of a deficiency of **folic acid, vitamin B6, vitamin B12 and choline.** Homocysteine can be converted in the body to a harmless substance known as cystanthionine when adequate nutrients are available. Nutritionist, Patrick Holford says, "Homocysteine predicts heart disease risk better than cholesterol, blood pressure or smoking." (3)

Hypertension (high blood pressure) seems to be one of those issues upon which <u>doctors cannot agree.</u> I'm not going to enter the controversy except to say I feel it is ludicrous in this day of talking about individual differences to think that we should all have the same blood pressure readings or that we all fit into any other "box" that has been created by the medical business. Does it make sense that a 70 year old should have the same blood pressure as a teen-ager? In addition many factors can affect or even invalidate blood pressure readings.

Blood pressure that is normal for me is NOT 120/80; it is higher. At my age (75) if my blood pressure was 120/80, I might be in danger of stroke or other issues. My blood is pumping through vessels that are less elastic than when I was 16, and my heart valves may not work as easily as they once did. (4)

There are many factors involved with reading blood pressure.

1. The size of the blood pressure cuff: Will a reading be accurate if the <u>same size cuff is used for all adults whether they are 98 pound females or 240 pound males who have heavy arms</u>?

2. Many people become very stressed when their blood pressure is taken known as "white coat hypertension", so what would their normal blood pressure be?

3. Is the person's blood sugar low?

4. Has the person just exercised?

5. Is the person under acute stress?

That being said, **extremely high blood pressure is a sign of a problem,** so we need to <u>find what is causing the elevated blood pressure and solve **that** problem</u>, not just medicate to lower the symptom.

Despite over 100 antihypertensive drugs that have been approved as being safe and effective, the sad fact is that medical science has not been very successful in controlling hypertension. "More than 43 million Americans have high blood pressure (hypertension), but less than one third of them have achieved targeted levels of blood pressure." (5)

<u>Side effects</u>: What is the cost in side effects of taking anti-hypertensive drugs? Impotence in men is a common side effect when taking a blood pressure medication. When I take a prescription of hypertension, I often have blurry vision, brain fog, sometimes a headache, and sometimes my blood pressure becomes erratic. Depending on my stress level and kidney function, at times I can control my blood pressure with herbs and exercise.

I've said over and over that cholesterol is not the basic problem in heart disease, but remember, **there is one kind of cholesterol that is a problem—oxidized cholesterol**. (6) We've discussed it in the "Fats" section. Avoid processed food and hydrogenated oils. Include adequate omega-3 fatty acids and saturated fats in your diet.

Triglycerides - Another important factor to consider when monitoring cardiovascular health is your triglyceride level. <u>Triglycerides in the blood are not made from dietary fats but are made in the liver from excess sugars</u> which have not been used for energy. Eating more calories than your body can use for energy contributes to higher triglycerides. The excess fuel is converted to (triglycerides) that sometimes settles around the waist or other areas on the body but can also cling to artery walls. (7)

High blood sugar levels lead to high triglycerides levels. Sugars and refined grains stimulate insulin production. Insulin stimulates the liver to produce triglycerides.

Some of the factors that cause high triglycerides are:
- Being overweight
- Eating a diet high in simple carbohydrates and simple sugars
- Eating trans-fats in processed and fast foods
- Consuming alcohol in excess
- Consuming foods and drinks made with high fructose corn syrup (HFCS)
- Lack of activity (exercise) - We all need at least 30 minutes of significant motion like walking per day.
- High blood pressure
- Diabetes – out of control blood sugar
- Taking birth control pills, estrogen therapy, some diuretics, and certain other medications may cause a rise in triglycerides.
- Heredity - For some people, high triglycerides can be attributed to family history. (7)

Drinking even a small amount of alcohol can cause a significant increase in your triglyceride levels, and consuming large quantities of alcohol can cause a severe and long-term increase in the blood levels of this potentially dangerous form of fat. High blood triglyceride levels, also known as hyperlipidemia, have been linked with an elevated risk of developing coronary artery disease. (8)

A simple blood test can reveal whether your triglycerides fall into a healthy range.

High fructose corn syrup (HFCS) has been implicated in the rise of triglyceride levels. It's has been found that people who use HFCS as a sweetener increase their triglycerides 32 percent relative to people who use mostly sugar. (9)

Why is excess fructose such a culprit, even worse than glucose? Because the two are metabolized differently. Glucose is used by and metabolized in **all** body cells. It is an energy provider for your brain, muscles, and all body organs. Fructose is not a direct source of energy. (10)

The metabolism of excessive amounts of fructose leads to fatty liver, which is a key step in the development of insulin resistance. **Insulin resistance** has been found to be a factor in heart disease as well as other chronic disease. Insulin resistance is associated with inflammation, as reflected by increased levels of the inflammatory markers nuclear factor-kappa B, interleukin-6, and C-reactive protein (CRP).5,9 C-reactive protein is the blood test that is a valuable tool to gauge hidden, imperceptible inflammation. (11)

Peripheral muscular changes influence the progression of heart failure. This effect may be due to chronic disturbances of insulin and glucose metabolism that affect the energy status of skeletal and myocardial muscle. (12)

Foods and Nutrients for good cardiovascular health:

Beet root – betaine, glyconutrients, antioxidants, betalains which have been found to have outstanding anti-inflammatory, antioxidant, and detoxifying effects.

Kelp – glyconutrients, iodine and other trace minerals

Goji Berry – glyconutrients, betaine, essential fatty acids, antioxidant vitamins and phytonutrients

Food sources of each nutrient can be found in the "Understanding the Nutritional Jargon" section of the book.

B vitamins - (B-3 (Niacin), B-6 (Pyridoxine), Folate (folic acid), and B-12 (Cyanocobalamin or methylcobalamin) work together to help reduce harmful homocysteine. Homocysteine is an ugly amino acid that causes your body to lay down sticky, artery-hardening platelets in blood vessels. (13)

** I feel it is difficult to consume adequate levels of B-vitamins in foods, so I have supplemented with a B-50 complex for years. It is important when supplementing to use a B-complex, so you get the <u>synergy of all the B vitamins</u>.

Betaine, also known as trimethylglycine, is important in controlling homocysteine is produced by the body from choline and from the amino acid, glycine. (14)

Vitamin C, a potent antioxidant that strengthens the blood vessels, helps reverse clogged arteries, and may lower blood pressure by protecting the body's supply of nitric oxide. Nitric oxide relaxes blood vessels, contributing to healthy blood pressure levels." (15)

Vitamin D deficiency can affect any area of our bodies. Researchers say a growing body of evidence suggests that vitamin D deficiency increases the risk of heart disease and is linked to other well-known heart disease risk factors such as high blood pressure, obesity, and diabetes.When supplementing use Vitamin D3. (16)

Vitamin E is important in the formation of red blood cells and is a powerful antioxidant that protects your cells from damaging free radicals and anti-inflammation.

**I also feel that anyone over 40 needs to supplement with <u>natural vitamin E</u> at 400 IU per day, gradually increasing that to 800 IU as you age or if there are cardio issues.

Coenzyme Q10 in the form of Ubiquinol is crucial in promoting heart health, preventing cardiovascular disease, and may even reverse signs of cardiovascular disease. CoQ10 improves tissue oxygenation and increases circulation. Start with 30 mg daily and work up to 100 mg daily. (17)

Omega-3 fatty acids help prevent erratic heart rhythms, making blood less likely to clot inside arteries (which is the proximate cause of most heart attacks), and improving the ratio of good (HDL) cholesterol to potentially harmful

(LDL) cholesterol. Omega-3's also reduce inflammation of the vessels and the heart. (18)

Calcium – I do not take a calcium supplement because I have had too much calcium in my blood (hypercalcemia). Researchers are changing their viewpoint on calcium supplementation. So many packaged and processed foods are enriched with calcium, but not magnesium. We have learned that finding the right balance of calcium, magnesium, trace minerals such as boron, and vitamin D for the individual is the important factor. Levels of calcium and vitamin D can be evaluated through a blood test, but since very little magnesium is in the blood, a blood test is not a accurate determinate for magnesium. Unless the diet is high in foods high in magnesium, most people would benefit from supplementing with magnesium. (20)

Magnesium affects the creation of ATP (adenosine triphosphate) the energy molecules of the body, the action of the heart muscle, the proper formation of bones and teeth, relaxation of blood vessels, and the promotion of proper bowel function. <u>Adequate magnesium is a major factor in maintaining a healthy heart</u>. (19)

Potassium/salt ratio – We have previously discussed the important of both minerals being in balance in the body. They are important for blood pressure balance and healthy cellular interchange. Consuming natural fruits and vegetables will usually give you the salt/potassium balance your body requires. Consuming highly salted foods will upset the balance and require more potassium rich foods. Excess of anything can cause problems and there is a problem with consuming salty processed food which usually contains MSG and many other health disturbing ingredients. Recent research described in Nature Magazine points out the fallacy of the "no salt" philosophy. (21)

Phytonutrients - An array of phytonutrients is needed for health, the cardiovascular system is no exception.

Bioflavonoids promote healing and prevent bruising. They are essential for the absorption of vitamin C. Some vitamin C supplements contain a small amount of bioflavonoids. Rutin is a non-citrus bioflavonoid that helps maintain the strength of blood vessels.

Glutathione, a major antioxidant, is recommended to protect the heart, veins, and arteries from oxidant damage. It helps to defend the body against damage from cigarette smoking and many of other toxins.

Bromelain, an enzyme found in pineapple, breaks down fibrin. Supplements of bromelain would be necessary as you probably couldn't eat enough pineapple to get a significant amount. 500 mg three times a day is suggested. Quercetin is a bioflavonoid that is thought to work synergistically with bromelain to enhance absorption.

Herbs that help the cardiovascular system:

Hawthorn berry – acts as an ACE inhibitor, calcium channel blocker, vasodilator, diuretic, antioxidant, heart tonic and relaxant. (22) It has phytonutrients, vitamins and minerals.

Cayenne – to get an adequate amount it is best taken in capsule form with food. Cayenne:
- reduces congestion and inflammation
- thins the blood and improve circulation
- may help to clean out the arteries and reverse atherosclerosis
- reduces cholesterol and triglyceride levels
- acts as a catalyst for other herbs
- acts as a tonic for the heart, kidneys, lungs, pancreas, spleen, and stomach (23)

Garlic may prevent heart disease by:
  a. thinning the blood, reducing its tendency to clot.
  b. reducing blood pressure.
  c. opening the blood vessels.

d. lowering levels of fat and cholesterol in the blood.

e. lowering serum levels of homocysteine.

f. protecting the heart from infection because of the antibacterial and antiviral properties of the garlic. (24)

Ginger root - blood thinner, promotes circulation, and anti-inflammatory which improves vascular health. Ginger is one of the best foods in reducing the "stickiness" of blood platelets, lowering the incidence of clots. (25)

Motherwort - is effective when used for nervous heart problems, heart flutters, cardiac edema, and to lower blood pressure. (26)

Monitoring nitric oxide levels for heart health.

Nitric oxide:

- Reduces arterial plaque
- Expands blood vessels reducing blood pressure
- Controls platelet function so they don't clump together and cause blood clots
- Relieves impotence

Eating nuts and grass-fed meat will provide L-arginine, which, along with adequate vitamin C, will keep nitric oxide at a healthy level. Usually nitric acid from foods is not a problem, but using nitric acid supplements can have serious side effects. (27)

Exercise – Walking is one of the best habits for preventing cardiovascular problems. We all need a combination of aerobic and weight bearing exercise to maintain good circulation and strong muscular structure.

What we avoid is as important as what we eat.

Avoid hydrogenated fats (trans-fats) which destroy your blood vessels. That translates to NOT using hydrogenated vegetable oils, nut butters, white shortening, or eating bakery goods or most packed mixes. Use real butter, olive oil, coconut oil, or non-hydrogenated cold pressed nut oil. (28)

Avoid all sodas, as the phosphoric acid counteracts the calcium/magnesium balance in the body.

Avoid stress, which is considered one of the biggest factors in cardiovascular disease. There are dozens of books about it, but stress is such an individual factor that each person needs to evaluate his/her situation. Factors to consider:

- Becoming angry quickly is a serious factor. Deep breathing when you become irritated or angry will bring oxygen to the heart muscle to protect it.
- Relationships – family, work, friends, school
- Financial situation
- Addictions – sugar, alcohol, nicotine, drugs of any kind

Decide what you can change. Even simple changes may make a difference.

Blood viscosity and clotting

Blood coagulation can be easily tested and should fall within a desirable range. If it coagulates too easily, clots can form which in turn can lead to adverse health conditions such as heart attacks.

If blood doesn't clot enough, conditions such as extreme bleeding from a cut or small wound, nosebleeds, hemorrhages, heavy periods in women, and bleeding strokes may occur. If a person's blood isn't clotting enough and he has an accident such as a car accident, he could have a serious problem by losing too much blood. (29)

There is some evidence suggesting that people with thicker (or more viscous) blood have higher chances of developing heart disease or having a heart attack or stroke. (29)The more viscous the blood, the harder the heart must work to move it around the body and the more likely it is to form clots inside arteries and veins. Finding your best level of viscosity is important.

Vitamin K is used in the body to <u>control blood clotting</u>. It is essential in the creation of prothrombin in the body, which is the precursor to thrombin - a very important factor in blood clotting.

Caution: If you are taking any cardiac drugs, check with your doctor before making any diet or supplement modifications. Know that high vitamin K intake can interfere with anticoagulant medication. (30) Prescription blood thinners or aspirin seem to be very popular as blood thinners. One needs to be aware of the dangers involved, especially if blood thinning-foods or herbs are also consumed. Eating just the blood thinning foods and herbs is more desirable than using drugs. The combination can be dangerous. Many foods contain salicylates, aspirin-like substances which will thin the blood. Alcohol will also thin the blood. (31)

Foods and Herbs that Thin the Blood (32)

Blueberries	Grapes	Prunes
Cayenne pepper	Raw honey	Raisins
	Jicama	Strawberries
Cherries	Licorice	Tangerines
Chewing gum	Olive Oil	Thyme
Cider	Omega-3s	Turmeric
Cinnamon	Onions	Vinegar
Cranberries	Oranges	Vitamin E
Dill	Oregano	Wine
Garlic	Paprika	
Ginger	Peppermint	

Using herbs and natural foods can significantly decrease the risk of cardio-vascular disease. Some factors to note:

- Oils that help reduce blood clotting are black currant, borage, hemp and fish oils.
- Garlic and onions both have proven to be very effective in reducing blood clots. **Garlic contains nine different, naturally occurring, antiplatelet compounds.** (33)
- Reishi mushroom has been shown effective for reducing blood clots, for healthy blood pressure, lowering cholesterol and triglycerides, and improving HDL. (34)

Varicose veins are veins that have enlarged and twisted, often appearing as a bulging, blue blood vessel that is clearly visible through the skin.

Goals to prevent or eliminate varicose veins includes to:

1. Strengthen the blood with flavonoid-rich extracts and vitamin C. A tendency for weak blood vessels may be genetic, but a diet high in nutrients can be overcome some of the weakness.

2. Make sure bowel movements are soft, easy and regular (at least two a day). I recommend a colon cleanse followed by a liver cleanse for everyone once a year as a yearly tune-up to keep the bowels moving easily. Consider adding a bulking agent such as psyllium seed, pectin, or guar gum to your diet. These are mildly laxative as they attract water and form a gelatinous mass, making defecation easier. Usually add any of the above to a glass of water, mix well, drink, and then drink another glass of water as a chaser. Without adequate water, they won't work and can even add to the problem.

3. Fibrin is naturally produced in your body and gets deposited around varicose veins. You have an increased risk of thrombophlebitis, myocardial infarction, pulmonary embolism, or stroke if your body cannot break down fibrin. Pineapple and papaya are foods that contain enzymes which break down the fibrin.

4. Increase circulation (movement of blood) through exercise.

5. Foods like ginger, garlic, and green tea are good for blood thinning and cleansing. Other than these, the most commonly used supplements are Papain, Bromelain, Rutin, Coenzyme Q10 and Magnesium. (35)

Follow the above dietary guidelines for the cardiovascular system. To strengthen your veins, daily consume **dark red or purple berries** – hawthorn, blueberries, bilberries, black currants, blackberries, or even black cherries, which contain compounds that strengthen blood vessels. **Garlic, onions, ginger, and ground cayenne (red pepper)** contain compounds that tend to break down fibrin, increase circulation, lower blood pressure, and reduce congestion. Use these liberally in your diet.

Herbs: The following herbs are more specific for the veins.

Gotu kola (Centella asiatica) extract has been found to reinforce the "cement" that holds your veins and valves together so they work more efficiently. It seems to enhance connective tissue structure, reduce sclerosis, and improve blood flow. European studies have found the gotu kola is an effective treatment for venous insufficiency and varicose veins - 60 to 120 mg were taken daily. (36)

Horse chestnut (Aesculus hippocastanum) is known as a venotonic, meaning it improves venous tone by increasing the contractile potential of the elastic fibers in the vein wall. Horse chestnut has been found effective in the treatment of varicose veins by the German Commission E. Use only standardized extract. (37)

Butcher's broom (Ruscus aculeatus) has been used in combination with vitamin C by the Italians for varicose veins. Use in extract form. (38)

Other helpful information about varicose veins:

- Bathing the affected parts in white oak bark tea is suggested by several experienced practitioners to stimulate blood flow. Simmer (don't boil) a strong tea, soak cotton compresses in the tea, and apply to the affected area.
- Avoid sitting or standing in one position for extended lengths of time, which doesn't allow the leg muscles to contract and push the blood upward. Change positions and exercise those leg muscles as much as possible. Walking is great because it gets your blood moving.
- Elevate your legs whenever possible. Dangling legs put pressure on the area where your legs leave the chair.
- Acupressure or acupuncture treatment can be helpful in clearing congestion and improving circulation.
- Wearing elastic compression stockings is an option, though they can be hot and expensive. Even wearing lighter weight support hose may be helpful, especially if you are on your feet most of the time. (39)

2. BLOOD SUGAR ISSUES

Diabetes is rampant, and so are other blood sugar issues which can cause great distress to the body.

Diabetes is a disorder characterized by abnormally high blood glucose levels. People with diabetes cannot properly process glucose, a sugar the body uses for energy. As a result, glucose tends to move inefficiently from the bloodstream to the tissues of the body where it is needed. At the same time that blood glucose levels are elevated, the rest of the body can be starved for glucose. Diabetes can lead to poor wound healing, higher risk of infections, and damage to the eyes, kidneys, nerves, and heart.

There are risks with taking the usually prescribed diabetic drugs. It says right on the National Institutes of Health Medline Plus Web site, "The use of sulfonylurea anti-diabetic agents has been reported, but not proven in all studies, **to increase the risk of death from heart and blood vessel disease"**.

A person with diabetes has a 50 percent greater chance of having a heart attack than a person without diabetes, who has a 5% risk.

In my reading, I have found there have been significant deaths from sulfonylurea. (40)

**If you are taking any diabetes medication discuss the short and long term side effects of the drug with your pharmacist and/or doctor. Consider working with a natural practitioner to control your diabetes. In my experience, it is not difficult, and there will be fewer side effects.

The reality is that diabetes is a major industry.

As you have read, **I have controlled my diabetes for over thirty years with diet, exercise, and other natural options.** Considering my family history, if I had not made drastic changes in my lifestyle and diet, I would have followed my family on the insulin trail. People ask me why I think it is such a big deal to avoid insulin or other diabetic drugs, since many people use them.

There are many reasons:
- I've watched several people deteriorate, go blind, and die an early death because they could not discipline themselves to balance the insulin with the sugars they consumed.
- The side effects of diabetic drugs are unacceptable to me.
- Two of my siblings have died from diabetic complications.
- I don't like shots and I don't want my body to have to deal with drugs.
- I want to have total health, not just a series of band-aids to control symptoms.

How have I controlled my Borderline Diabetes for over 30 years? Here are the basics:
- Eat at the first sign of low blood sugar. For me signs are becoming light headed, dizzy, and/or extreme hunger pangs.
- Drink plenty of water.
- Eat high-protein foods at every meal and snack. I find eating meat helps me control my blood sugar much better than vegetables proteins.
- Eat several servings of a variety of complex carbohydrate vegetables and greens and a couple of raw fruits each day.
- Avoid refined sugar, white flour, and all processed foods.
- Avoid all sodas and fruit drinks.
- Hardly ever eat desserts. When I eat nutritious food I don't need anything else. If I want fruit or a simple, healthful dessert, I eat it alone, not after a big meal.
- Avoid artificial sweeteners, as they are harmful and often cause food cravings.
- Exercise, especially walking, resets my metabolism to be more efficient.

The first step to managing diabetes is to <u>believe you can</u> make some changes that will help lower your insulin intake in Type I, or totally control other forms of diabetes naturally.

For forty years, medical research has consistently shown with increasing clarity that Type II diabetes is a degenerative disease directly caused by an engineered food supply focused on profit instead of health. (41) If not curable, Type II diabetes can often be managed naturally without the side effects involved with drug therapy.

It is ironic that often physicians suggest patients use artificial sweeteners to avoid consuming sugar, especially in sodas. I wish they understood the dangers of artificial sweeteners. Why don't they recommend people drink water? We have already discussed the dangers of using HFCS (high fructose corn syrup), Aspartame, and Sucralose (Splenda). Research shows these sweeteners are factors involved in the increase of diabetes. (42)

Often people are told to avoid meat, especially red meats. We need the specific amino acids that meats provide. We also need fats. When the doctor diagnosed my diabetes he told me I needed to eat meat at every meal. When I eat meat at every meal, I'm satisfied so I don't need to eat as often.

Insulin resistance - We need to understand the role of insulin in the body before we can discuss insulin resistance. Insulin is a hormone produced by the beta cells in the pancreas. When the beta cells detect that food has been eaten, the cells release insulin into the bloodstream. Insulin triggers the body's cells to allow glucose to enter them. Glucose is broken down (metabolized) to produce the energy needed for the cells to work properly. When we eat foods high in refined carbohydrates, insulin levels surge to remove the sugar from the blood and get it into your cells. This mechanism works very well for the most part. However, if insulin spikes too often from a diet rich in the high-carb foods that trigger insulin secretion, your cells respond by decreasing the acceptance of insulin receptors on their surfaces. Eventually, this prevents glucose from getting into your cells. Insulin:

- regulates the cellular absorption and utilization of glucose

- is needed for to regulate the cellular absorption and utilization of <u>amino acids and fatty acids</u>
- activates and inactivates enzymes (the protein catalysts for the body's biochemical reactions)
- directly affects certain genetic processes including protein synthesis (43)

Insulin resistance happens when the cells begin to resist the insulin that transports blood sugar throughout the body for use by the cells. Eventually the body tries to compensate for the cells' inability to use insulin by overproducing it. Insulin resistance by the cells activates insulin receptors in the liver, which in turn activates cholesterol and triglyceride production. (44)

Insulin resistance is associated with inflammation, as reflected by increased levels of the inflammatory markers nuclear factor-kappa B, interleukin-6, and C-reactive protein (CRP).5,9. The C-reactive protein blood test is a valuable tool to gauge hidden inflammation.

Take charge of blood sugar issues including diabetes.

1. Do not go longer than three hours without eating!
2. In the morning avoid foods that cause your blood sugar levels to spike and then crash which includes: simple sugars (including candy), cookies, many processed foods, sodas, white/refined bread, and products containing them.
3. Eat an animal protein like eggs or a small piece of meat early in the day (breakfast), which helps stabilizeblood sugar levels. Protein should be eaten with every meal and with most snacks. Good protein foods include free-range eggs, poultry and other lean naturally grown animal protein, legumes, nuts, and seeds. Quality protein drinks with low sugar levels may be acceptable occasionally in emergency situations but not as a regular replacement for protein.
4. Avoid alcohol.
5. Avoid artificial sweeteners.
6. Eat essential fats incouding saturated fats and a balance of omega 3 and 6 by eating fish (including

347

salmon), nuts, and seeds. Use olive, coconut, avocado, and flax seed oils.

7. Eliminate trans-fats completely from your diet.
8. Consume plenty of soluble fiber, which will reduce inflammation and help balance blood sugar. Choose vegetables, nuts, beans, seeds and whole grains, especially ground flaxseed, oat bran, and apples. When increasing fiber it is very important to increase the amount of water you drink. For example, drink a cup of water for every tablespoon of flaxseed eaten.
9. Eat ground flaxseed, which contains essential fatty acids that protect against nerve damage and keep the blood supply of the arteries consistent. Flaxseed also works to lower cholesterol, thereby protecting against heart disease.
10. Consider chia seed gel. It supplies all the essential amino acids and essential fatty acids plus a myriad of other nutrients. I add it to drinks, cereal, yogurt, uncooked concoctions.
11. Use phytonutrients to provide basic nutrients for all cells and body systems. Emerging research suggests some flavonoids enhance insulin response and reduce insulin resistance.
12. Choose green or white tea, dark cocoa, and apples, whose polyphenols are emerging as powerful facilitators of insulin responses as well as being potent anti-inflammatory compounds.
13. Eat bilberries, blueberries and other dark berries, which are sources anthocyanins. The antioxidant properties may contribute to improved insulin sensitivity. Plus they are factors for a healthy vascular system. Blood vessel integrity is important in avoiding neuropathy and in protecting the eyes. (45)

Cautions: If you are currently taking insulin or any diabetic drug, consult your diabetes care team before starting any nutritional supplements or herbals. Take into consideration that many conventional physicians know little about nutritional supplements or herbs.

• When using supplements or herbs, blood glucose levels should be checked more often to determine the

348

effectiveness of whatever changes you make and to determine if medication changes are necessary. **Blood sugar issues are serious, so don't play with this without proper counsel.**

To a carefully planned natural dietary plan practitioners may add supplements to balance blood sugar and insulin. Below are some examples:

Vitamins A, B, C, D, and E – Adequate consumption of these vitamins is basic to all cellular structure and activity. A good multiple will have these. Vitamin B Complex helps produce enzymes that convert glucose to energy and may also aid in preventing diabetic nerve damage. Scientists have found a link between high levels of homocysteine and diabetic retinopathy. B vitamin deficiency is found in high levels of homocysteine. (46)

Alpha lipoic acid (ALA) a major antioxidant, is useful to curtail inflammatory responses and improve insulin responses. Alpha lipoic acid helps regulate glucose levels by protecting cell membranes and blood lipids against oxidative damage. ALA also does something that no other antioxidant is known to do, it has the unique capacity to actually recycle vitamins C and E from their molecular building blocks. For this reason, it is sometimes referred to as the "mother" antioxidant. In addition, ALA can help your body better utilize coenzyme Q10 and glutathione." (47)

Coenzyme Q10 (ubiquinol form) is often thought of as a heart health supplement, but it also plays an important role in regulating insulin levels. (17)

DHEA –Using DHEA may be something you want to discuss with your holistic practitioner. My holistic doctor prescribed a DHEA gel made at a compounding pharmacy which I find much more effective than taking a DHEA oral supplement.

Resveratrol, a flavonoid found in grape skins and concentrated in red wine, has been found to improve insulin responses in people with diabetes; however, the sugars in red wine will warrant low consumption.

349

Chromium is one of the basic building blocks of all things, both living and non-living. Chromium participates in the metabolism of glucose by enhancing the effects of insulin. Without chromium, the hormone insulin would not be able to perform its functions. It has been found that chromium strengthens certain effects of insulin on the body's cells more effectively. Using chromium supplements should be discussed with your health practitioner. (48)

Magnesium: It has been found that magnesium can improve regulation of blood sugar levels. Low magnesium is common in both Type I insulin-dependent and Type II non-insulin-dependent diabetics. The body needs magnesium to secrete enough insulin to regulate blood sugar, and insulin helps transport magnesium into your cells. (49)

Zinc is an essential mineral that is a component of enzymes needed to repair wounds, maintain fertility in adults, help cells reproduce, preserve vision, boost immunity, and protect against free radicals, among other functions. Copper is needed with long-term use of zinc, because zinc inhibits copper absorption. (50)

Vanadium - Small doses of this trace mineral are essential for body function and repair. Human studies suggest that vanadium may reduce blood sugar levels and improve sensitivity to insulin in people with type 2 diabetes. Foods rich in vanadium include: black pepper, dill, parsley, radishes, eggs, cold pressed vegetable oils, buckwheat, and oats. (51)

Aloe vera – Preliminary trials have found that aloe vera effectively lowers blood sugar in people with type 2 diabetes. The typical amount used in this research was 1 tablespoon (15 ml) of aloe gel per day. (52)

Cinnamon - Researchers have found the water-soluble polyphenols in cinnamon help to diminish the dangerous after-meal surge in blood glucose. In my case, cinnamon lowers my blood sugar too much. You will need to experiment; it is best not to take more than one teaspoon of cinnamon per day until your research is more complete. (53)

Garlic helps control blood sugar and improves blood flow, reducing the risk of circulatory disorders.

According to Dr. Joseph E. Pizzorno Jr., a naturopathic physician and author of The Clinician's Handbook of Natural Medicine, before insulin was invented diabetes was treated with botanical medicine; helpful herbs for diabetes include garlic, onion, bitter melon, gymnema, fenugreek, bilberry, ginkgo and ginseng. Licorice and stevia, which may help reduce sugar cravings and serve as sugar substitutes, may also help diabetics control their blood sugar levels. (54)

Panax Ginseng berries (American) - Several studies showed that American Ginseng stimulates insulin production, reduces pancreatic beta cell loss and helps control of Type II diabetes. (55)

**Whenever you can consume nutrients in foods, the risk of reaching toxic levels is practically eliminated.

Diabetic neuropathy is a type of nerve damage that can occur if you have diabetes. High blood sugar can injure nerve fibers throughout your body, but diabetic neuropathy most often damages nerves in your legs and feet.

Control your blood sugar to avoid neuropathy

- Controlling your blood sugar with foods as described above will lower the risk of neuropathy.
- Exercise to keep your weight optimal and increase circulation. Foot reflexology is very effective in keeping circulation in the feet.
- Supplement with nutrients and herbs as needed.
- Drink adequate water. (56)

Diabetic Retinopathy is a serious eye disease which can occur in people with diabetes. It may result in poor vision and even blindness.

Diabetes affects many parts of our body, such as the small blood vessels around your eyes. Diabetes can damage the small blood vessels inside the retina, causing blood to leak into the eye. This causes blurred vision or partly blocked images. This is called diabetic retinopathy and can lead to poor vision and blindness.

- Early symptoms include blurriness, hazy images, and seeing spots
- Once bleeding in the eye occurs, you will see spots floating. If this happens, see your doctor for treatment right away, even if the spots go away. If not treated, vision loss and blindness can occur. The earlier you get treatment, the more likely the treatment will be effective.
- If you have diabetes, you should get an eye exam at least once a year.
- Early detection and treatment are the best protection against blindness.

Your diet can protect your eyes from diabetic retinopathy. The diet described above for diabetics will also help protect the eyes. Most important is to **avoid all refined sugars and artificial sweeteners**. Consume foods high in lutein, zeaxanthin, Vitamins A, C, E, and the B-complex vitamins, as well as zinc and selenium. Supplementing these nutrients may be necessary. As a diet-controlled diabetic I supplement all of the above except zinc, of which I get plenty in my food. If you have space to raise herbs and flowers, calendula petals are a **great source of lutein and zeaxanthin. Bioflavonoids,** especially those from bilberry, grape seed extracts, and pine bark based pycnogenol, have long been known to normalize blood vessel permeability and reduce hyperglycemia in diabetic patients. The bioflavonoids actually improved retinal health in 79% of the patients who took them. (57)

Low blood sugar and susceptibility to viral infections:

Dr. Benjamin P. Sandler, in researching the connection between blood sugar and infection, noticed that many patients who had symptoms of low blood sugar also had poor resistance to infections such as colds, sore throat, grippe, influenza, bronchitis, and pneumonia. By increasing the protein content of their diet and by reducing the sugar and starch content, they improved considerably. They became stronger, and had fewer infections. (58)

It has been found by investigators that a meal consisting of protein, fat, and complex carbohydrates, but with no simple sugars or starches, NEVER caused low blood sugar. I find it interesting that when I eat a meal of protein, fat, and complex carbohydrates, my blood sugar remains stable. (58)

Anyone with blood sugar issues is familiar with the glucose tolerance test and the fasting blood sugar test, but there is also another test, the Hemoglobin A1c test, which shows the average amount of sugar (glucose) that has been in your blood over the last 2 or 3 months. It does this by measuring the amount of glucose that's attached to your red blood cells. The higher the level of your blood sugar, the more sugar will be attached to your red blood cells. The glucose stays attached to the hemoglobin for the life of the red blood cell, which is 2 or 3 months. I find the A1c test to be the most helpful for me.

If your blood sugar is high, start working with a good nutritionist or holistic practitioner to help you make positive changes to control your blood sugar.

Some interesting sources to read are:

http://www.womentowomen.com/insulinresistance/default.aspx, http://www.jonbarron.org/topic/diabetes

"Insulin Resistance—A Lethal Link Between Metabolic Disease and Heart Attack" by William Davis, MD

http://www.lef.org/magazine/mag2008/aug2008_Insulin-Resistance-A-Lethal-Link-between-Metabolic-Disease-and-Heart-Attack_01.htm, http://altmedicine.about.com/cs/conditionsatod/a/Diabetes.htm

3. __AUTOIMMUNE DISEASES__

Have you wondered why in the last decade so many people are being diagnosed with an autoimmune disease? What has caused this sudden proliferation of symptoms which the medical profession calls autoimmune disease? Are the factors involved in causing autoimmune disease similar to those causing cancer? The functioning of the immune system is central to both as well as other disease.

Many medical diagnoses see the various autoimmune diseases as individual conditions, such as MS, lupus, or fibromyalgia, which need specific treatment. From my personal experience and years of study, I tend to see the causes of cancer, most of the autoimmune syndromes, and most other chronic diseases are the same: a toxic body and nutrient deficiency.

The simplest explanation for what happens in autoimmunity is when the immune system is bombarded with so many foreign invaders it becomes unable to distinguish Self from the invaders and starts attacking Self – its own cells and organs. Why is this happening?

- The cells are starving for the entire array of vitamins, minerals, and phytonutrients.
- The body is toxic and needs to be cleansed by nutrient dense protocols.
- The body is damaged from infections which alter the body's ability to heal. Underlying infections may be constantly drawing on the immune system.
- The body records the effect of unresolved emotions which produce stress in all parts of the body and create free radicals.

I finally found someone who sees auto-immune disease as I do. Dr. Ronald P. Drucker in an article entitled "What Caused my Autoimmune Disease, and where is the Successful Path Back to Health?" has validated my understanding of how auto-immune disease might develop. Thank you, Dr. Drucker for sharing this with us online. For the whole story please read http://www.thecodeoflife.info/causes/

To quote Dr. Drucker, "I am of the opinion that most autoimmune diseases are triggered by the traumatic suppression of healthy immune system response. Once immunity has been compromised by these triggers, bacterial, fungal, parasitic, viral, and/or yeast infections or infestations may take hold (usually in the digestive tract initially), causing further deteriorating health conditions in virtually every system of the body. I am also of the opinion that Resistance to the devastation of these immune suppressing triggers may be compromised by a weakened physiological environment, encumbered by stress, and in some cases poor nutrition and/or assimilation. (59)

My conclusions:

1. The immune system and digestive system become damaged by:
   - Toxic drug use causing allergic reactions
   - Antibiotics given without restoring the balance of bacteria in the intestines
   - NSAIDs, anti-inflammatory medications which can lead to intestinal permeability and/or gastric bleeding
   - Surgeries and accidents causing physical trauma
   - Chronic emotional and/or physiological stress
   - Physical exhaustion
   - Poor nutrition and assimilation
   - Chemicals and heavy metals in our environment
   - Toxic chemicals in food supply

2. We know that much of the immune system functions within the digestive system, so when the intestinal environment is not working properly, the immune system will be suppressed and nutrients will not be absorbed into the blood stream.

3. If the body's environment (cellular terrain) is compromised, the territory is vulnerable to bacterial, fungal, viral infections, parasites, or the development of yeast overgrowth. These will cause many symptoms if the immune system fails to protect the body.

4. If the intestinal environment is damaged, yeasts can change into an invasive mycelial fungus with rhizoids that penetrate the protective mucosal lining of the intestinal tract. Fungus and negative bacteria invade the intestinal wall causing permeability causing leaky gut. The lining of the digestive tract becomes permeable and leaks undigested food molecules, proteins, and toxins (antigens) that may cause chronic inflammation. Various conditions can now develop, such as intestinal permeability, which is associated with such illnesses as rheumatoid arthritis, food allergies, Crohn's disease, ulcerative colitis, ankylosing spondylitis, eczema, chronic fatigue, irritable bowel syndrome, diverticulitis, cystic fibrosis, chronic hepatitis, and an entire list of autoimmune diseases.

Digestive failure cripples the immune system. The immune system can no long recognize its body's parts as Self and allows an immune response to attack its own cells and tissues, culminating in autoimmune disease. Inflammation becomes rampant. Multiple systems fail as they are not getting the nutrients they need and are being attacked by the immune system:

- Gastrointestinal: Bloating, excess gas, diarrhea, abdominal pain, gastritis, gastric ulcers, constipation, and many other problems may emerge.
- Enzyme destruction: Enzymes are the key to breaking down foods in the body so that they can be utilized as nourishment.
- Fatigue is extremely common, as impaired metabolism doesn't enable the body to get enough fuel and impaired enzyme functioning inhibits energy production.
- Weight gain is common, although when chronic diarrhea is present, unwanted weight loss can be life threatening.
- Respiratory system problems: sore throat, sore mouth, contributing to sinus infections, bronchial infections, and pneumonia
- Cardiovascular system: palpitations, rapid pulse rate, pounding heart

- Genitourinary system: vaginitis, frequent urination, lack of bladder control, itchy rashes
- Musculoskeletal system: muscle weakness, joint pain, leg pains, muscle aches, stiffness, slow coordination
- Central nervous system: headaches, poor brain function, poor short-term memory, fuzzy thinking
- Adrenal system: abnormal hormone responses
- Immune system: autoimmune and allergic reactions

Penetration by fungus and the resulting intestinal permeability cause a disruption in the absorption of nutrients into the bloodstream, and finally nutritional deficiencies on the cellular level. Deficient cellular nourishment leads to reduced immunity, premature cellular aging, and further weakening of the body's defense systems. This can lead to fatigue, allergies, decreased immunity, chemical sensitivities, depression, poor memory, digestive complaints, and many other conditions.

The liver and adrenals struggle setting the stage for environmental sensitivities. As the liver and adrenal glands become chronically overwhelmed, tolerance to the fumes of certain environmental chemicals is reduced. These may include gasoline, diesel, other petrochemicals, formaldehyde, perfumes, cleaning fluids, insecticides, tobacco, pesticides, household cleaners, and potentially many other triggers not listed here.

The liver is the principle organ responsible for detoxification. When functioning properly, the liver filters two quarts of blood every minute, removing unwanted toxins and bacteria. The liver also secretes a quart of bile each day. Bile is necessary for fat dissolution. An optimally functioning detoxification system is necessary for providing good health and preventing disease. Many diseases, including cancer, rheumatoid arthritis, lupus, Alzheimer's, Parkinson's, and other chronic age-related conditions are linked to a weakened detoxification system. It can also contribute to allergic disorders, asthma, hives, psoriasis, and eczema and is associated with CFS, FMS, depression, and systemic candidiasis.

357

Antigens trigger complex allergic reactions. Toxins from microorganisms and undigested food molecules (antigens) enter the blood stream & body cavities. (To review, an antigen is a substance that, when introduced into the body, elicits an immune response simulating the production of an antibody. When antibodies attack allergens but don't manage to kill them, a new antigen-antibody complex is created which the body does not recognize. Antigens can include toxins, bacteria, foreign blood cells, and the cells of transplanted organs.

Antigens set up residence in cells and body tissues and are recognized as foreign invaders. Intestinal permeability allows antigens to leak out of the digestive tract and into the bloodstream. This triggers an autoimmune reaction and can create pain and inflammation in any of the body's tissues. Pain and inflammation can occur anywhere unprocessed proteins are deposited, including muscles, tissues, joints, and organs—nearly everywhere.

Allergic reactions can manifest in a variety of symptoms: fatigue, brain fog, depression, joint and muscle pain, digestive disorders, headache, rash, breathing problems, and inflammation of the nose, throat, ears, bladder, and intestinal tract. It can lead to infections of the sinus, respiratory, ear, bladder and intestinal membranes. In an attempt to arrest these infections, doctors might prescribe a broad spectrum antibiotic. Such antibiotics promote yeast and fungal overgrowth and often additional symptoms.

At any juncture in the line of sequential events, allopathic disease treatment (the treatment of symptoms via drugs) may, and often does, exacerbate the overall deterioration of the body's terrain. Many times these toxic synthetic chemical compounds directly cause disease, and/or function as triggers in the promotion of disease. The overwhelming majority of these substances cause short and long term cellular damage to varying degrees, without addressing root causes of disease.
(59)http://www.thecodeoflife.info/causes/.

I am NOT going to discuss the many autoimmune diseases individually, as I feel the underlying causes are basically the same. After reading about the process of developing an autoimmune disease, I think you will recognize how to turn it around. **You've heard it before:**

Nutrify the body.

Detoxify the body.

Deal with your emotional baggage.

Nutrients, not drugs, are needed to heal all disease. Drugs have their place in critical illness, but only nutrients can heal the body.

There is not enough room in this book to deal specifically with each malady that may exist. However, it is my belief, that if you follow the dietary information and use detoxifying procedures as indicated in this book, you may find your disease and risk of disease lessened.

4. WHAT HAS SOCIETY DONE TO OUR CHILDREN?

Why do children have maladies like autism, ADD, and ADHD? The causes are likely multiple-faceted: including: excitotoxins, pesticides, mercury in vaccines, and other heavy metals; aluminum and formaldehyde; damaged guts and immune systems; and nutritional deficiencies. (60) (61)

I get very angry when I hear people blaming the kids and the schools for the many dysfunctional youth we have today. I believe their behavior is usually NOT their fault but the result of a toxic world which has developed out of a society that:

- Discouraged breastfeeding for many years, so babies received toxic formulas and didn't receive the nutrients and natural antibodies in breast milk.
- Accepted that whatever foods or formulas were in the store were safe.
- Wanted fast food, which is nutritionally dead and full of additives such as MSG, to accommodate their busy lives.
- Accepted vaccinations without understanding the ramifications.
- Encouraged whatever industrial production is necessary to accommodate their busy lives. This production often introduced a wide variety of toxins into our systems - antibiotics and hormones given to feedlot cattle, toxins from industry going into the air and water, GMOs being created to increase agricultural production, and drugs and vaccinations being used indiscriminately, their residue being found in our water supplies.
- Put so much pressure on couples to keep up materialistically that no one had time or energy to prepare real food and provide a healthy environment for their families.

Too often schools are blamed. Schools take the children they are given and try to educate them. Often children have neither been nurtured nor properly fed, nor received the basic training needed to function in life.

Why doesn't society say NO to toxins in our foods?

There is a ton of research on the role excitotoxins (MSG, Aspartame, etc.) play in causing massive behavioral problems in kids. Why are they still in our foods, drinks, vaccines, and so many other products? There is much research indicating that "Attention Deficit Disorder" (ADD) may in part be caused by MSG and other excitotoxins. (62)

Exposure to sugar and chemicals will disrupt the gut microflora and contribute to long term illness. In one study, it was noted that by the age of 2 years, 35% of the children studied had developed allergic eczema, a condition in which the skin becomes irritated, red and itchy. Giving the pregnant mother probiotics often prevents eczema in children. Giving a probiotic in the formula or sprinkling it on food of infants will often prevent any type of yeast infection. (63)

Too often children are put on drugs when they really need good nutrition and a properly functioning digestive system. In the following references people who have successfully dealt with autism or other neurological damage by thinking out of the box.

"How a Physician Cured Her Son's Autism" at www.Mercola.com tell us how Dr. Natasha Campbell-McBride, M.D. cured her son of autism. Dr. Campbell-McBride has also written an amazing book, Gut and Psychology Syndrome, and trains others to duplicate her success. (64)

Impossible Cure: The Promise of Homeopathy is the amazing story of how Amy Lansky's son was cured of autism with homeopathy. Impossible Cure: The Promise of Homeopathy by Amy Lansky, R.L. Ranch Press, Portola Valley, CA 2003

Children with Starving Brains, by Jaquely McCandless, MD is a great book about how her focus changed after her granddaughter was diagnosed with autism. Her devotion, insights, and discoveries will help anyone working to help an autistic child. (65)

At this point I ask you to go to your computer and read a very poignant article by my friend Tim Bolen. Tim has been a leader in health freedom and a champion of the rights of individuals and groups who are being attacked for their work in "alternative healing". This article says more than I have room to say, so please read "Why Autism is Still With Us..."December 16th, 2012 http://bolenreport.com/ Thank you, Tim!

Earlier we discussed at great length that health begins before conception and is very crucial during infancy and childhood. I think most of the health problems of our children could be avoided if we were aware of our toxic environment. We need to educate our young people so they know what is needed to give birth to healthy children.

I feel many of the afflicted children can be helped if we are willing to think out of conventional medicine strategies. We need to concentrate on:

- Providing a toxic- free environment.
- Provide the best organic fruits, vegetables and herbs as the basis of the diet.
- Avoiding processed foods, sodas, and sugar.
- Providing the good quality protein and fats needed for proper growth.
- Building the child's immune system by replanting good bacteria and feeding them with prebiotics.
- Eating a healthful diet to model for children.
- Understanding that vaccines with toxic ingredients may not be the answer to avoiding disease and advocating against the pressure put on parents to vaccinate.
- Spending time in the sun so natural vitamin D is absorbed.
- Spending quality time with our children.
- Working with a natural practitioner who is willing to understand our children's issues.
- Assessing which nutritional supplements needed.

According to a study found in *Pediatrics* magazine, many toddlers are eating inappropriately low-fat diets. (66) Approximately 60 percent of the human brain is composed of fatty material, and 25 percent of that material is DHA. Since humans cannot produce DHA, they must consume it. What happened to giving infants and children cod liver oil? When you give your children cod liver oil you will also be supplying them with essential omega-3 fats that will maximize their brain development and help prevent ADHD. **Use caution**, as overdosing with cod liver oil could give the child too much vitamin D. (67)

Charles Gant, M.D., Ph.D., a New York physician, believes ADD/ADHD is likely caused by an imbalance in **dopamine.** This vital neurotransmitter helps integrate thoughts, feelings, and sensory information in the frontal lobes as well as updates feedback about current motor activity. He elaborates, "In evolutionary terms, this is the last part of the human brain to develop and is one of the first parts to lose its function when there is a generalized stress or injury to the central nervous system." When dopamine activity is compromised, Gant says people become unfocused and distractible because they have difficulty coordinating all this information and choosing the next task. (69)

Dopamine is made from two essential amino acids, tyrosine or phenylalanine, in the presence of adequate amounts of folic acid, iron, vitamins C, B3, and B6. Therefore, it could be a dietary deficiency of these necessary nutrients that is causing the dopamine deficiency, says Dr. Gant. He has found that ADD can be treated with nutrients and amino acids, the raw materials the brain uses naturally to synthesize this neurotransmitter. Dr. Gant says, "Nutritional supplementation will virtually erase symptoms of garden variety, uncomplicated ADD." (70)

ADHD may be caused by allergies to a wide range of possible substances, from chemical additives, preservatives, and artificial colorings to foods such as dairy, chocolate, wheat, soy, etc. We don't have conclusive evidence.

Chemicals and behavior.

In a Rachel's Environment & Health Weekly report, "ADHD and Children's Environment," Peter Montague points to the role of prenatal exposures to lead, cigarette by-products, alcohol, and pesticides, and even low levels of industrial chemicals, in interfering with hormones, especially thyroid hormones. Previous studies have shown that combinations of chemicals can increase the toxicity of a single poison by a factor of 160 to 1600. (71) Montague concludes: "At a time when Americans are searching for causes of **aggression and violence** among children, it would make sense to consider malnutrition, food additives, tobacco additives, toxic metals, pesticides and other endocrine-disrupting industrial toxicants — all of which many U.S. children are exposed to from the moment of conception onward." (71)

B1, Thiamine, is called the "nerve vitamin." We now know that thiamine is necessary for proper functioning of the nervous system and good mental health. Among other things, it is needed to create myelin, the protective sheath that insulates nerve fibers. Even a mild B1 deficiency can cause nerves to become hypersensitive and an individual to become irritable, apathetic, and forgetful. Many infants and children rarely eat foods that contain the B vitamins, so they may be very deficient. (72)

Magnesium - In the cerebrospinal fluid that bathes the brain and spinal cord, magnesium is present in higher concentrations than in the blood plasma. More than 300 different enzymes in the human body require magnesium to function, and many are crucial to cerebral metabolism and cognitive function.

Biochemist James South, M.A., a leading expert on brain nutrition, has noted a remarkable similarity between the symptoms of ADD and the symptoms of chronic magnesium deficiency. These include difficulty concentrating and remembering, confusion and disorientation, irritability and apathy, and muscular restlessness. He points out magnesium's many roles in mental function. (73)

364

In a 1997 study, Polish researchers found that 95% of the ADHD children they examined were deficient in magnesium. Magnesium activates vital structural components of brain cell membranes which are essential for proper mental function. (74)

Numerous studies suggest that the risk for ADHD cluster around at least eight risk factors:
- food and additive allergies
- heavy metal toxicity and other environmental toxins
- low-protein/high-carbohydrate diets
- mineral imbalances
- essential fatty acid and phospholipid deficiencies
- amino acid deficiencies
- thyroid disorders
- B-vitamin deficiencies (75)

I feel these factors are an underlying cause of many diseases today.

Water - Children may often replace drinking water with sodas or juice drinks which are laden with artificial preservatives, sweeteners, and colors which are toxic. Lack of drinking pure water can lead to dehydration, which depletes the brain and other organs of fluids. (Remember, the brain is more than 75% water.)

Several prestigious doctors believe ADHD arises from a combination of immunologic, allergic, and digestive dysfunction that begins with damage to the child's immune system early in development. The injury may be due to environmental toxin exposure, but in the majority of cases, he believes mercury-containing vaccines do play a role. Thimerosal and aluminum in vaccines are intrinsically neurotoxic, and they can also modulate immune function.(75)

Management of the complex multi-system problems characteristic of ADHD, autism, and other developmental problems is a major challenge for physicians and families of these children. Dr. Bradstreet centered his approach on the following goals:

365

- improvement of GI function (digestion, absorption of nutrients, and elimination)
- restoration of normal immune function
- elimination of heavy metals and other toxins
- supplementation to optimize hepatic, immunologic, neurologic, and cognitive function

Detoxification may be necessary depending on what is found during testing. Any detoxifying protocol used in children needs to be supervised by a qualified physician.

Spirulina and chlorella often bring quick recovery from malnutrition and this is **crucial in chelation of autistic children**. (76) (77)

A dietary plan of foods and supplements including vitamins, minerals, phytonutrients, amino acids, essential fatty acids, phospholipids, and probiotics is in order not only for children, but for all of us.

5. ALZHEIMER'S DISEASE

What if Alzheimer's is preventable? (79)

By taking action now, you can stack the odds in your favor, keeping your brain healthy to enjoy the years ahead.

There is also much evidence that in many cases Alzheimer's can be reversed. (80) Like most other diseases we have discussed, increasing nutrients and detoxifying the body are the basic protocols.

There are many factors involved in the development of Alzheimer's disease.

Our elderly are deficient in many nutrients.

Most people suffering from Alzheimer's are the generation that was told not to eat eggs because of cholesterol. (We've already learned what a nutritional powerhouse the "magnificent egg" is.) They were the margarine generation. They were told butter was bad and to eat the new hydrogenated fats. They were the generation that learned to use the quick mixes and processed foods which contain oxidized cholesterol and additives. They were the first generation whose bodies had to deal with tens of thousands of new chemicals in their air, food, and water.

They were encouraged to eat soy products because production of soy was plentiful and easy, and the new products could bring a handsome profit. We didn't know then that unfermented soy is not a good food.

This generation also has very high numbers of cardiovascular problems and cancer. It is no accident that these diseased states started during the times when newly-created foods and a plethora of chemicals and heavy metals were found in our foods and environment.

Alzheimer's patients tend to have low levels of DHA and other good fats. They ate foods mostly made with hydrogenated vegetable oils. They were told not to eat saturated fats like butter and coconut oil which the body needs.

When eating processed food they were both getting a dose of newly-created additives and missing the nutrients that had been processed away.

Raw vegetables, greens, herbs and fruit were absent in the diets of many people in the last 40 years as they embraced the new packaged foods. These generations have become deficient in antioxidants, vitamins, and minerals.

Vitamin B complex deficiencies exist as well. People were told not to eat red meat and few ate whole grain products, which are sources of B vitamins. Folate and other B vitamins will lower homocysteine levels, and researchers have found a link between high homocysteine and impaired memory. (81)

As you can see, many toxins of our new fast lifestyle are implicated in the development of Alzheimer's.

Aspartame, glutamate (MSG), & other excitotoxins are implicated in Alzheimer's Disease.

Scientists have learned from many studies that certain parts of the brain are especially sensitive to excitotoxins. Glutamate (MSG and various other forms) added to foods as a flavor enhancer is one the most serious toxins, along with aspartate.

A blood-brain barrier helps protect some of the brain from free radical damage and exposure to excitotoxins, however, some parts of the brain have no blood-brain barrier. These include the hypothalamus, circumventricular organs, pineal gland and a small nucleus of the brain stem. Where the barrier does exist, it can also become damaged and develop leaks. This can happen when there has been a stroke, head injury, degenerative disease, infection, fever, or low blood sugar (hypoglycemia). When a leak develops, toxins can enter the brain and cause damage. (62)

Xylene and **toluene** are pollutants found in popular beverages, decaffeinated powders, carbonated drinks, and many household and industrial substances. Toluene and xylene are commonly found in:

- Fingernail polish and remover
- Glues/adhesives
- Lacquers
- Octane booster in gasoline
- Paints
- Paint thinners
- Printing & leather tanning processes
- Rubber and plastic cements
- Wood stains (62) (82)

Dr. Hulda Clark considered the presence of certain parasites in combination with toluene or xylene as the cause of Alzheimer's disease. In Dr. Hulda Regehr Clark's The Cure For All Cancers she says, "Fasciolopsis buskii is the fluke (flatworm) that I find in every case of cancer, HIV infection, Alzheimer's, Crohn's disease, Kaposi's, endometriosis, and in many people without these diseases."

It is interesting that these two pollutants are solvents that seek the brain, inviting the common fluke parasite to a location it would not normally be and where it can multiply. Undercooked meats and your pets are sources of the common fluke. (82)

Aluminum - Starting in the 1940s new products containing aluminum were introduced into our lives. These included antiperspirants, baking powder, and antacids, among others. Aluminum cookware and bakeware became the standard because it conducted heat so evenly. Aluminum isalso an adjunct ingredient in many vaccines.

Aluminum is very toxic to the nervous system. It is implicated as one of the primary causes of Alzheimer's disease. "Researchers have found Aluminum buildup in all Alzheimer's sufferers." (83)

Mercury – Mercury toxicity has been linked to Alzheimer's disease. Listed below is just some of the evidence:

369

- Alzheimer's disease was first described in 1906, just a few decades after the widespread introduction of amalgam fillings.
- Alzheimer's disease sufferers have two to three times the brain mercury levels found in unaffected people.
- People with more amalgam fillings have been shown to have significantly more neurological, memory, mood, and behavioral problems than control groups.
- Exposure to mercury has also been shown to cause subtle deterioration in memory.
- Mercury has been used a preservative in vaccines since the 1930s. (84)

Other toxins such as freon, thallium, and cadmium have been found to be factors in Alzheimer's.

High-Sugar Consumption Raises Your Risk of Alzheimer's

High blood sugar may cause Alzheimer's. Some researchers think insulin resistance contributes to the development of Alzheimer's. The healthy brain uses insulin to make a critical nerve chemical called acetylcholine. If the brain cells become insulin-resistant, then they can no longer make acetylcholine. As the acetylcholine levels drop, the brain gets inflamed and grows amyloid plaques, which are found in Alzheimer's patients. Insulin resistance affects the amount of insulin that gets to the brain cells. It has been found insulin concentrations in the brain drop significantly in early Alzheimer's and continue to fall as the disease worsens.

Statin drugs – Cholesterol plays a crucial role in the brain, first by enabling signal transport across the synapse, and second by encouraging the growth of neurons through healthy development of the myelin sheath. Therefore, it makes sense to me, since statin drugs are known to cripple the liver's ability to synthesize cholesterol, causing the LDL levels in the blood to plummet, that cognitive problems would occur. Because cholesterol works to ensure the integrity of the myelin sheath (responsible for carrying electrical messages throughout the brain for memory and focus), it seems logical that lowering cholesterol can have a negative impact on memory and focus.

Your body knows how much cholesterol it needs and will tell the liver. When we mess with the body's natural process we cause havoc.

HRT - A connection has been found between Hormone Replacement Therapy (HRT) and Alzheimer's and dementia in women. (85)

Many herbs have been found to aid in preventing and reversing Alzheimer's.

Turmeric: For example, a recent study of patients with Alzheimer's found that less than a gram of **turmeric** daily, taken for three months, resulted in "remarkable improvements." (86) Research indicates that turmeric has many neuroprotective physiological actions that are anti-Alzheimer's disease properties. (86)

Turmeric contains a variety of compounds (curcumin, tetrahydrocurcumin, demethoxycurcumin, and bisdemethoxycurcumin) which may strike at the root pathological cause of Alzheimer's disease by preventing β-amyloid protein formation. (86)

Curcuminoids appear to rescue long-term potentiation (an indication of functional memory) impaired by amyloid peptide, and may reverse physiological damage by restoring distorted neurites and disrupting existing plaques. (86)

Other foods, nutrients and herbs that have been found to help with Alzheimer's: (86) (87) (88)

- **Sage**: A 2003 study found that sage extract has therapeutic value in patients with mild to moderate Alzheimer's disease.
- **Gingko biloba** is one of the few herbs proven to be at least as effective as a common pharmaceutical drug in treating and improving symptoms of Alzheimer's disease.
- **American ginseng:** In a 2008 article published in the Journal of Chinese Medicinal Materials, claims that

American ginseng extracts reduced cell death in Alzheimer's disease in animal studies.

- **Melissa offinalis,** also known as lemon balm, has been found to have therapeutic effect in patients with mild to moderate Alzheimer's disease. (88)
- **Coconut Oil:** Containing approximately 66% medium chain triglycerides, coconut oil is capable of improving symptoms of cognitive decline in those suffering from dementia by increasing brain-boosting ketone bodies.
- **Cocoa**: A 2009 study found that cocoa procyanidins may protect against lipid peroxidation associated with neuronal cell death in a manner relevant to Alzheimer's disease.
- **Resveratrol** is mainly found in the Western diet in grapes, wine, peanuts, and chocolate.

- **Alpha lipoic acid** (ALA) is a powerful antioxidant and one of the most effective free radical scavengers. Perhaps more importantly, it's the only one known to be easily transported into your brain, where it offers dramatic benefits for people with brain diseases like Alzheimer's disease.

- **Folic acid**: Many people are deficient in B vitamins, Also, the entire B group of vitamins, especially including the homocysteine-modulating B6 and B12, may have the most value in Alzheimer's disease prevention and treatment.

Let's review some things we can do to prevent Alzheimer's.
- Consume essential fatty acids, especially Omega-3s; supplement if needed.
- Eat a diet high in phytonutrients, vitamins, minerals, and essential fatty acids.
- Avoid excitotoxins such as MSG and Aspartame.
- Avoid xylene, toluene, cadmium, lead, freon, thallium, and other toxic metals.
- Avoid mercury - no amalgam fillings, no flu shots.
- Avoid aluminum – cookware, cans, antiperspirants, and other personal products.

372

- Avoid drugs such as statins, HRT, or anything else that will disturb cognitive functioning.
- Exercise regularly.
- Keep challenging your mind. Do puzzles, read, and/or build things, which are all calisthenics for the mind.

Free downloadable book (pdf) <u>What Really Causes Alzheimer's Disease</u> by Dr. Harold D. Foster

PART E. HOW TO EXERCISE WHEN YOU HATE TO

Our bodies need to move. The lymph system is almost totally dependent on moving our arms and legs. The body needs to move for several other reasons.

- To strengthen your heart.
- To maintain strong bones and muscles.
- To trigger the metabolism for weight management.
- To help the body relax for better sleep.
- To stimulate the release of endorphins to elevate your mood.
- To help the lungs to breathe deeply thus providing more oxygen to the cells.
- To sweat to remove toxins from the body.

http://www.mayoclinic.com/health/exercise/HQ01676

We have an interesting paradox in our society. We hire someone to clean the house and mow the lawn, then we go to the gym to exercise. It's all about preferences. I don't like to clean house, but personally would rather push the vacuum cleaner or mop the floors than go to a gym.

Choose a form of exercise you enjoy doing, so you will do it regularly.

Do you like to dance? Dancing is great exercise and a great release from the worries of the day. Line dancing works for singles or for someone whose significant other doesn't like to dance. I found square dancing to be great fun, good exercise, and a great mental release. How about dance lessons to get started?

If you like to walk, golf, or play tennis or squash, find an exercise buddy. You'll do it more consistently.

Be practical. Cardiovascular exercises like running, swimming, cycling, and aerobics are especially good for the heart, but to be strong our bodies need a balance of aerobic and weight training

PART F. THE POWER OF HOMEOPATHY

It is exciting to me that more and more people are taking my homeopathy classes. Most of them have incorporated nutrition and using herbs in their daily lives, but realized they needed to know something more if they were to be in charge of their own health.

So, what is homeopathy?

Homeopathy is a safe, low-cost, nontoxic system of medicine used by an estimated 500 million people worldwide. It is particularly effective in treating chronic illnesses that fail to respond to conventional treatment, and is also a great method of self-care for minor conditions such as insect bites, colds, stomach upset, and flu.

Homeopathy was founded in the late 1700's in Germany by Samuel Hahnemann who was also known for his work in pharmacology, hygiene, public health, industrial toxicology, and psychiatry. Dr. Hahnemann was very frustrated with the practice of medicine of his day which he felt was barbaric and ineffective.

Homeopathy is based on the principle of "likes cures likes". Remedies are used that specifically match the symptom patterns of an illness and act to stimulate the body's natural healing process.

Practitioners of Classical Homeopathy take a detailed health history of the patient as well as the patient's family history thereby looking at a picture of the patient's health, not only the immediate symptoms. He will then consult repertories and materia medicas to determine the remedy that most closely matches the total picture of the patient's symptoms. Homeopathy treats the whole individual. It seeks to assist the body's own healing energies rather than override them with powerful medicines.

In homeopathy the process of healing begins by eliminating the immediate symptoms, then progressing to the older underlying symptoms. Many of these underlying layers are residues of fevers, trauma, or chronic disease that were unsuccessfully treated or suppressed by conventional medicine.

There are more than 3,000 known homeopathic remedies which are prepared from mostly natural sources.

Homeopathic remedies are based on the Law of Infinitesimal Dose. Whereas conventional treatment feels that larger doses are more effective, homeopathy dilutes and potentizes a medicine to release its energy and make it more effective. Remedies of 3X or 3C to 12X or 12C are commonly used for acute conditions whereas the higher potencies of 30C and 200C are most effective for chronic disease

Acute remedies can be the basis of self-care, but chronic remedies should be used only through a qualified homeopath.

If you are interested in learning more about homeopathy you might want to see if anyone in your area is giving classes or find classes online. Basic books to help you understand homeopathy include:

The Complete Book of Homeopathy by Dr. Michael Weiner
Homeopathic Remedies by Asa Hershoff, MD 2000 Avery
Impossible Cure: The Promise of Homeopathy by Amy L. Lansky, PhD 2003 RL Ranch Press
Practical Homeopathy by Vinton McCabe 2000 St. Martin's Griffin, NY

George Vithoulkas, Director, Athenian School of Homeopathic Medicine says, "The long-term benefit of homeopathy to the patient is that it not only alleviates the presenting symptoms, but it reestablished internal order at the deepest levels and thereby provides a lasting cure."

Homeopathy is not new to the United States. The first homeopathic medical school was established in the US in 1835 in Allentown, PA. From the beginning of homeopathy there was tremendous opposition from the conventional medical practitioners of the time, so it is also today in the U.S. In spite of opposition by the year 1900 there were twenty-two homeopathic medical schools and nearly one hundred homeopathic hospitals in the United States. With the coming of test tube drugs came the financial incentives for practitioners to use them. Science also discredited homeopathic remedies as having no value.

According to Dr. Trevor Cook, President of the United Kingdom Homeopathic Medical Association, "The explanation of the therapeutic action of the highly dilute homeopathic remedies appears to lie in the domain of quantum physics and the emerging field of energy medicine. A study using nuclear magnetic resonance (NMR) imaging demonstrated distinctive readings of subatomic activity in twenty-three different homeopathic remedies. This potency was not demonstrated in placebos." Source: Alternative Therapies: The Definitive Guide by Burton Goldberg

"The World Health Organization (WHO) has cited homeopathy as one of the systems of traditional medicine that should be integrated worldwide with conventional medicine in order to provide adequate global health care." Source: http://www.aimcenteraz.com/homeopathy.asp

In the United Kingdom homeopathic hospitals and out-patient clinics are part of the national health system, and homeopathy is recognized as a postgraduate medical specialty by virtue of an act of Parliament. Homeopathy has been used by the British royal family for the past four generations. Source: Alternative Therapies: The Definitive Guide

FINDING A HOLISTIC PRACTITIONER

Finding a holistic practitioner who looks at all facets of the body is very helpful medicine. Many of us are dealing with autoimmune issues and have found the drugs offered did not help long term and often caused new debilitating symptoms.

Below are some websites that provide names of various holistic practitioners in your area.

http://www.functionalmedicinedoctors.com/

http://www.naturopathic.org/AF_MemberDirectory.asp?version=1

http://www.cancure.org/10-list-of-clinics-in-the-united-states-offering-alternative-therapies/

http://www.homeopathycenter.org/find-homeopath

Often visiting with people who work in health food stores will give you names of local holistic practitioners. Always interview a new practitioner to see if he (she) is a good fit for your situation.

To continue your studies with the author follow her website: www.holisticmamalinda.com

Part A References

1The Paleo Diet, by Loren Cordain, Ph.D., John Wiley & Sons, Inc., Hoboken, NJ, 2002

2 http://articles.mercola.com/sites/articles/archive/2012/05/21/fluoride-health-hazards.aspx

3 Detoxify or Die, Sherry A. Rogers, MD, Sand key company, Inc. 2002

4https://www.urmc.rochester.edu/encyclopedia/content.aspx?ContentTypeID=1&ContentID=994

5"U.S. Death Rate From Infectious Diseases Started Rising 25 Years Ago, As the Economy Tanked,
http://archive.larouchepac.com/node/10781

6 "Degenerative disease is avoidable" http://healthy-living.org/html/

7 www.aarda.org/autoimmune-information/autoimmune-statistics

8 http://www.naturalnews.com/048706_autoimmune_disease_Candida_natural_remedies.htm

9. http://www.disabilityscoop.com/2013/03/20/autism-rate-1-in-50/17540/

10 http://www.nbcnews.com/id/44350075/

11 [QuarterWatch, May 2012
http://www.ismp.org/quarterwatch/pdfs/2011Q4.pdf] see www.ahrp.org

12 http://www.photius.com/rankings/healthranks.html

13 "Infectious Causes of Chronic Fatigue Syndrome", Holtorf Medical Group

14 Fight for Your Health, Byron Richards, Truth in Wellness, LLC, 2006, p 11-12

15 www.healthranger.org/ Thursday, July 22, 2004 by: Mike Adams

16 http://www.pdrhealth.com/drug_info/rxdrugprofiles/drugs/cym1693.shtml

17 http://www.ratical.org/radiation/CNR/RMP/execsumm.html

18 Canadian columnist Dr. W. Gifford–Jones

19 Peter Gotzsche, M.D. - a researcher at the Nordic Cochrane Center in Denmark

20 Breast Cancer Detection Demonstration Project

21 "Mammograms offer no health benefits whatsoever, doctors conclude" by David Gutierrez

22 http://breastthermography.com/

23 "How Do MRIs Aid in Breast Cancer Diagnosis and Screening?" By Yasmine Ali, MD http://breastcancer.about.com

24 "Breast Ultrasound - Imaging for Breast Abnormalities" By Pam Stephan
http://breastcancer.about.com/od/diagnosis/a/ultrasound.htm

25 Ralph W. Moss, http://www.alkalizeforhealth.net/Lneedlebiopsy.htm

26 Our Toxic World–A Wake Up Call, by Doris J. Rapp, M.D., Environmental Research Foundation, 2003

27 http://humrep.oxfordjournals.org/content/early/2012/12/02/humrep.des415.abstract

28 Centers for Disease Control report on chemical exposure in U.S., October 18, 2000

29 The Battle For Health Is Over pH, by Gary Tunsky

30http://www.barrypopik.com/index.php/new_york_city/entry/death_begins_in_the_colon

31 Natural Strategies for Cancer Patients by Russell Blaylock, M.D., Kensington Publishing Corp., New York, NY

32 http://www.relfe.com/wp/health/electromagnetic-ionizing-radiation-stress/

33 http://www.upi.com/Health_News/2012/10/16/Half-a-night-sleep-loss-affects-brain/UPI

34 www.health.harvard.edu/press_releases/importance_of_sleep_and_health.htm

35 https://www.urmc.rochester.edu/news/story/3584/scientists-discover-previously-unknown-cleansing-system-in-brain.aspx

36 "Most Vaccines Contain Cancer-Causing Ingredients, But What More...?" By Christina Saric, http://naturalsociety.com/vaccines-contain-carcinogens/#ixzz3OFOWrfKc

37 "Infections that lurk in your body" Blaylock, Dec 2008 newsletter

38 "Biofilms and Recurring infections" By Michelle Moore, http://www.staph-infection-resources.com/recurring/biofilms/

39 http://www.ncbi.nlm.nih.gov/pmc/articles/PMC3970805/ and Peter D'Adamo, ND MIFHI http://www.4yourtype.com/herbs_biofilm.asp

40 http://beyondpesticides.org/assets/media/documents/antibacterial/triclosan-williams.pdf

41 "Microbial Reproduction" http://www.microbeworld.org/interesting-facts/microbial-reproduction

42 The Cure for All Diseases by Hulda Regehr Clark, Ph.D, N.D.

43 Leo Galland, M.D. Townsend Letter for Doctors, 1988 as found on http://www.pestdepot.addr.com/parasitic_problem.htm

44 Hazel Parcells, D.C., N.D., Ph.D. quoted from http://www.gseinformation.com/parasites.htm

45 http://www.diagnose-me.com/treatment/berberine-containing-herbs.html

46 http://www.globalhealingcenter.com/benefits-of/grapefruit-seed-extract

47 "Discover the Underlying Cause" http://candidafree.net/

48 "Candida, Fungal-Type Dysbiosis, and Chronic Disease: Exploring the Nature of the Yeast Connection", the Townsend Letter, June 2012
49 "Candida Cleanse Food List" by Cathy Wong, http://altmedicine.about.com/od/popularhealthdiets/a/candida_foods1.htm
50 http://www.naturalnews.com/033459_candida_natural_remedies.html
51 http://www.aspergillus.org.uk/
52 http://www.toxic-black-mold-info.com/moldhealth.htm
53 http://www.survival-center.com/foodfaq/ff14-mol.htm
54 www.cdc.gov/nceh/hsb/chemicals/aflatoxin.htm
55 Dr. Christopher's 3 Day Cleansing Program, Mucusless Diet, and Herbal Combinations, Christopher Publications,2002
56 http://www.herbal-treatment-remedies.com/antiviral-herbs.html
57 "Nephritis", Merck Manual, Home Edition, p 601-608
58 "Mechanism of Vaccine Induced Diabetes and Autoimmunity" at www.vaccines.net/mechanis.htm
59 "The Killer Vaccines An Honest Physician Warns of Serious Dangers" by Dr. Russell Blaylock
60 "The Truth about Gardasil" http://truthaboutgardasil.org/
61 http://www.newsmax.com/Health/Health-News/doctor-shortage-physician-crisis/
62 Paraphrase taken from Jefferson's Notes on Virginia, Query XVII (1781-1785).
63 The Natural Physician's Healing Therapies, by Mark Stengler, N.D., Prentice Hall, USA 2001
64 "The Cancer Business" by Patrick Rattigan ND, http://www.theforbiddenknowledge.com/hardtruth/cancer_business.htm
65 "Free Radicals: A Major Cause of Aging and Disease"bySharma, Hari, M.D.,http://www.consumerhealth.org/articles/display.cfm?ID=19990303172533
66 Cancer is not a Disease-It's a Survival Mechanism byAndreas Moritz, Ener-chi.com, 2008
67 "How do healthy cells become cancerous?"http://www.sciencemuseum.org.uk/ 2003
68 Natural Strategies for Cancer Patients, Russell L. Blaylock, MD, Kensington Publishing Corp., 69
69 Dismantling Cancer by Francisco Contreras, MD, Jorge Barroso-Aranda, MD, PhD, & Daniel E. Kennedy Interpacific Press, 2004
70 "Cancer's Sweet Tooth" by Patrick Quillin, PHD, RD, CNS, Nutrition Science News, April 2000
71 "Vegetable Oils: Beware of Common Fats That Are Even More Dangerous Than Trans Fats" http://articles.mercola.com/sites/articles/archive/2014/08/31/trans-

fat-saturated-fat.aspx

72 "InfectionsThat Lurk in Your Body — What You Must Know",
Russel Blaylock MD. *The Blaylock Wellness Report*, Vol. 5 No.12

73 Dr. William Li, M.D on http://doctornalini.com/foods-that-starve-cancer/

74 Angiogenisis Foundation, www.angio.org

75 The Optimum Nutrition Bible by Patrick Holford, Judy Piatkus
Publisher, London p 81

76 "Understanding Free Radicals and Antioxidants"
http://www.healthchecksystems.com/antioxid.htm

77 "Food Sources of Glutathione" Erica Wickham,
http://www.livestrong.com/article/335859-food-sources-of-glutathione/

78 http://www.antioxidants-for-health-and-longevity.com/glutathione-food-sources.html

79 Transdermal Magnesium Therapy by Mark Sircus, AC., O.M.D.,
Phaelos Books,Chandler, AZ 2007

80 "Isothiocyanates"
http://lpi.oregonstate.edu/infocenter/phytochemicals/isothio/

81 "Lycopene",
www.whfoods.org/genpage.php?tname=nutrient&dbid=121Cached

82 "What are ORAC Units?"http://oracvalues.com/sort/orac-value

83 "Several culinary and medicinal herbs are important sources of
dietary antioxidants",
http://www.phytochemicals.info/research/antioxidants-herbs.php

84 Research on Antioxidants, ORAC and Whole Foods
Source:
http://hometown.aol.com/omarxango/myhomepage/resume.html

85 "ORAC VALUES OF FRUITS & VEGETABLES" Agriculture Research,
February 1999,
http://www.drdavidwilliams.com/nc/ORAC_values.asp

86 ORAC levels of some common
foods:http://optimalhealth.cia.com.au/OracLevels.htm

87 "Plant Sterols – Super Nutrients from Nature" by Julie Daniluk,
http://vitalitymagazine.com/food-features/plant-sterols-super-nutrients-from-nature/71

88 http://undergroundhealthreporter.com/beets-as-a-leukemia-natural-treatment/#axzz3mtHO5j3r

89 "What's New and Beneficial About Beets"
http://www.whfoods.com/genpage.php?tname=foodspice&dbid=49

90 "Asparagus Cures Cancer",
http://www.goodhealthwellnessblog.com/210/asparagus-cures-cancer/

92 "Ann Wigmore Wheatgrass Treatment For Cancer"
http://www.cancertutor.com/Cancer/Wheatgrass.html

93 "Dirty Dozen",
http://www.ewg.org/foodnews/dirty_dozen_list.phphttp

94 "Clean Fifteen",
http://www.ewg.org/foodnews/clean_fifteen_list.php
95 "Organic Foods Have More Antioxidants, Minerals",
http://www.drweil.com/drw/u/WBL02077/Organic-Foods-Have-More-Antioxidants-Minerals.html
96 How to Fight Cancer & Win by William L. Fischer, Agora Books, 2000
97 "The costly war on cancer", The Economist, May 26, 2011
98 "The Man Who Questions Chemotherapy: Dr. Ralph Moss",
     http://www.mercola.com/article/cancer/cancer_options.htm
99 "Gardasil - 18 Dead, Thousands Suffer Complications"
https://www.lifesitenews.com/news/gardasil-18-dead-thousands-suffer-complications
100 "11 Deaths, 28 Miscarriages, 3461 Adverse Reactions: HPV Vaccine's Dark Side" from
http://www.betterhealthnews.com/2008/01/29/hpv-vaccines-dark-side/
101 "Dangers of Cancer Radiation",
http://encognitive.com/node/1575
102 Cancer: Why We're Still Dying to Know the Truth by Philip Day, Credence Publications 2003
103 "Here Are 11 Effective, Natural Strategies To Kill Your Cancer"
http://www.cancer-prevention.net/
104 "Garlic consumption and cancer prevention",
http://ajcn.nutrition.org/content/72/4/1047
105 Artemisinin: Extract of Chinese Herb Fights Cancer,By Robert Jay Rowen M.D.,
http://www.springboard4health.com/notebook/nutrients_artemisinin.html
106 http://naturalsociety.com/artemesinin-iron-causes-98-reduction-breast-cancer/
107 "Biological Activites For Extracts of Taxus Brevifolia",
 http://www.bighornbotanicals.com/Biological_Activities.htm
108 "Pacific Yew Taxus brevifolia"
http://www.herbs2000.com/herbs/herbs_pacific_yew.htm
109 Curcumin Research Suggests Effect on Melanoma, Breast and Lung Cancers
http://www.mdanderson.org
110 "Cancerous Cells Cannot Thrive Without This" www.mercola.com
111http://www.naturalnews.com/042577_cancer_treatment_hydrogen_peroxide_alternative_medicine.html
112 Feed Your Genes Right, by Jack Challem, John Wiley & Sons, Inc.
113 The Battle For Health Is Over pH, by Gary Tunsky, New Century Press 2005
114 Your Body's Many Cries for Water by F. Batmanghelidj MD, Global Health Solutions 1997

115 "THE IMPORTANCE OF WATER",
http://www.laleva.cc/environment/water.html
116 "Functions of water in the body", http://www.mayoclinic.org/
117 "Dehydration Caused by a Medicine"
http://www.webmd.com/fitness-exercise/dehydration-caused-by-a-medicine
118 "Time to End the War on Salt",
http://www.scientificamerican.com/article/its-time-to-end-the-war-on-salt/
119 You're Not Sick, Your're Thirsty by F. Batmanghelidj MD, Aarnwe Books 2003
120 "Why High Salt Consumption Alone Will Not Increase Your Heart Disease Risk"
April 04, 2013, www. Mercola.com
121 http://lpi.oregonstate.edu/infocenter/minerals/potassium/
122 Prescription for Nutritional Healing, Fifth Edition by Phyllis A. Balch, CNC p 39-40
123 Low Potassium (Hypokalemia) Overview",
http"://www.emedicinehealth.com/low_potassium/article_em.htm
124 "Paleolithic Nutrition — A Consideration of Its Nature and Current Implications",
http://www.nejm.org/doi/full/10.1056/NEJM198501313120505
125 The pH Miracle by Dr. Robert Young, Ph.D., D.Sc. and Shelley Redford Young, L.M.T., Grand Central Life & Style, revised 2010, page 13
126 http://www.alkalizeforhealth.net/
127 The UV Advantage by Dr. Michael F. Holick,
www.VitaminDHealth.org
128 http://www.vitamindcouncil.org/about-vitamin-d/
129 "Bone Health Co-factors",
http://www.nutritionaloutlook.com/jointbone-health/bone-health-cofactors-new-science-vitamin-d-k2-magnesium-and-zinc
130 "Document on Vitamin D", National Institute of Health,
http://ods.od.nih.gov/factsheets/vitamind.asp
131 "Vitamin D Treats Congestive Heart Failure" Dr. Joseph Mercola,
3/5/03, mercola.com   132http://www.webmd.com/multiple-sclerosis/news/20100823/vitamin-d-linked-to-autoimmune-diseases
133 Bone-Health Cofactors: New Science on Vitamin D, K2, Magnesium, and Zinc
134 www.orthomolecularhealth.com/nutrients/vitamin-d
135 http://www.inquisitr.com/1656231/vitamin-d-deficiency-causes-depression-and-sad/
136 Dr. Michael F. Holick, www.VitaminDHealth.org
137 http://news.ku.dk/all_news/2010/2010.3/d_vitamin/,
www.homefirst.com.
138 http://www.hsph.harvard.edu/nutritionsource/vitamin-d/
139 "Vitamin D myths, facts and statistics",
http://www.naturalnews.com/003069.html

140 "The sunscreen myth: How sunscreen products actually promote cancer" by Mike Adams, http://www.naturalnews.com/021903_sunscreen_skin_cancer.html

141 http://www.ewg.org/2015sunscreen/report/the-trouble-with-sunscreen-chemicals/

142 http://www.hsph.harvard.edu/nutritionsource/what-should-you-eat/vitamin-d/index.html

143 http://www.diseaseeducation.com/science/Stem-Cells.php

144 Prescription for Nutritional Healing, Fifth Edition by Phyllis A. Balch, CNC, Avery, New York, p 776

145 "Vaccines and Immune Depression", Dr Joseph Mercola,http://www.mercola.com/article/vaccines/immune_suppression.htm143

146 "Anatomy and Physiology of the Immune System, Part 1" by Jon Barron - http://www.jonbarron.org/immunity/anatomy-physiology-immune-system-antibodies

147 "Strengthen Your Immune System and Fight Colds, Infections, Flu, & Cancer" http://www.jonbarron.org/immunity/health-program-boost-immune-system-flu-1

148 Gut and Psychology Syndrome, Dr. Natasha Campbell-McBride M.D., Medinform Publishing, 2010

149 http://www.medicinenet.com/liver/article.htm

150 http://kidshealth.org/parent/general/body_basics/endocrine.html

151http://sciencewithme.com/science-article-for-kids-learn-about-the-human-nervous-system/

152 http://www.innerbody.com/image/urinov.html

153 http://www.webmd.com/lung/how-we-breathe

154 http://www.healthpages.org/anatomy-function/musculoskeletal-system-bones-joints-cartilage-ligaments/

155 http://www.human-body-facts.com/muscular-system.html

156 https://www.perio.org/consumer/perio_cardio.htm

157 "2006 Biggest Health Threat to the United States - US Dentistry.." http://www.bolenreport.net/feature_articles/feature_article030.htm

158 Fluoride Action Network, www.FlourideAlert.org

159http://www.fda.gov/MedicalDevices/ProductsandMedicalProcedures/DentalProducts/DentalAmalgam/ucm171094.htm

160 http://www.toxicteeth.org/mercuryFillings.aspx

161 "Banning Amalgams", http://www.holisticdentistry.ie/mercury-fillings-banned.html

162 Gray's Anatomy 29th Edition page 4

163 www.echiropractic.net

164 http://www.echiropractic.net/what_is_a_subluxation.htm

165 "Preconception health", http://www.womenshealth.gov/pregnancy/before-you-get-pregnant/preconception-health.html

166"Damage from toxins can pass to offspring" By Elizabeth Weise, USA TODAY, 6/2/2005

167 "What Every Girl & Woman Needs to Know NOW if They Ever Want to Have a Baby" http://www.bodyecology.com/07/01/11/woman_needs_to_know_have_a_baby.php

168 Your Body's Many Cries for Water by F. Batmanghelidj MD, Global Health Solutions 1997

169 "Dietary Recommendations for Children" by Mary G. Enig, PhD http://www.westonaprice.org/childrens-health/dietary-recommendations-for-children-recipe-for-future-heart-disease

170 The Omega-3 Connection by Dr. Andrew Stoll, Free Press, 2002

171 http://authoritynutrition.com/canola-oil-good-or-bad/

172 Fats that Heal Fats that Kill by Udo Erasmus, pages 100-112

173 "The best health-boosting supplements to take during pregnancy" http://www.naturalnews.com/035730_prenatal_nutrition_pregnancy_supplements.html

174 "Magnesium Baths for Safer Pregnancy and Birth", http://drsircus.com/medicine/magnesium/magnesium-baths-for-safer-pregnancy-and-birth-2/

175 "Folic Acid and Pregnancy" http://www.webmd.com/baby/folic-acid-and-pregnancy?page=2

176 "Folate" http://www.whfoods.com/genpage.php?tname=nutrient&dbid=63

177 "Preconception Health", http://www.womenshealth.gov/pregnancy/before-you-get-pregnant/preconception-health.html\

178 "Homocysteine" by C. Norman Shealy, M.D., Ph.D., Youthful Aging Newsletter

179 "More Vitamin D, No Vaccines, Virtually No Autism" by Mayer Eisenstein, MD, JD, MPH. http://www.autismone.org/content/more-vitamin-d-no-vaccines-virtually-no-autism-0

180 "Pregnancy Alters Gut Bacteria", http://www.livescience.com/36589-pregnancy-changes-gut-bacteria.html

181 "The Medical Denial of Environmental Illnesses" by Harold E Buttram, MD from http://curezone.com

182 Excitotoxins: The Taste That Kills by Russell Blaylock, p 73.

183 "Commonly Prescribed Antibiotic Implicated in Autism" http://www.prweb.com/releases/2005/1/prweb194276.htm

184 "MMR vaccine, autism, CDC coverup" https://jonrappoport.wordpress.com/2014/08/20/breaking-mmr-vaccine-autism-cdc-coverup/

185 Gut and Psychology Syndrome by Natasha Campbell-MdBride, MD

186 "Thimerosal Linked To Autism: New Clinical Findings",

187 "Autism and Mercury",
http://articles.mercola.com/sites/articles/archive/2001/02/24/autism-mercury-part-two.aspx
188 "Health Risks of Mercury",
https://www.scdhec.gov/HomeAndEnvironment/Mercury/HealthRisks ofMercury/
189"The Dangers of Drinking Soda Pop",
http://dherbs.com/articles/dangers-drinking-soda-127.html
190 "Pregnant Women Should Not Eat Soy Products."
www.mercola.com
191 US government scientists, Drs. Daniel Doerge and Daniel Sheehan, The Guardian August 13, 2000
192 The Proven Dangers of Microwave Ovens
    http://www.globalhealingcenter.com/microwave-ovens-the-proven-dangers.html
193 "Why We Should All Get Rid of Our Microwave Ovens" by: Sheryl Walters http://www.naturalnews.com/023103.html
194 "Damage From Toxins Can Pass to Offspring", by Elizabeth Weise, USA TODAY, 6/2/05
195 "Chlorinated Water Yields 14% Increase In Still Births And Birth Defects"
Jacqui Thornton and Martyn Halle - The UK Telegraph,
http://www.telegraph.co.uk/
196 "The Tragic Troubles with Chlorine and Pregnancy - Doubles Risk of Birth Defects" http://www.healthylivingtalk.com/the-tragic-troubles-with-chlorine-and-pregnancy-doubles-risk-of-birth-defects/
197 http://www.ewg.org/research/pfcs-global-contaminants/pfc-health-concerns
198 "Case Study: Phthalates"
http://www.chemicalbodyburden.org/cs_phthalate.htm
199 "Phthalate Plasticizers Dangerous, Especially to Children"
www.Mercola.com #207
200 "Body Burden — The Pollution in Newborns",
http://www.prescriptionbeds.com/new_research_march_2005.htm
201"Tests Find More Than 200 Chemicals in Newborn Umbilical Cord Blood",http://www.scientificamerican.com/article/newborn-babies-chemicals-exposure-bpa/
202 "These Over-The-Counter NSAIDs Double the Risk of Miscarriage", Mercola.com
203 "Common Antibitoics Tied to Birth Defects",
http://www.nbcnews.com/id/33588427/ns/health-pregnancy/t/common-antibiotics-tied-birth-defects/#.VjqP-Gt6KDM
204 "Pregnancy and Baby Protection",
http://emfradiationprotection.org/pregnancy-protection
205 Your Body's Many Cries for Water, by F.Batmanghelidj, MD p 15
206 "Herbal Allies for Pregnancy Problems By Susun Weed",
http://herbalgardens.com/articles/herbs-for-pregnancy.html

207 <u>Feed Your Genes Right</u> by Jack Challem, John Wiley & Sons, Inc. 2005

Part B References

1 <u>The False Fat Diet,</u> Elson Haas, MD, The Ballantine Publishing Group, 2001, p 3
2 http://www.webmd.com/allergies/foods-allergy-intolerance
3 http://www.drlwilson.com/articles/food_intolerance.htm
4 "Humans ar Omnivores", http://www.biology-online.org/articles/humans-omnivores.html
5 *Dr. Gabriel Cousens M.D.,* http://www.veganmainstream.com/dr-gabriel-cousens-on-diet-deficiencies-for-vegans-and-meat-eaters
6 http://www.instah.com/miscellaneous-problems/are-glycosylation-and-ageing-related/
7 Nutrition and Physical Degeneration 6th Edition, by Weston Price, Price-Pottenger Nutrition Foundation, 2000
8 <u>The Paleo Diet,</u>Loren Cordain, Ph.D., John Wiley & Sons Inc., Hoboken, NJ, 202, pages 9-10
9 "Blood Groups and the History of Peoples", <u>The Eat Right 4 Your Type Encyclopedia,</u> http://www.dadamo.com/
10 <u>Eat Right 4 Your Type</u> by Dr. Peter J. D'Adamo with Catherine Whitney, G.P. Putnam's Sons, 1996
11 <u>The Metabloic Typing Diet</u> by William Wolcott and Trish Fahey, Random House, NY 2000
12 "How to Combine Foods for Optimal Health", http://articles.mercola.com/sites/articles/archive/2013/10/27/food-combining.aspx
13 "CONGRESSIONAL RECORD, DR. RICHARD WURTMAN, ASPARTAME
"http://www.wnho.net/congressionalrecord.htm
14 "Iron and Cancer" http://ejtcm.com/2011/03/18/iron-and-cancer-2/
15 "All About Endocrine Disruptors" by Ryan Andrews, http://www.precisionnutrition.com/all-about-endocrine-disruptors
16 "Understanding brain damage and endocrine disorders caused by MSG,"http://www.truthinlabeling.org/Dang.html
17 <u>Excitotxoins: the Taste that Kills,</u> Russell L. Blaylock M.D. Health Press, Santa Fe, NM, 1997 Introduction
18 <u>Excitotxoins: the Taste that Kills,</u> Russell L. Blaylock M.D. p 33-36
19 <u>Excitotxoins: the Taste that Kills</u> by Russell Blaylock p 143-144
20 "The truth about MSG and its addictive, neurotoxic side effects", by Joel Edwards http://www.naturalnews.com/048414_MSG_side_effects_monosodium_glutamate.html
21 http://www.truthinlabeling.org/Milk%20and%20MSG.html

22 <u>Excitotoxins:The Taste that Kills</u>, by Russell L. Blaylock, M.D. pages 195-197

23 "Types of products that contain MSG", http://www.truthinlabeling.org/II.WhereIsMSG.html

24 "The Danger of MSG and How it is Hidden in Vaccines", www.Mercola.com

25 Information provided by the Truth in Labeling Campaign, www.truthinlabeling.org

26) "Aspartame: By Far the Most Dangerous Substance Added to Most Foods Today", http://articles.mercola.com/sites/articles/archive/2011/11/06/asp artame-most-dangerous-substance-added-to-food.aspx

27 "Aspartame... the BAD news!"http://www.dorway.com/badnews.html#symptoms

28 <u>Excitotxins: The Taste that Kills,</u> Russell Blaylock, MD, P 254

29 <u>Excitotxins: The Taste that Kills</u>, Russell Blaylock M.D., P37

30 "Sudden Cardiac Death: The Role of Aspartame, MSG and Other Excitotoxins" by Russell L. Blaylock, M.D http://beyondhealth.com/media/wysiwyg/kadro/articles/SuddenCard iacDeath.pdf

31 http://www.examiner.com/kids-nutrition-exercise-in-fort-worth/can-a-little-food-additive-like-msg-really-kill

32 "Aspartame Even More Toxic When Mixed with Food Coloring", www.Mindingtheplanet.net, 12/23/05

33 "The Bitter Truth about Aspartame and Neotame", *Aspartame Consumer Safety Network Fact Sheet*

34 "Flying Safety", May 1992 as found on http://www.dorway.com/betty/ntsbmsg.txt

35 "New Guide Warns of 'Dirty Dozen' Food Additives", http://www.ewg.org/release/new-guide-warns-dirty-dozen-food-additives

36 "Pouring It On: Health Effects of Nitrate Exposure" http://www.ewg.org/research/pouring-it/health-effects-nitrate-exposure

37 "Nitrate Health Effects" by Bruce A. Macler Ph.D http://www3.epa.gov/region09/ag/workshop/nitrogen/2013/macl er-nitrate-released.pdf

38 "Processed Meats Cause Cancer" http://www.organicconsumers.org/foodsafety/processedmeat050305 .cfm

39 "Are Nitrates and Nitrites Bad for You?" http://nutritiondiva.quickanddirtytips.com/nitrates-and-nitrites.aspx

40 "Don't Use Foods or Products Made with Coal Tar Dyes", http://www.healthychild.org/easy-steps/dont-use-products-made-with-coal-tar-dyes/

41 "Food Dyes Linked to Cancer ADHD Allergies" by Laurel Curran, http://www.foodsafetynews.com/2010/07/popular-food-dyes-linked-to-cancer-adhd-and-allergies/#.VkSu1-J6KDM

42 http://dherbs.com/articles/dangers-drinking-soda-127.html
43 "Are You Still Drinking Soda Pop?"
http://thealkalineway.blogspot.com/2012/12/are-you-still-drinking-soda-pop.html
44 "10 Diseases Linked To Soda",
http://articles.mercola.com/sites/articles/archive/2009/02/10/10-diseases-linked-to-soda.aspx
45 "Dangers of High Fructose Corn Syrup – HFCS" at
http://www.femhealth.com/DangersofHFCS.html
46 "16 Reasons To Stop Drinking
Soda"http://www.emedexpert.com/tips/soft-drinks.shtml
47 "Too Much Soda & Potassium Levels" Jan 19, 2014 by Victoria
Weinblatt http://www.livestrong.com/article/544525-too-much-soda-potassium-levels/
48 "Soda Manufacturers Attempt to Downplay Sodium Benzoate Link
to Hyperactivity" by David Gutierrez – NewsTarget, Friday,
January 04, 2008
49 "Beer and coke cans are killers",
http://helpfreetheearth.com/news496_aluminum.html
50 "Does Your Favorite Soda have BPA in It?"
http://thepeopleschemist.com/does-your-favorite-soda-have-bpa-in-it/
51 "Sucralose", http://tuberose.com/Sucralose.html
52 Dr. Janet Starr, *Hull's Health Newsletter*, December 2003
53 Sucralose Toxicity Information Center,
http://www.HolisticMed.com/splenda/
54 "Do Sweet 'N Low Dangers Still Exist?", http://www.lifescript.com
55 Acesulfame-K Toxidity Information Center,
http://www.holisticmed.com/acek/
56 Death by Modern Medicine, by Dr. Carolyn Dean and Trueman
Tuck, Matrix Verite, Inc, Belleville, ON, 2005, p256
57*Journal of the National Cancer Institute*February 4, 2004;
96(3):229-233
58 Lick the Sugar Habit by Nancy Appleton, Avery Trade, Second
Edition, 1988.
59 "The Murky World of High-Fructose Corn Syrup" at
http://www.westonaprice.org/motherlinda/cornsyrup.html
60 "Fructose Sets Table For Weight Gain Without Warning"
http://www.sciencedaily.com/releases/2008/10/081016074701.htm
61 "Increased dietary fructose linked to elevated uric acid levels and
lower liver energy stores",
http://www.sciencedaily.com/releases/2012/09/120913104121.htm
62 "What Is Metabolic Syndrome?"
http://www.webmd.com/heart/metabolic-syndrome/metabolic-syndrome-what-is-it
63 "Fructose Raises Triglyceride Levels",
http://articles.mercola.com/sites/articles/archive/2001/01/14/fructose-part-one.aspx#!

64 "Triglycerides: Why do they matter?"
http://www.mayoclinic.org/diseases-conditions/high-blood-cholesterol/in-depth/triglycerides/ART-20048186
65 "Soda Warning? High-fructose Corn Syrup Linked To Diabetes, New Study Suggests"
http://www.sciencedaily.com/releases/2007/08/070823094819.htm
66 http://www.huffingtonpost.com/dr-mercola/agave-this-sweetener-is-f_b_537936.html
67 "Honey Composition and Properties" by J. W. White, Jr. and Landis W. Doner
http://www.beesource.com/resources/usda/honey-composition-and-properties/
68 "HEALTH BENEFITS OF HONEY"
http://www.beesonline.com/HealthBenefitsOfHoney.htm
69
http://kidshealth.org/parent/pregnancy_newborn/feeding/honey_botulism.html
70 "Stevia: Sweeten Your Life With Out The Weight Gain",
http://vitanetonline.com/forums/1/Thread/1137
71 "7 Things You Didn't Know About Stevia" by Kate Bratskeir
http://www.huffingtonpost.com/2014/10/16/stevia-what-is-it_n_5983772.html
72 Sugar Alcohols: Good or Bad?
http://authoritynutrition.com/sugar-alcohols-good-or-bad/
73 http://www.ific.org/publications/factsheets/sugaralcoholfs.cfm
74 Xylitol - Is It Safe or Effective? by: Rami Nagel
http://www.naturalnews.com/022986_xylitol_health_sugar.html
75 "Xylitol: Should We Stop Calling It Natural?"
http://www.crunchybetty.com/xylitol-should-we-stop-calling-it-natural
76 Definition of Food, http://www.thefreedictionary.com/food
77 "B3" http://www.umm.edu/altmed/articles/vitamin-b3-000335.html
78 "B3" www.whfoods.com/genpage.php?tname=nutrient&dbid=83
79 "Pantothenic acid"
http://www.whfoods.com/genpage.php?tname=nutrient&dbid=87
80 "B5 Pantothenic acid"
http://www.healthy.net/scr/article.aspx?id=2127
81 "B6 Pyridoxine"
http://www.whfoods.com/genpage.php?tname=nutrient&dbid=108
82 "Biotin" http://www4.ncsu.edu/~knopp/BCH451/Biotin.html
83 "Folate"
http://www.whfoods.com/genpage.php?tname=nutrient&dbid=63
84 "Folate" Prescription for Nutritional Healing, Fifth Edition, Phyllis A. Balch p 24
85 http://www.webmd.com/baby/news/20090302/birth-defects-linked-to-low-vitamin-b12.

86 "Vitamin B12" Prescription for Nutritional Healing, Fifth Edition by Phyllis A. Balch p23
87 http://lpi.oregonstate.edu/infocenter/othernuts/choline/
88 http://www.vitguide.com/inositol-benefits/
89 http://www.buzzle.com/articles/inositol-benefits.html
90 "Vitamin C" http://www.whfoods.com/genpage.php?tname=nutrient&dbid=109
91 http://www.benefitsofvitaminc.com/
92 http://www.globalhealingcenter.com/natural-health/10-foods-containing-vitamin-d/
93 "Natural vs. Synthetic Vitamin E" by Jack Challem, The November 2001 Issue of *Nutrition Science News*
94 http://www.anyvitamins.com/vitamin-k-info.htm
95 "Betaine" http://eprints.iisc.ernet.in/12077/
96 "Betaine reverses toxic effects of aluminium: Implications in Alzheimer's disease (AD) and AD-like pathology" http://core.ac.uk/display/11610154
97 "Calcium" http://www.organicfacts.net/health-benefits/minerals/health-benefits-of-calcium.html
98 "Calcium" http://www.whfoods.com/genpage.php?tname=nutrient&dbid=45
99 "Chromium" http://www.drkalsweightlosstips.com/the-benefits-of-chromium.html
100 "Copper" http://www.whfoods.com/genpage.php?tname=nutrient&dbid=53
101 "Copper" http://www.healthaliciousness.com/articles/high-copper-foods.php
102 "Iodine" http://www.organicfacts.net/health-benefits/minerals/health-benefits-of-iodine.html
103 "Iron" http://www.organicfacts.net/health-benefits/minerals/health-benefits-of-iron.html
104 "Iron: The Hidden Truth About Enriched White Flour" http://www.globalhealingcenter.com/natural-health/enriched-white-flour/
105 The Miracle of Magnesium by Carolyn Dean, MD, ND
106 "Magnesium: The Forgotten Miracle Nutrient", The Blaylock Wellness Report June 2011
107 "Magnesium" http://www.whfoods.com/genpage.php?tname=nutrient&dbid=75
108 "Manganese" http://www.whfoods.com/genpage.php?tname=foodspice&dbid=128 #healthbenefits
109 "Manganese" http://www.healthaliciousness.com/articles/foods-high-in manganese
110 "Molybedenum" http://www.realtime.net/anr/minerals.html
111 "Molybedenum" Prescription for Nutritional Healing, 5th Edition, Phyllis A. Balch, p 39

112 "Potassium"
http://www.whfoods.com/genpage.php?dbid=95&tname=nutrient
113 "Health Benefits of Phosphorus"
http://www.organicfacts.net/health-benefits/minerals/health-benefits-of-phosphorus.html
114 "Selenium"
http://www.whfoods.com/genpage.php?dbid=95&tname=nutrient
115 "The mineral selenium proves itself as powerful anti-cancer medicine"
http://www.naturalnews.com/016446_selenium_nutrition.html
116 "Can Silica Help Prevent Alzheimer's Disease"
http://www.naturalheavymetaldetox.com/best-prevention-against-alzheimers-disease
117 "Silica and the importance of this mineral"
http://www.amoils.com/health-blog/silica-and-the-importance-of-this-mineral/
118 "Sulfur Sets the World of Nutrition on Fire" by Earl L. Mindell, R.P, PhD http://ahha.org/articles.asp?Id=58
119 "Minerals: Sulfur" by Elson Hass,
http://www.healthy.net/scr/Article.aspx?Id=2066
120 "Zinc: The Immune System Nutrient" by Christopher Hobbs and Elson Haas from http://www.dummies.com/how-to/content/zinc-the-immune-system-nutrient.html
121 "Zinc"
http://www.whfoods.com/genpage.php?tname=nutrient&dbid=115
122 "ORAC"
http://hometown.aol.com/omarxango/myhomepage/resume.html
123 "Antioxidant Enzymes" http://biotecfoods.com/enzymes.htm
124 "The Ultimate Guide to Antioxidants",
http://articles.mercola.com/antioxidants.aspx
125 "List of antioxidants in food",
https://en.wikipedia.org/wiki/List_of_antioxidants_in_food
126 "Alpha lipoic acid (ALA)"
http://www.wholehealthmd.com/refshelf/substances_view/1,1525,10002,00.html
127 "Bioflavonoids" Frank M. Painter, D.C.,
   http://www.chiro.org/nutrition/ABSTRACTS/bioflavonoids.shtml
128 "Bioflavonoids",
http://www.susunweed.com/herbal_ezine/September04/menopausal.htm
129 "The Importance of CoQ10 Levels in Human Health" by Dr. David Jockers
   http://www.naturalnews.com/046350_CoQ10_food_sources_heart_health.html
130 "Possible Health Benefits of Coenzyme Q10" by Roland Stocker, Ph.D.
https://www.grc.com/sr6dev/misc/coq10/Coenzyme%20Q10a.pdf

131 "Alleviating Congestive Heart Failure with Coenzyme Q10" by Peter H. Langsjoen, MD, FACC, http://www.lifeextension.com/magazine/2008/2/Alleviating-Congestive-Heart-Failure-With-Coenzyme-Q10/Page-01

132 "Glutathione: The Mother of All Antioxidants" http://www.huffingtonpost.com/dr-mark-hyman/glutathione-the-mother-of_b_530494.html

133 "Glutathione Food Sources", www.antioxidants-for-health-and-longevity.com/glutathione-food-sources.html

134 "The Glutathione-Rich Lifestyle" http://www.iherblibrary.com/glutathione-book/the-glutathione-rich-lifestyle

135 "Milk Thistle Detox for Heavy Metals, Chemotherapy, and Radiation",http://draxe.com/milk-thistle-detox-for-heavy-metals-chemotherapy-and-radiation/

136 "Glutathione Food Sources" www.antioxidants-for-health-and-longevity.com/glutathione-food-sources.html

137 "Foods that Contain Melatonin", http://www.livestrong.com/article/279680-food-containing-melatonin/

138 "Quercetin", http://www.umm.edu/altmed/ConsSupplements/Quercetincs.html

139 "Health benefits of Quercetin and its role in human nutrition", http://www.nutriherb.net/quercetin_health_benefits.html

140 "Lutein for Your Eyes and Your Health" http://www.mdidea.com/products/herbextract/marigold/data08.html

141 "What are lutein and zeaxanthin?" http://top200foodsources.com/Nutrients/Lutein

142 "Astaxanthin", http://www.phytochemicals.info/phytochemicals/astaxanthin.php

143 "Phytochemicals in Foods - 7 Health Benefits of Canthaxanthin" http://womenhealth-phytochemicals.blogspot.com/2012/02/phytochemicals-in-foods-7-health_18.html

144 "Epicatechin gallate" http://en.wikipedia.org/wiki/Epicatechin

145 "Ellagic Acid", http://www.phytochemicals.info/phytochemicals/ellagic-acid.php

146 "Ellagic acid", Dietary Wellness, Phyllis A. Balch, CNC, Avery, 1992 p51

147 "Lycopene's Effects on Health and Diseases" http://www.naturalmedicinejournal.com/journal/2011-03/lycopenes-effects-health-and-diseases

148 "Lycopene Potent Antioxidant Protection" http://worldshealthiestfoods.com/genpage.php?tname=news&dbid=19

149 http://worldshealthiestfoods.com/genpage.php?tname=news&dbid=19150

http://worldshealthiestfoods.com/genpage.php?tname=news&dbid=
40Lycopene: A Woman's Heart's Best Friend
151 "Lycopene Fights Infertility"
http://worldshealthiestfoods.com/genpage.php?tname=news&dbid=
59
152"Top 10 Foods Highest in Lycopene"
http://www.healthaliciousness.com/articles/high-lycopene-foods.php
153 "Isothiocyanates"
http://lpi.oregonstate.edu/infocenter/phytochemicals/isothio/
154 "I3C and DIM for Breast & Prostate Cancer Prevention" by Byron
J. Richards, http://www.wellnessresources.com/
155 "The Benefits of Pterostilbene" by Cathy Wong, ND
http://altmedicine.about.com/od/herbsupplementguide/a/Pterostilbe
ne.htm
156 "Plant Sterols – Super Nutrients from Nature" by Julie Daniluk,
R.H.N.
   http://vitalitymagazine.com/food-features/plant-sterols-super-
   nutrients-from-nature/
157 "Beta-Sitosterol"
http://altmedicine.about.com/od/healthconditionsdisease/a/Beta-
Sitosterol.htm
158 "Top High Lignan Foods that Lower Breast Cancer Risk"
http://doctornalini.com/top-high-lignan-foods-that-lower-breast-
cancer-risk/
159 "Lignans"
http://www.lef.org/magazine/mag2010/apr2010_Lignans_01.htm
160 "All About Enzymes" http://lifewithnature.com/detox-foods/all-
about-enzymes/
161 "Enzymes: The Energy of Life"
http://www.enzymedica.com/what_are_enzymes.php
162 "Enzymes Nature's Life Preservers"
http://www.hum.org/enzyme_health.html
163 "Enzymes" Prescription for Nutritional Healing, Fifth Edition, by
Phyllis A. Balch,
CNC p.72-73
164 "Probiotics: The Answer to Many Mystery Illnesses", The
Blaylock Wellness Report, Vol. 3, No.10
165 "The Good Bacteria Story" http://www.rgarden.com/49.html
166 The Natural Physician's Healing Therapies by mark Stengler, ND,
Ptrentic Hall, 2001
167 "The Healing Power of Foods" by Edward Bauman, Ph.D.
168 "The Medical Features of the papyrus Ebers",
http://archive.org/stream
169 Holistic Woman's Herbal, Kitty Campion, Barnes & Noble Books,
New York, 1995, p 5
170 "Cancer's Secret Weakness"
http://articles.mercola.com/sites/articles/archive/2010/01/30/intervi
ew-donnie-yance.aspx

171 Today's Herbal Health, Third Edition, Louise Tenney, M.H., Woodland Books, Pleasant Grove, UT, 1992, p 41

172 Edible and Medicinal Plants of the West, by Greg Tilford, Mountain Press Publishing Co, Missoula, MT, 1997, p. 1

173 "Surgery Patients Unaware of Herbal Risk", http://www.webmd.com/news/20090416/surgery-patients-unaware-of-herbal-risk

174 http://altmedicine.about.com/od/druginteractions/p/chamomile.htm

175 "10 Common Herb Mistakes and How to Avoid them" http://altmedicine.about.com/od/herbsupplementguide/a/herb_mistakes.htm

176 "Dr. Lita Lee on microwaves" http://organicblue.pbwiki.com/litalee

177 "Garlic" http://www.anniesremedy.com/herb_detail128.php

178 "Garlic" www.whfoods.com/genpage.php?tname=foodspice&dbid=60

179 The Garlic Book: Nature's Powerful Healer, by Stephen Fulder, Ph.D., Avery Publishing Group, Garden City Park, New York

180 "Onions" http://www.whfoods.com/genpage.php?tname=foodspice&dbid=45

181 "Health Benefits of Onions" http://www.foods-healing-power.com/health-benefits-of-onions.html

182 "Onion" http://www.webmd.com/vitamins-supplements/ingredientmono-643-ONION

183 "Basil" http://www.anniesremedy.com/herb_detail4.php

184 "Basil Nutrition Facts" http://www.nutrition-and-you.com/basil-herb.html

185 "Basil" http://www.whfoods.com/genpage.php?tname=foodspice&dbid=85

186 "Health Benefits of Marigold Flowers" http://www.livestrong.com/article/444206-health-benefits-of-marigold-flowers/

187"Calendula" http://www.anniesremedy.com/herb_detail145.php

188 "Marigold, Calendula officinalis" http://www.mdidea.com/products/herbextract/marigold/data01.html

189 Calendula Safety, http://www.herbs-info.com/calendula.html

190 http://www.anniesremedy.com/herb_detail122.php?gc=b122Cayenne pepper pods

191 "The Healing Power of Cayenne Pepper" by Dr. Patrick Quillin http://www.thewomenwarriors.net/phpbb2/viewtopic.php?t=220

192 "How To Use Cayenne Pepper To Stop A Heart Attack Fast!" http://www.naturalnews.com/030566_cayenne_pepper_heart_attack.html

193 "The Health Benefits of Cilantro" http://www.globalhealingcenter.com/cilantro.html

194 "Cilantro Research" http://www.pectin-plus.com/cilantro.html

195 "MEDICINAL QUALITIES OF DANDELION" by Yashpal

196 "Benefits of Organic Dandelion Leaf" on http://www.globalhealingcenter.com/benefits-of/organic-dandelion-leaf

197 "Dandelion gets scientific acceptance as an antioxidant and 'novel' cancer therapy" by: Donna Earnest Pravel http://www.naturalnews.com/035418_dandelion_cancer_therapy_herbs.html

198 "Dill benefits health" http://www.zhion.com/herb/Dill.html

199 "Dill weed (herb) nutrition facts" http://www.nutrition-and-you.com/dill-weed.html

200 "Ginger" root http://www.anniesremedy.com/herb_detail27.php

201 "Medicinal Properties of Ginger" http://www.botanicalonline.com/medicinalsgengibreangles.htm

202"Ginger is an amazing wide spectrum tonic and remedy" by Paul Fassa http://www.naturalnews.com/033562_ginger_health_remedy.html

203 "Natural ginger is up to 10,000 times more effective than chemotherapy drugs at treating cancer, study shows" by David Gutierrez, staff writer http://www.naturalnews.com/052009_ginger_chemotherapy_cancer_treatment.html

204 "Nutrition & Health Benefits Of Eating Horseradish" on http://lifestyle.iloveindia.com/lounge/benefits-of-horseradish-8298.html

205 "Horseradish" http://www.botanical.com/botanical/mgmh/h/horrad38.html

206 "Horseradish nutrition facts" http://www.nutrition-and-you.com/horseradish.html

207 "Horseradish Protection Against Cancer and More" by Steve Goodman, http://www.lifeextension.com/magazine/2009/11/Horseradish-Protection-Against-Cancer-And-More/Page-01

208 "Oregano" http://www.anniesremedy.com/herb_detail163.php

209 "What Are the Health Benefits of Oregano?" www.mercola.com

210 "Oregano Shown to be the Most Powerful Culinary Herb" by Sheryl Walters http://www.naturalnews.com/024627_oregano_oil_food.html

211"Oregano nutrition facts" http://www.nutrition-and-you.com/oregano.html

212 "Parsley "http://www.anniesremedy.com/herb_detail108.php

213 "Parsley" http://www.whfoods.com/genpage.php?tname=foodspice&dbid=100

214 "Parsley" http://www.herbs2000.com/herbs/herbs_parsley.htm

215 "The Power of One" http://www.naturalplantation.com/purslane_facts.html

216 "Purslane" https://www.organicfacts.net/health-benefits/vegetable/purslane.html

217 "Purslane nutrition facts" http://www.nutrition-and-you.com/purslane.html
218 "Roemary" http://www.anniesremedy.com/herb_detail51.php#medicine
219 "Rosemary" http://www.nutrition-and-you.com/rosemary-herb.html
220 "Health Benefits of Rosemary" http://www.healthdiaries.com/eatthis/16-health-benefits-of-rosemary.html
221 "Sage" http://www.globalherbalsupplies.com/herb_information/sage.htm
222 "Sage" http://www.nutrition-and-you.com/sage-herb.html
223 "Savory herb nutrition facts" http://www.nutrition-and-you.com/savory.html
224 "Health benefits of Savory" http://www.nutrition-and-you.com/savory.html
225 "Chinese tea consumption is associated with longer telomere length in elderly Chinese men" http://www.ncbi.nlm.nih.gov/pubmed/19671205
226 "Why Asians Get So Old & Wise", Wednesday, September 21, 2005, http://www.unknowncountry.com/news/?id=4868
227 "Health Benefits Of White Tea" http://www.whiteteaguide.com/whiteteahealthbenefits.htm
228 "Thyme" http://www.anniesremedy.com/herb_detail57.php
229 "Thyme herb nutrition facts" http://www.nutrition-and-you.com/thyme-herb.html
230 "Thyme" http://www.whfoods.com/genpage.php?tname=foodspice&dbid=77
231 "What are the benefits of thyme?" http://www.medicalnewstoday.com/articles/266016.php
232 "Turmeric Produces 'Remarkable' Recovery in Alzheimer's Patients"http://www.greenmedinfo.com/blog/turmeric-produces-remarkable-recovery-alzheimers-patients?page=2
233 "Turmeric" http://www.anniesremedy.com/herb_detail239.php
234 "20 Health Benefits of Turmeric" http://www.healthdiaries.com/eatthis/20-health-benefits-of-turmeric.html
235 "3 Reasons to Eat Turmeric"http://www.drweil.com/drw/u/ART03001/Three-Reasons-to-Eat-Turmeric.html
236 "Curcumin Protects the Brain and Fights Cancer", Dr. Russell Blaylock in his August 2011 Wellness Report
237 "Curcumin Story" Professor, Bharat Aggarwal at http://www.curcumin.co.nz/curcumin-story.htm
238 "Turmeric and black pepper fight cancer stem cells" http://www.anticancerbook.com/post/Turmeric-and-black-pepper-fight-cancer-stem-cells.Html,

239 "Turmeric"
http://www.whfoods.com/genpage.php?tname=foodspice&dbid=78
240 "Blueberries"
http://www.whfoods.com/genpage.php?tname=foodspice&dbid=8#summary
241 http://www.womenfitness.net/blueberries.htm
242 http://drbenkim.com/articles-antioxidants.html
243 "Raspberries"
http://www.whfoods.com/genpage.php?tname=foodspice&dbid=39#summary
244 http://www.antioxidants-for-health-and-longevity.com/benefits-of-goji-berries.html
245 http://www.gojiberries.us/gojiberrybenefits.aspx
246 "Chinese Herbalism: Goji Berries"
http://blog.aoma.edu/blog/bid/307565/Chinese-Herbalism-Goji-Berries
247 The Health Benefits of Goji Berries
http://www.olaalaa.com/health-tips/the-health-benefits-of-goji-berries-anti-bacterial-anti-fungal-kidney/
248 "The Top Six Reasons Why Cherries are Naturally Good for You" by Dr. Joseph Mercola and Sara Potts
249 "What are Tart Cherries?
"http://altmedicine.about.com/od/completeazindex/a/tart_cherry_2.htm
250 "Prunes and Plums"
http://www.whfoods.com/genpage.php?tname=foodspice&dbid=35
251 "Nutrition Information on Prunes"
http://www.livestrong.com/article/247550-nutrition-information-on-prunes/
252 "Apple Nutrition"
http://extension.illinois.edu/apples/nutrition.cfm
253 Apple phytochemicals and their health benefits
http://nutritionj.biomedcentral.com/articles/10.1186/1475-2891-3-5
254 "Health Benefits of Apple Pectin: Apples for Health"
http://the-insomnia-video-stash.blogspot.com/2010/05/apple-pectin-for-health-apple-detox.html
255 "Apple Pectin for Health"
http://zerodisease.blogspot.com/2010/05/wonderful-benefits-of-apple-pectin.html
256 "Leafy Greens -- Ranked and Rated"
http://www.webmd.com/diet/healthy-kitchen-11/leafy-greens-rated
257 Green Leafy Vegetables - Nutritional Powerhouses
http://lowcarbdiets.about.com/od/lowcarbsuperfoods/a/greensnutrition.htm
258 "Spinach"
http://www.whfoods.com/genpage.php?tname=foodspice&dbid=43
259 "What's New and Beneficial About Swiss Chard?"
http://www.whfoods.com/genpage.php?tname=foodspice&dbid=16

260 "Beets"
http://www.whfoods.com/genpage.php?tname=foodspice&dbid=49
261 "Arugula" http://www.nutrition-and-you.com/arugula.html
262 http://www.growwheatgrass.com/aboutwheatgrass.html
263 "Barleygrass" http://www.gogreen.net.nz/barleygrass-nutrients.html
264 "Barley Grass"http://www.purehealingfoods.com/barleyGrassInfo.php
265 http://celiacdisease.about.com/od/everydaymedicalissues/f/Are-Wheat-Grass-And-Barley-Grass-Gluten-Free.htm
266 "Health Benefits of Blue Green Algae"
http://www.globalhealingcenter.com/natural-health/benefits-of-blue-green-algae/
267 "How does Spirulina differ from Chlorella and other blue-green algae?" http://www.nutrex-hawaii.com/how-does-spirulina-differ-from-chlorella-and-other-blue-green-algae
268 "Eating Healthy with Cruciferous Vegetables"
http://www.whfoods.com/genpage.php?tname=btnews&dbid=126
269
http://www.naturalnews.com/033548_watercress_cruciferous_vegetables.html
270 http://jonnybowden.com/high-carb-diets-and-breast-cancer-risk/
271 "Cabbage"
http://www.whfoods.com/genpage.php?tname=foodspice&dbid=19
http://www.naturalnews.com/052009_ginger_chemotherapy_cancer_treatment.html
273 Nutrients in cruciferous vegetables found to induce death of cancer cells http://www.naturalnews.com/020839.html
274 "Kale"
http://www.whfoods.com/genpage.php?tname=foodspice&dbid=38
275 "Kale nutrition facts" http://www.nutrition-and-you.com/kale.html
276 "Broccoli"
http://www.whfoods.com/genpage.php?tname=foodspice&dbid=9
277 "Beets"
http://www.whfoods.com/genpage.php?tname=foodspice&dbid=49
278 "Beet" http://fruitsnvegetables.com/beetroot.html
http://undergroundhealthreporter.com/vegetables-for-cancer-beetroot
279 "Avocados"
http://www.whfoods.com/genpage.php?tname=foodspice&dbid=5
280 http://www.avocado.org/avocado-nutrients/
281 "Quinoa"
http://www.whfoods.com/genpage.php?dbid=142&tname=foodspice
282"Quinoa" http://www.nutrition-and-you.com/quinoa.html
283 "Natural Sources of Beta-Sitosterol"

http://www.livestrong.com/article/219561-natural-sources-of-beta-sitosterol/
284 http://www.webmd.com/diet/features/benefits-of-flaxseed
285 "Anti-Cancer Breakthrough Discovered In The Hull of Flaxseeds" https://www.247wereport.com/health-news/whole-foods/2262-anti-cancer-breakthrough-discovered-in-the-hull-of-flaxseeds.html
286 "Health Benefits of Omega-3 in Flaxseeds" http://www.naturalnews.com/024359_flax_flaxseed_omega-3.html
287 "Flaxseeds Protect Against Radiation Exposure" http://www.greenmedinfo.com/blog/protect-yourself-radiation-flaxseeds
288 "Chia: 10 Health Benefits of This Superfood" http://whatscookingamerica.net/CharlotteBradley/Chai-Seeds.htm
289 "Chia" http://www.chiaforhealth.com/
290 "Sesame seeds" http://www.whfoods.com/genpage.php?tname=foodspice&dbid=84
291"Health benefits of sesame seeds" http://www.nutrition-and-you.com/sesame-seeds.html
292 "Lignans" http://www.lifeextension.com/magazine/2010/4/Lignans/Page-01
293 "Hemp Seeds" http://www.innvista.com/health/foods/hemp/hempseed.htm
294 "Treating Tuberculosis with Hemp" http://hemphealer.wordpress.com/category/hemp-and-health/hemp-and-tuberculosis/
295 "7 Heroic Benefits of Hemp Seed" http://draxe.com/7-hemp-seed-benefits-nutrition-profile/
296 "Pumpkin seeds" http://www.whfoods.com/genpage.php?tname=foodspice&dbid=82
297 "13 Health Benefits of Pumpkin Seeds" http://www.care2.com/greenliving/13-health-benefits-of-pumpkin seeds.html#ixzz2dhKOetNV
298 "Role of nutritional zinc in the prevention of osteoporosis" http://www.ncbi.nlm.nih.gov/pubmed/20035439
299 "Raw Pumpkin Seeds Nutrition" http://superfoodprofiles.com/raw-pumpkin-seeds-nutrition
300 "Amaranth as a rich dietary source of beta-sitosterol and other phytosterols" http://www.ncbi.nlm.nih.gov/pubmed/15366261
301 "Nutritional Benefits of Eating Amaranth" Dr. Michael T Murray on http://www.sharecare.com/question/what-nutritional-benefits-eating-amaranth
302 https://www.organicfacts.net/health-benefits/seed-and-nut/health-benefits-of-cumin.html
303 "Cumin seed nutrition facts" http://www.nutrition-and-you.com/cumin.html
304 "Cumin seed" https://www.mountainroseherbs.com/products/cumin-seed/profile

305 "Cumin Herb Profile" http://wellnessmama.com/5607/cumin-herb-profile/

306 "Beans and Legumes for Your Blood Type" http://www.mercola.com/forms/beans_legumes.htm

307 "Legumes Health Benefits, Nutrition Facts" http://www.diethealthclub.com/health-food/legumes-health-benefits.html

308 'Musical Fruit' Rich Source Of Healthy Antioxidants; Black Beans Highest http://www.sciencedaily.com/releases/2003/12/031205053236.htm

309 "Buckwheat" http://www.whfoods.com/genpage.php?tname=foodspice&dbid=11

310 Dr. Perricone, http://www.oprah.com/presents/2005/young/life/life_buckwheat.jhtml

311 http://www.antioxidants-for-health-and-longevity.com/nutrients-in-chocolate.html

312 "Natural Sources of Beta sitosterol" by Shelley Moore on http://www.livestrong.com/article/219561-natural-sources-of-beta sitosterol/

313 "Weston Price, The World's Greatest Dentist" http://www.curetoothdecay.com/Dentistry/weston_price_dentist.htm

314 "Psychobiotics: Can Stomach Bacteria Change Your Brain?" http://commonhealth.wbur.org/2013/11/psychobiotics-stomach-bacteria-change-your-brain

315 Gut and Psychology Syndrome, by Dr. Natasha Campbell-McBride, MD

316 "Taking the Mystery Out of Culturing Your Own Superfoods" http://nutritionaltherapy.com/taking-the-mystery-out-of-culturing-your-own-superfoods-by-caroline-barringer-ntp-chfs-fes/

317 http://www.rejuvenative.com/pages/Raw-Cultured-Vegetables.html

318 Eat right for Your Type, by Dr. Peter J. D'Adamo and Catherine Whitney.

319 The Miracles of Apple Cider Vinegar Health System by Paul and Patricia Bragg

320 http://www.immunesupport.com/message/malic.htm

321 http://www.homeremediesweb.com/apple_cider_vinegar_health_benefits.php

322 "Blackstrap Molasses Health Benefits" http://www.bodybydesignonline.com/diet/blackstrap-molasses-health-benefits/

323 http://www.health4youonline.com/newsletter_5-superfoods.htm

324 "15 Health Benefits of Blackstrap Molasses" http://www.healthdiaries.com/eatthis/15-health-benefits-of-blackstrap-molasses.html

325 http://articles.herballegacy.com/blackstrap-molasses/
327 "The Many Health Benefits of Raw Honey"http://draxe.com/the-many-health-benefits-of-raw-honey/
328 "HEALTH BENEFITS OF HONEY" http://www.bees-online.com/HealthBenefitsOfHoney.htm
329 "Chemical Composition of Honey" http://www.chm.bris.ac.uk/webprojects2001/loveridge/index-page3.html
330 "Bee Pollen, Honey, Propolis and Royal Jelly: Nature's Perfect Foods" http://www.beepollenhub.com/
331 "Royal Jelly" http://www.webmd.com/vitamins-supplements/
332 "Royal Jelly: A Superfood Fit for a Queen (or King!)" http://www.healthyanswers.com/nutrition/2013/12/royal-jelly-a-superfood-fit-for-a-queen-or-king/
333 "Antibacterial, antifungal and antiviral activity of propolis of different geographic origin" http://www.sciencedirect.com/science/article/pii/S0378874198001317
334 "Propolis" http://supplementpolice.com/propolis/
335 Heal with Amino Acids and Nutrients by Bill J. Sahley, Phd., CNC and Katherine M. Birkner, CRNA, PHD
336 "An alternative to antibiotics" on http://www.eurekalert.org/pub_releases/2011-06/f-aat060811.php
337 "8 Plant Foods that Contain Complete Proteins" http://www.revmodo.com/organic-food/8-plant-foods-that-contain-complete-proteins-for-vegans/
338 "Dietary magnesium and C-reactive protein levels." King D, Mainous A 3rd, Geesey M, Woolson R. J Am Coll Nutr. 2005 Jun 24(3):166-71 at http://www.lef.org/magazine/
339 "L-lysine - Helps the Immune System" on http://www.articlesbase.com/health-articles/llysine-helps-the-immune-system-69108.html
340 http://www.umm.edu/altmed/articles/lysine-000312.htm
341 "L −Tryptophan - nature's answer to Prozac" by James South MA at http://intelegen.com/nutrients/ltryptophan__natures_answer_to_p.htm
342 "Carnosine" http://en.wikipedia.org/wiki/Carnosine
343 "Carnosine, Still the Best for Anti-Aging" by: Jon Barron,onbarron.org/article/carnosine-still-best-anti-aging#.Vq-egdB6KDM
344 "Glutamine for Intestinal and Immune Health" byC. Norman Shealy, M.D., Ph.D. https://normshealy.com/glutamine-for-intestinal-and-immune-strength/
345 "Glutamine" http://umm.edu/health/medical/altmed/supplement/glutamine

346 "Taurine"
http://www.springboard4health.com/notebook/proteins_taurine.html
347 "Taurine – THE Hidden Deficiency" by C. Norman Shealy, M.D.,
Ph.D.
https://www.normshealy.com/taurine-the-hidden-deficiency/
348 *The FASEB Journal,* http://www.fasebj.org/content/18/3/511.ful
349 "Vegan Protein sources"
http://www.naturodoc.com/library/nutrition/protein.htm
350 The Paleo Diet by Loren Cordain, PhD. John Wiley & Sons, Inc.
2002
351 "Discover How Your Beef is Really Raised" by Michael Pollan on
http://articles.mercola.com/sites/articles/archive/2002/04/17/cattle
1.aspx
352 "Oxycholesterol versus Cholesterol" by Gabe Mirkin, M.D,
http://www.coconutresearchcenter.org/ind...
353 Wm Campbell Douglass II in his newsletter Daily Dose:
November 14, 2003
354 "Raw Eggs for Your Health -- Major Update"
http://articles.mercola.com/sites/articles/archive/2002/11/13/eggs-
part-two.aspx#!
355 "Eggs"
http://www.whfoods.com/genpage.php?tname=foodspice&dbid=92
356 "What Are the Health Benefits of Free-Range Hens' Eggs?" by
Dawn Walls-Thumma
http://homeguides.sfgate.com/health-benefits-freerange-hens-eggs-
79219.html
357 "Newest Research On Why You Should Avoid Soy"
http://www.mercola.com/article/soy/avoid_soy3.htm
358 "Soy" http://www.westonaprice.org/Soy-Alert/
359 www.herpes.org/10-things-you-need-to-know-about-
preventing-outbreaks-without-d
360 Legumes Health Benefits, Nutrition Facts
    http://www.diethealthclub.com/health-food/legumes-health-
    benefits.html
361 "The Best Antioxidant Beans"
    "http://www.livestrong.com/article/318039-the-best-antioxidant-
    beans/
362 "The Truth About Saturated Fat" by Mary Enig and Sally Fallon
on www.mercola.com
363 "Cholesterol-The Essential Nutrient" from *Youthful Aging* by
Norm Shealy www.selfhealthsystems.com
364 http://www.westonaprice.org/moderndiseases/statin.html
365 "Cholesterol is NOT the Cause of Heart Disease"
http://drrosedale.com/Cholesterol_is_NOT_the_cause_of_heart_dise
ase#axzz3LpCXgL98
366 https://chriskresser.com/still-think-low-fat-dairy-is-the-
healthy-choice-think-again/

367 "Oxycholesterol versus Cholesterol" by Gabe Mirkin, M.D and http://www.coconutresearchcenter.org/ind...

368 Fats that Heal Fats that Kill by Udo Erasmus, Alive Books, Burnaby, BC, Canada 1986

369 http://www.whfoods.com/genpage.php?tname=foodspice&dbid=81

370 https://draxe.com/omega-3-foods/

371 "Anticancer Research"2002 March April;22(2A):537-43, www.mercola.com

372 https://chriskresser.com/how-too-much-omega-6-and-not-enough-omega-3-is-making-us-sick/

373 Essential Fatty Acids by Deborah Lee, Woodland Health Series

374 http://www.lef.org/magazine/mag2010/apr2010_Lignans_01.htm

375 "Krill Oil supplement health benefit" by Ray Sahelian, M.D. at http://www.raysahelian.com/krilloil.html

376 http://www.raysahelian.com/currant.html

377 http://www.theherbsplace.com

378 "Hemp compared to other oils" http://www.hempseed.ca/compare-efas.ihtml

379 Prescription Nutritional Healing, Third Edition, Balch & Balch, p 75-76

380 The Optimum Nutrition Bible by Patrick Holford

381 "Trans Fat Much Worse for You Than Saturated Fat", www.mercola.com382 http://www.nutritionmd.org/nutrition_tips/nutrition_tips_understand_foods/carbs_versus.html

382 http://www.columnfivemedia.com/work-items/infographic-carbs-are-killing-you-eating-fat-doesnt-make-you-fat

383"Carbohydrates" http://www.nutritionmd.org/nutrition_tips/nutrition_tips_understand_foods/carbs_versus.html

384 Dangerous Grains, James Braly, MD and Ron Hoggan, M.A., Avery Books, New York, 2002

385 http://paleoleap.com/what-is-wrong-with-grains/

386 http://www.mindbodygreen.com/0-9739/how-gluten-wreaks-havoc-on-your-gut.html

387 http://thepaleomama.com/2014/01/eating-can-tear-holes-gut/

388 "What is Wrong with Grains" at http://paleoleap.com/what-is-wrong-with-grains/

389 http://www.thehealthyhomeeconomist.com/

390 "Wheat and a Refined Western Type Diet" by Stewart Hare http://www.grainmiller.com/Wheat-and-a-Refined-Western-Type-Diet.html

Part C References

1 Colon Health: the Key to a Vibrant Life by Norman W, Walker, Norwalk Press, 1979.
2 "Beyond Antibiotics" by Lawrence Wilson, MD http://www.drlwilson.com/articles/antibiotics.htm
3http://www.medicinenet.com/inflammatory_bowel_disease_intestinal_problems/article.htm
4 Tissue Cleansing Through Bowel ManagementbyDr. Bernard Jensen, Bernard Jensen International, 1981
5 "Scientist May have Discovered Appendix's Purpose" http://www.nbcnews.com/id/21153898/ns/health-health_care/t/scientists-may-have-found-appendixs-purpose/#.Vi0S4Gt6KDM
6 http://www.news-medical.net/news/2007/10/08/30907.aspx
7 http://articles.mercola.com/sites/articles/archive/2007/10/23/is-your-appendix-really-a-useless-organ.aspx
8 Blaylock Wellness Report, Vol 5, No.6.
9 The Inflammation Syndrome by Jack Challem, p 44.
10 http://www.patrickholford.com/index.php/blog/blogarticle/171/
11 Detoxify or Die by Sherry A. Rogers, M.D. Sand Key Company, Inc.
12 http://www.naturalhealth365.com/beets_liver.html/
13 http://robertvon.com/mbp.html.
14 "Cancer, Sulfur, Garlic & Glutathione" by Dr.Mark Sircus, http://drsircus.com/medicine/cancer/cancer-sulfur-garlic-glutathione/
15 http://undergroundhealthreporter.com/get-rid-of-toxins-in-the-body/
16 http://www.globalhealingcenter.com/natural-health/foods-that-detox-the-body/
17 http://www.doctorshealthpress.com/food-and-nutrition-articles/turmeric-tea-liver-detox
18 www.antioxidants-for-health-and-longevity.com/glutathione-food-sources.html
19 http://www.globalhealingcenter.com/benefits-of/organic-milk-thistle-seed
20 http://www.theherbprof.com/vitSelenium.htm
21http://www.naturalnews.com/047895_glutathione_antioxidants_free_radicals.html
22 http://www.naturodoc.com/library/treatments/removing_heavy_metals.htm
23http://www.diabetesselfmanagement.com/blog/juicing-is-it-for-you/
24 http://www.curezone.org/schulze/herbal_colon_cleanse_1_2.asp

25 http://www.curezone.org/schulze/herbal_colon_cleanse_1_2.asp
26 http://altmedicine.about.com/od/coloncleanse/a/colonic_enema.htm
27 http://personalliberty.com/2010/06/17/what-your-overworked-liver-is-dying-to-tell-you/
28 http://herballegacy.com/Dr._Christopher_Formulas.html
29 http://www.wikihow.com/Do-an-Apple-Cleansing-Fast
30 http://thedetoxspecialist.com/blog/cleansing/2-day-apple-detox-diet/
31 EWG's 2015 Shopper's Guide to Pesticides in Produce™
32 http://curezone.com/cleanse/liver/huldas_recipe.asp
33 http://herbsfirst.blogspot.com/2010/05/is-candida-causing-your-health-problems.html
34 http://www.naturalnews.com/033459_candida_natural_remedies.html
35 http://undergroundhealthreporter.com/vegetables-for-cancer-beetroot#axzz1qFHJVkuc
36 http://altmedicine.about.com/od/therapiesfrometol/a/hydrotherapy.htm
37 "The Science of Far Infrared Therapies" by Dr. Toshiko Yamazaki, http://www.immunematrix.com/joomla-dist/index.php?option=com_content&view=article&id=49&Itemid=59
38 http://www.the-infrared-sauna-effect.com/dangers-of-the-infrared-sauna.html
39 http://www.the-infrared-sauna-effect.com/dangers-of-the-infrared-sauna.htm

Part D References

1 http://www.mayoclinic.org/diseases-conditions/heart-disease/in-depth/heart-disease/ART-20046167
2 http://www.nhlbi.nih.gov/health/health-topics/topics/heartattack/signs.html
3 https://www.patrickholford.com/blog/homocysteine-does-it-predict-heart-disease
4 "6 Medical Myths That Can Threaten Your Life", Blaylock Wellness Report Vol.10, No.1
5 "Blood Pressure Treatment Usually Fails" Meeting of the American Society of Hypertension, May 2000
6 http://www.drmirkin.com/heart/8097.htm
7 "Sugars and Triglycerides" http://www.thewayup.com/newsletters/061510.htm
8 http://healthguides.healthgrades.com/article/how-does-alcohol-affect-triglyceride-levels
9 John Bantle, Professor, University of Minnesota http://www.femhealth.com/DangersofHFCS.html

10 http://www.thewayup.com/newsletters/061510.htm

11 http://www.livescience.com/34757-insulin-resistance-develop-diabetes-heart-disease.html

12 http://www.ncbi.nlm.nih.gov/pubmed/9247528

13 http://www.drsinatra.com/vitamin-b-benefits-for-your-heart/

14 http://www.umm.edu/altmed/articles/betaine-000287.htm

15 *The Lancet,* December 18, 1999 ;354. Stress depletes vitamin C.

16 "Too Little Vitamin D Puts Heart at Risk" http://www.webmd.com/heart-disease/news/20081201/too-little-vitamin-d-puts-heart-at-risk

17 http://www.mayoclinic.org/drugs-supplements/coenzyme-q10/evidence/hrb-20059019

18http://www.mayoclinic.org/diseases-conditions/heart-disease/in-depth/omega-3/art-20045614

19 http://www.lifeextension.com/magazine/2014/12/magnesium-the-missing-link-to-a-healthy-heart/page-01

20 https://health.clevelandclinic.org/2014/05/supplements-taking-many-can-hurt/

21 http://www.scientificamerican.com/article.cfm?id=review-adds-salt-to-a-familiar

22http://www.dynamicchiropractic.com/mpacms/dc/article.php?id=536

6123 http://www.heart-health-guide.com/benefits-of-cayenne-pepper.html

24 http://www.healwithfood.org/cardiovascular/raw-garlic-benefits.php

25 http://nstarzone.com/FOURSPICES.html

26 http://www.redrootmountain.com/motherwort-healing-the-anxious-heart-and-mind/53

27 http://www.drugs.com/sfx/nitric-oxide-side-effects.html

28 http://www.mayoclinic.org/diseases-conditions/high-blood-cholesterol/in-depth/trans-fat/art-20046114

29 Patrick Holford, http://www.ctds.info/natthinners.html

30 http://www.anyvitamins.com/vitamin-k-info.htm

31 http://www.med-health.net/Natural-Blood-Thinners.html

32 http://www.ctds.info/natthinners.html

33 http://www.ctds.info/natthinners.html

34 Terry Willard in Herbs for Health Dec. 04 p. 7

35 http://www.thrombocyte.com/what-is-fibrin/

36 http://www.healthline.com/health/gotu-kola-varicose-veins#Overview1

37 www.pfaf.org/user/plant.aspx?LatinName=Aesculus+hippoc a..
38 Encyclopedia of Natural Medicine, Second Edition, by Michael Murray, N.D & Joseph Pizzorno, N.D. p.1998, p 830.
39 Holistic Woman's Herbal by Kitty Campion, p 129
Prescription for Nutritional Healing, 3rd Edition, by Balch & Balch, p 672-674
40 http://www.pharmacytimes.com/news/Sulfonylureas-Associated-With-Increased-Risk-of-Death
41 http://www.healingmatters.com/deception.htm
42 http://healthland.time.com/2011/06/29/studies-why-diet-sodas-are-no-boon-to-dieters/
43 http://customers.hbci.com/~wenonah/hydro/crbacker.htm
44 The Natural Physician's Healing Therapies by Mark Stengler, N.D.p 157-158
45 "A Natural Approach to Insulin Resistance"
http://www.womentowomen.com/insulinresistance/default.aspx
46 "Homocysteine and diabetic retinopathy", by Liama Brazionis and colleagues. Diabetes Care 31:50-56, 2007
47Care.diabetesjournals.org
48 "Dietary Chromium: An Overview" by Barry Mennen, M.D.,
http://lpi.oregonstate.edu/infocenter/minerals/chromium/
49 The Miracle of Magnesium by Carolyn Dean
50http://www.whfoods.com/genpage.php?tname=nutrient&dbid=11 5
51 http://www.umm.edu/altmed/articles/vanadium-000330.htm
52 "Aloe Vera & Gibberellin, Anti-Inflammatory Activity In Diabetes" Davis RH; Maro NP J Am Podiatr Med Assoc 79(1):24-6 1989 Jan
53 http://www.life-enhancement.com/magazine/article/914-cinnamon-reduces-blood-sugar-and-cholesterol-levels
54 The Clinician's Handbook of Natural Medicine; Joseph E. Pizzorno Jr., N.D.; 2002
55 https://www.ncbi.nlm.nih.gov/pmc/articles/PMC3659577/
56 "Ways to Make Nutritional Progress Against Diabetes" by Andrew W. Saul at
http://www.doctoryourself.com/diabetes.html
57 http://www.eyenutrition.info/diabetes.html
58 https://www.seleneriverpress.com/historical/low-carb-diet-that-prevented-polio/

59 http://www.thecodeoflife.info/causes/
60 "What Causes ADHD/ADD: Genetics, Lifestyle,
Environment ..."
www.webmd.com/add-adhd/guide/adhd-causes
61http://articles.mercola.com/sites/articles/archive/2013/1
2/05/adhd-glyphosate.aspx?e
62 Excitotoxins: The taste That Kills by Russell Blaylock,
MD
63 The Lancet April 7, 2001;357:1076-1079 Mercola 211
64 www.gutandpsychologysyndrome.
65 Children with Starving Brains by Jaquely McCandless,
MD, Bramble Books, 2007
66 PediatricsJuly 2000;106:109-114
67 Mollie Martin, WorldNetDaily.com at Mercola.com.
68 Arch Gen Psychiatry. 2007;64(8):932-940.
69 "What Causes ADHD/ADD: Genetics, Lifestyle,
Environment ..."www.webmd.com/add-adhd/guide/adhd-
causes
70 "ADHD Appears To Be Associated With Depressed
Dopamine Activity In The Brain" Science Daily Magazine,
Aug. 14, 1998
71 Science, June 7, 1996
72
http://umm.edu/health/medical/altmed/supplement/vitami
n-b1-thiamine
73 http://smart-nutrition.net/JamesSouth-ADHD.htm
74http://www.nutritionalmagnesium.org/index.php?page=
Childrens+ADD+%26+
75http://articles.mercola.com/sites/articles/archive/2013/1
2/05/adhd-glyphosate.aspx
76http://www.naturalnews.com/027361_chlorella_natural_
detox.html
77 http://spirulinathegreat.com/taking-spirulina-for-
autism-is-this-a-good-treatment-or-just-a-fluke
78 http://drsircus.com/medicine/magnesium/magnesium-
chloride-benefits
79) http://abcnews.go.com/Health/Wellness/ways-
prevent-alzheimers-disease/story?id=2008615780
80http://drhyman.com/blog/2010/06/14/9-steps-to-
reverse-dementia-and-memory-loss-as-you-age-2/
81 "Plasma Total Homocysteine and Memory in the Elderly: The
Hordaland Homocysteine Study" Annals of Neurology, Vol. 58, No. 6,
December 2005, ncbi.nlm.nih.gov
82 The Cure for All Diseases by Hulda Clark
83 http://www.livingnetwork.co.za/drclarknetwork/common-
ailments/alzheimers-dementia-memory-loss/
84 http://www.thenaturalrecoveryplan.com/articles/Alzheimers-
Autism-The-Mercury-Connection.html

85 Contributing Editor: Health Sciences Institute e-Alert, 5/29/2003
86 http://www.greenmedinfo.com/blog/turmeric-produces-
remarkable-recovery-alzheimers-patients?page=2
87http://articles.mercola.com/sites/articles/archive/2011/0
7/23/this-antioxidant-dramatically-inhibits-alzheimers-
disease-progression.aspx
88http://www.soilandhealth.org/02/0201hyglibcat/020184.Foster.Alz
heimers.pdf

INDEX

228, 230, 241,
243, 246, 247,
256, 257, 258,
260, 261, 263,
268, 269, 270,
274, 284, 337,
338, 339
cancer, 9, 10, 15,
16, 17, 21, 22,
25, 27, 28, 31,
34, 48, 49, 50,
51, 52, 53, 54,
55, 59, 61, 62,
64, 65, 66, 67,
68, 69, 70, 71,
72, 80, 82, 83,
84, 85, 86, 89,
98, 114, 115,
141, 142, 148,
149, 156, 164,
165, 167, 173,
176, 186, 188,
190, 192, 193,
196, 197, 207,
208, 210, 212,
213, 216, 217,
219, 221, 222,
224, 226, 227,
228, 229, 230,
231, 232, 233,
237, 238, 239,
240, 242, 244,
245, 247, 248,
249, 250, 251,
253, 254, 261,
275, 282, 284,
290, 293, 302,
304, 306, 311,
329, 354, 357,
367, 369
Candida, 24, 31,
126, 208, 222,
322, 324
Canthaxanthin,
189

carbohydrates, 20,
33, 92, 112, 150,
154, 156, 158,
173, 184, 186,
195, 197, 199,
255, 263, 269,
296, 297, 321,
334, 346, 353
carcinogen, 89,
145, 147, 148
cardiovascular, 14,
16, 23, 55, 59,
88, 108, 123,
151, 152, 165,
186, 190, 209,
210, 260, 265,
280, 281, 286,
287, 294, 329,
331, 333, 335,
336, 337, 338,
339, 340, 342,
367
carnosine, 122
Carotenes, 156
carrageenan, 22,
132
cataracts, 59, 149,
156, 189, 190,
212, 225, 238,
275
catechins, 37, 190,
265, 311
Cayenne, 3, 59,
213, 214, 215,
317, 338, 341
celiac disease, 246,
298
cell phones, 4, 23,
117, 307
cellular terrain, 19,
25, 27, 80, 81,
355
chelate, 313
Chelation Pesto,
216, 313

417

420